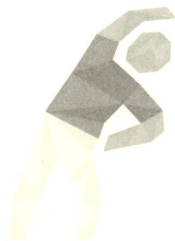

The Stretching Sidekick
Journal

VOLUME 1

Increase Flexibility & Mobility.
Live More Comfortably.

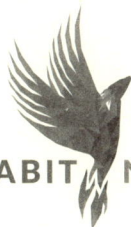

HABIT NEST

Your home for building healthy lifestyle habits.

habitnest.com

For information about permission to reproduce elections from this book,
email **team@habitnest.com**

Visit our website at **habitnest.com**

Publishers Disclaimer

While the publisher and author have used their best efforts in preparing this book, they make no representations or warranties with respect to the accuracy or completeness of the contents of this book. The advice and strategies contained herein may not be suitable for your situation. You should consult with a professional where appropriate. Neither the publisher nor the author shall be liable for any loss of profit or any other commercial damages, including but not limited to special, incidental, consequential, or other damages. The company, product, and service names used in this book are for identification purposes only. All trademarks and registered trademarks are the property of their respective owners.

Special Thanks

We'd like to extend a wholehearted, sincere thank you to the Habit Nest team for all their help in bringing this project to life. Learn more about us here: **habitnest.com/pages/about-us**

We love ya!

Exercises Disclaimer

The exercises provided by Habit Nest™ (and habitnest.com) are meant to serve as a general guide and are not to be interpreted as a recommendation for a specific treatment plan, product, or course of action. The exercises provided are not without their risks, and this or any other exercise program may result in injury. They include, but are not limited to: risk of injury, aggravation of a pre-existing condition, or adverse effect of over-exertion such as muscle strain, abnormal blood pressure, fainting, disorders of heartbeat, and very rare instances of heart attack. To reduce the risk of injury, before beginning this or any exercise program, please consult a healthcare provider for appropriate exercise prescription and safety precautions. While this is an exercise guide, it is not intended to be a direct fit for each person. It is imperative that each person tweaks the program to work for them in a way that suits their personal needs best, especially from a safety standpoint. Do not perform any exercises that cause you pain in any way. Consult with a certified personal trainer to help guide you through each exercise in person to assure they are all being done properly and in ways that will minimize injury.

The exercise instruction and advice presented are in no way intended as a substitute for medical consultation. Habit Nest™ disclaims any liability from and in connection with this program. As with any exercise program, if at any point during your workout you begin to feel faint, dizzy, or have physical discomfort, you should stop immediately and consult a physician.

Information Disclaimer

The information provided by Habit Nest™ (and habitnest.com) is for educational and entertainment purposes only, and is not to be interpreted as a recommendation for a specific treatment plan, product, or course of action. Habit Nest™ does not provide specific medical advice, and is not engaged in providing medical services. Habit Nest™ does not replace consultation with a qualified health or medical professional who sees you in person, for the health and medical needs of yourself or a loved one. In addition, while Habit Nest™ frequently updates its contents, medical, health and fitness information changes rapidly, and therefore, some information may be out of date. Please see a physician or health professional immediately if you suspect you may be ill or injured. Before implementing any nutritional information provided, consult with a nutritionist as well to make sure you can fit your personal health and nutrition needs.

ISBN: 9781950045273   First edition

The Habit Nest Mission

We are a team of people obsessed with taking ACTION
and learning new things as quickly as possible.

We love finding the fastest, most effective ways to build
a new skill, then systemizing that process for others.

With building new habits, we empathize with others every step
of the way because we go through the same process ourselves.
We live and breathe everything in our company.

We use our hard-earned intuition to outline beautifully designed,
intuitive products to help people live happier, more fulfilled lives.

Everything we create comes with a mix of bite-sized information,
strategy, and accountability. This hands you a simple yet
drastically effective roadmap to build any skill or habit with.

We take this a step further by diving into published scientific
studies, the opinions of subject-matter experts, and the feedback
we get from customers to further enhance all the products
we create.

Ultimately, Habit Nest is a practical, action-oriented startup
aimed at helping others take back decisional authority over
every action they take. We're here to help people live wholesome,
rewarding lives at the brink of their potential!

– Amir Atighehchi, Ari Banayan, & Mikey Ahdoot. Cofounders of Habit Nest

Contents

Page

Our Mission in Creating This Journal

Our body is the vehicle through which we experience life.
We all want a body that is apt to perform in our day-to-day lives,
is healthy, fit enough to exercise, doesn't experience random pain,
and simply feels good to be in.

Finding yourself in a body like the one described above takes work.

Of course, diet and exercise are believed to play the largest roles in how your body feels. Without diet and exercise, you cannot possibly optimize your experience of your body. There is also a growing collection of research about the significant impact of stress on the body.

A few often neglected, yet incredibly important aspects of how we experience ourselves in our bodies are *flexibility*, and *range of motion*.

We've all run into physical pain, tension, or discomfort at some point or another. Most of us (yes, really) likely even have chronic discomfort we experience in one or part of our body or another on a day-to-day basis.

Much of our physical discomfort is a result of lack of flexibility and range of motion, both of which are critical to *mobility*.

This journal is all about taking a proactive approach to flexibility and range of motion through *devoting time to stretching.*

Why? Because stretching keeps muscles more flexible, stronger, and healthier. We need flexibility to maintain a range of motion in the joints.

Without it, muscles become tight. When muscles are tight and you call on them for activity, they're weak and unable to extend, putting you at risk for joint pain, strains, and muscle damage.

Simply put, when your muscles and joints are less tense, your body is happier and can more readily perform in your daily life.

We're not physical therapists, and we don't have the ability to diagnose or treat you for any physical issues you may be experiencing, but we do want to provide you with a general stretching regimen and information you can act on, that can help make your body feel better on a daily basis through an increase in flexibility and range of motion, which will improve mobility and the way your body feels in your daily life.

The What

Stretching: What It Is & Why We Need To Do It

We've gone over what mobility, joint range of motion, and flexibility are, and now it's time to get into how we're going to help you improve your flexibility and range of motion, which will in turn positively impact your mobility.

So, *what is stretching?*

Stretching is any physical exercise that involves elongating muscles to the point of feeling significant tension for at least several seconds. **It is a form of exercise** in which muscle groups are deliberately flexed or stretched to improve elasticity.

Chances are that you already perform some sort of stretching routine on a daily basis. Little things like twisting your body, or lifting your arms up when yawning are stretches. Think about how many animals you've seen stretch. Dogs, cats, bears... even birds stretch!

We stretch because it feels good. It feels good because it increases activity in the parasympathetic nervous system (resulting in relaxation), stimulates the release of endorphins, improves blood circulation, and reduces muscle tension.

All of this together gives us the sensation relaxation and and comfort in the body. After a good stretch your body feels longer, more relaxed, and limber. Many animals naturally stretch, like we do, after waking up from sleep, before moving, etc.

Here, in this journey, we'll be focusing on intentional daily stretching for an extended period of time, specifically to improve flexibility and range of motion.

The benefits of increased flexibility and range of motion:

- Increased blood supply and nutrients to joint structures
- Increased quantity of synovial joint fluid
- Increased neuromuscular coordination
- Increased range of motion, more freedom of movement
- Improved performance in physical activity and activities of daily life
- Increased blood flow to muscles
- Improved posture
- Can help heal or prevent pain
- Stress relief, calm mind, decreased tension headaches
- Can improve sleep quality

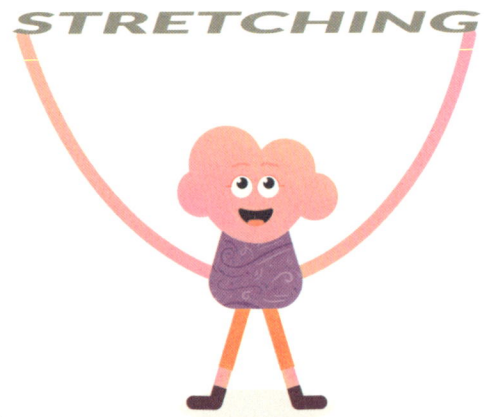

STRETCHING

Understanding Mobility, Flexibility, & Range of Motion

As humans, what sets us apart from other animals is our desire to be great as opposed to simply surviving. We all have a vision of what our ideal life might look like.

Mobility

Every day of our lives, our bodies perform a whole host of physical actions. We wake up, get out of bed, brush our teeth, tie our shoes, walk around, sit, stand, bend, twist, turn, lift things, carry things, exercise, etc.

We're, quite literally, always using our body in some way or another, even if we're simply sitting or lying still. From a very young age, we build physical habits for every action and possible circumstance we find ourselves in.

When it comes to physical movement, we don't think about how *to do* anything that requires us to move, we simply perform the movements.

You can think of **mobility** as 'readiness to move.'

It's the ability to move your whole body freely and normally without restraint (meaning discomfort, tension, or pain).

You can understand your own mobility better by asking yourself what daily activities you perform that you find even the slightest bit uncomfortable.

For example: getting into or out of bed, sitting in or getting up from a chair, picking something up off the floor, or certain exercises. Any movement or physical action which leads to strain, pain, or unnecessary tension or discomfort **may** have to do with limited mobility.

A person with **great mobility** is able to move functionally and efficiently, with little to no restrictions or difficulty.

Less mobility means it's harder to move or perform certain movements without difficulty.

Note: As stated in the disclaimer (we will continue to repeat this), if you have poor mobility, pain, or discomfort anywhere in your body, we recommend speaking to a trained professional to address, diagnose, and treat any issues you may be having. Decreased mobility is caused by many factors. It should be diagnosed and treated by trained professionals, like physical therapists, who have the experience and education necessary to find the underlying causes.

Factors ***beyond our control*** that affect mobility:

Here are a few examples:

- The shape of your particular body

- Age

- Disease

- Physical disability

Factors that, to a certain extent, ***can be regulated by oneself***:

Note: The following can still be influenced by factors beyond our control, which is why it is essential to speak to trained professionals if you are experiencing any symptoms.

1. Muscle weakness

2. Muscle/joint flexibility

3. Muscle imbalances

4. Improper alignment and posture

5. General physical health

6. Injury (either a current injury, or one that either never fully healed or wasn't properly rehabilitated)

Improving mobility requires enhancing muscular flexibility, stability, strength, and joint mobility.

Flexibility vs. Range of Motion

Range of motion is the available amount of movement of a joint, whereas *flexibility* is the ability of soft tissue structures, such as muscle, tendon, and connective tissue, to elongate through the available range of joint motion.

In other words, a muscle can stretch and elongate to the extent that the range of motion of a joint allows for.

Reasons for limited range of motion and flexibility:

Many variables affect the loss of normal joint range and muscular flexibility.

For example:

1. Injury

2. Inactivity – lack of use

3. Poor physical daily habits formed over time

4. Lack of stretching – the range of motion is influenced by the soft tissues that surround the joints like muscles, ligaments, and tendons

5. Medical conditions (including, but not limited to, those that impact the spine, wear and tear of the joints, or cause stiff muscles/muscle spasms)

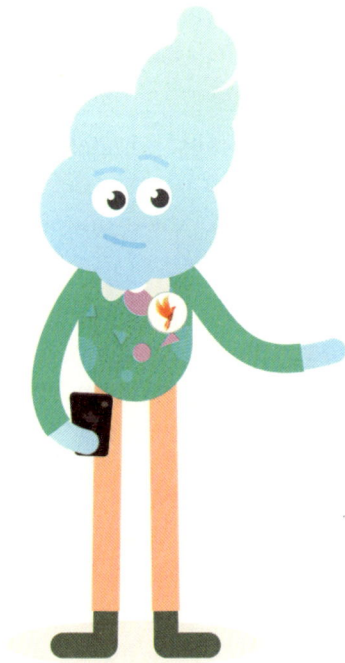

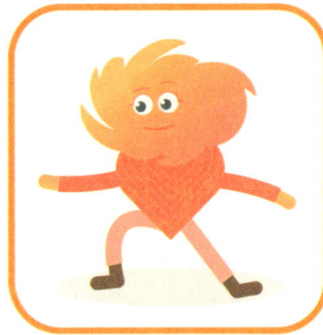

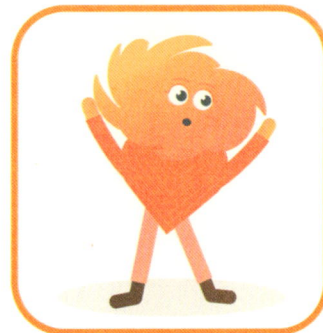

Symmetry & Muscle Imbalances

Physical symmetry is incredibly important to functional mobility, and avoiding injury and pain.

The majority of us have large discrepancies in strength and flexibility from one side of our body compared to the other, which ,over time, can lead to premature, uneven, and unnatural wear and tear.

Muscle Imbalances

In the discussion about **mobility**, we mentioned that one of the primary factors impacting our mobility is muscle imbalances.

We'd like to explain a little bit more about what muscle imbalances are and the most common types of muscle imbalances.

Muscle imbalance is a pretty easy concept to understand.

Every joint in the body is surrounded by muscles that produce and control movement. The muscles around the joint work together as opposing forces that keep the joint centered for optimal movement. If muscles on one side of a joint become too tight from overuse, they could cause the muscles on the other side to become too weak from lack of use. This is called a muscle imbalance - where one set of muscles is stronger, weaker, or higher than its opposing group of muscles.

If a group of muscles is being overworked while its opposite muscle group isn't working enough, there's a higher risk of injury as a result of an altered path of motion for a joint during movement.

For example, if your quadriceps and hamstrings are unequal (both sides of your upper legs), it can cause stress on the knee joint.

This sort of muscle imbalance between the quads, hamstrings, and hips can lead to the knee pulling to one side or the other rather than staying in line.

The imbalance can limit mobility, which ultimately affects alignment, posture, and proper movement, which all lead to increased risk of injury and pain over time.

Some of the most common causes
of muscle imbalances are:

1. Natural development.

2. Certain activities of daily life (overuse of certain muscle groups at the expense of others, based on the way you live).

3. Lack of flexibility (if muscles are shortened due to repetitive motions or sustained positioning, it can change the way a joint moves).

4. Injury leading to compensating with incorrect muscle groups for certain movements.

5. Inactivity.

6. Poor posture.

7. Unbalanced exercise (exercising one muscle group while neglecting or not balancing it with opposing muscle groups).

8. Exercise with improper form.

Muscle imbalances usually occur around joints - areas of the body that are the most mobile. That's why **muscle imbalances most commonly occur at the hips, shoulders and knees**.

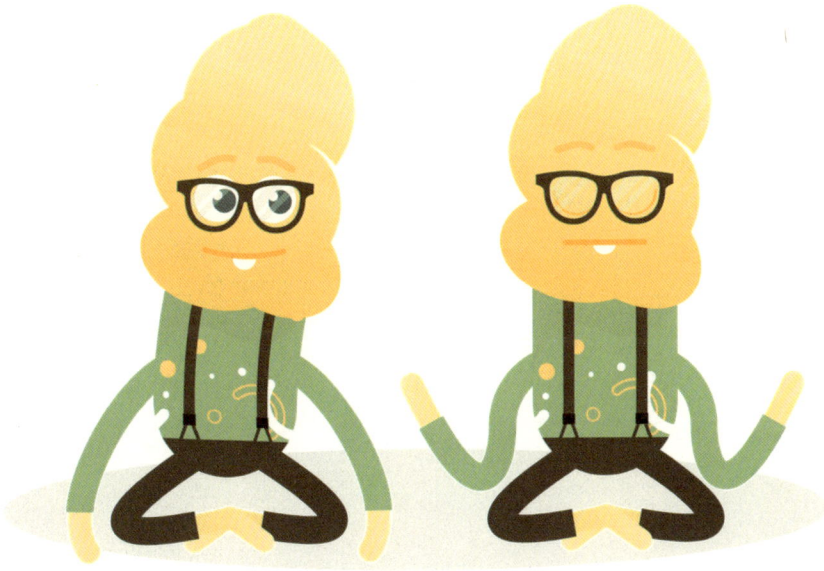

Types of Stretching

The most common types of stretching are:

1. Dynamic (active)

2. Static (passive)

3. PNF ('Proprioceptive Neuromuscular Facilitation')

4. Ballistic (a subset of dynamic stretching)

Dynamic Stretching

What it is:

Dynamic stretching involves stretching your muscles while actually performing movement (think Yoga). Actively moving muscles and joints while stretching them to their full range of motion and repeating several times without holding it at any point.

For example, swinging your leg back and forth to its maximum possible range of motion, repeatedly, without stopping when you feel the maximum stretch.

What it's best for:

Dynamic stretching is thought to be best used as a warm-up to exercise, because it not only elongates muscles and pushes the boundaries of range of motion, but it also stimulates the working of muscles as you stretch, preparing them for exercise. Sort of like activating the muscle to prepare it for exercise while also loosening it up.

Static Stretching

What it is:

Static stretching is what most people know as traditional stretching. You stretch a muscle or group of muscles to the maximum possible range of motion , then hold it there for an extended period of time.

What it's best for:

Static stretching is **awesome for increasing flexibility and range of motion** because it allows you to focus on the single point of maximum range of motion and hold it there while trying to relax in order to extend the range. Static stretching can also facilitate muscle recovery after a workout, leading to less pain and stiffness. For that reason, static stretching is ideal **after you exercise**, not before.

There is a lot of contradictory information about how static stretching prior to exercise impacts the body, but one line of research shows that static stretching as part of a warm-up immediately prior to exercise can be detrimental to muscle strength, and performance in running and jumping. Of course, this is all dependent on how much stretching you do, whether you include other warmup exercises in your routine, and the type of exercise you get. In general, it may be better to save static stretching for after your workouts to avoid any possible detriment to performance and strength.

Proprioceptive Neuromuscular Facilitation

What it is:

PNF or 'Proprioceptive Neuromuscular Facilitation' is a type of stretching that involves contracting and relaxing muscles as you stretch them.

The most common type of PNF stretch is the '**Contract-Relax Method.**' You begin by performing a static stretch of a muscle group, then contracting the muscle group against resistance (flexing or activating the muscle) while it's still in the stretching position, and then repeating the static stretch again while trying to deepen the stretch.

What it's best for:

PNF has gained a lot of popularity as a way to increase flexibility, range of motion, and strength. Many believe it is *optimal prior to exercise,* similarly to dynamic stretching, as it also involves stimulating the working of muscles as they're being stretched, preparing them for use.

Ballistic Stretching

What it is:

Ballistic stretching is a form of dynamic stretching that forces muscle groups into an extended range of motion, even if the muscles haven't relaxed enough to enter that range, by performing bouncing movements. For example, rather than slowly stretching your hamstring, you bounce up and down to force the stretch more quickly.

What it's best for:

Ballistic stretching **isn't widely recommended** for the vast majority of people, as there is an increased risk of injury. It's thought that ballistic stretching should only be utilized by athletes who know their bodies' limits extremely well, while under the supervision of a trainer.

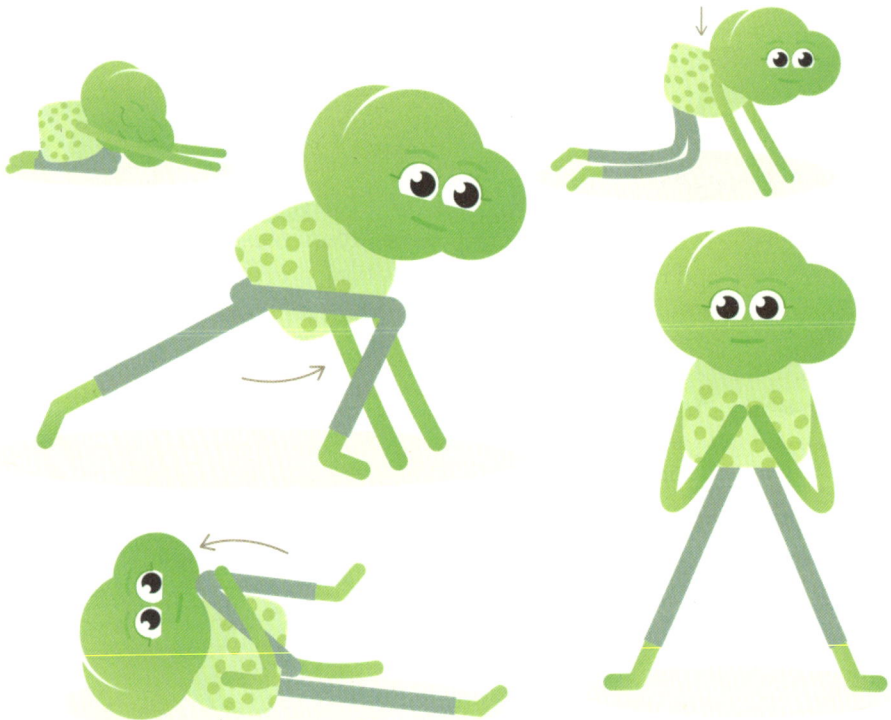

The Who & Why

The Three Factors of Behavior Change

James Clear, author of *Atomic Habits*, writes that there are essentially three parts to behavior change (we love your work, James!).

1. The Outcomes

The **first** is the outside layer: The Outcomes. This is synonymous with your goals. An example of setting your outcomes is:

> *"I want to be super flexible and experience less physical pain."*

Outcomes are most useful at setting a larger, over-arching vision for where you want to go. The downsides of over-focusing on your outcomes are relying on hitting your goals to bring you happiness instead of enjoying the process, and a lack of practicality for what to do day-to-day.

Your outcomes are likely to change over the course of your life to match your ever-evolving goals and needs.

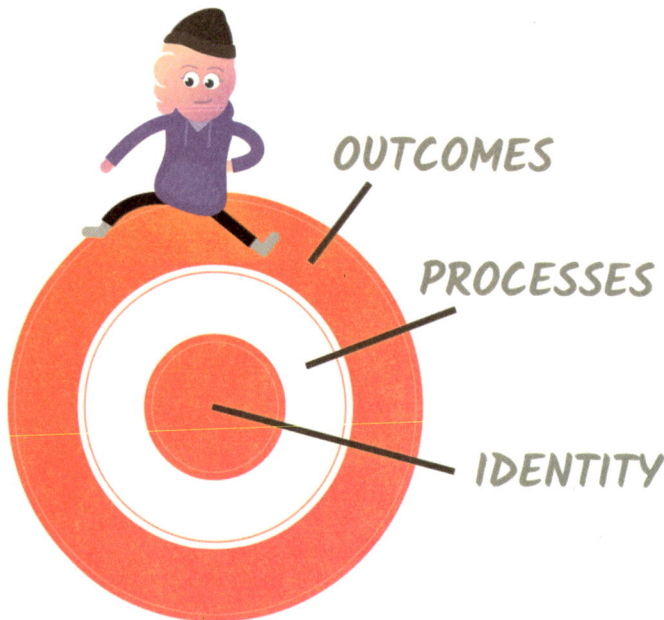

OUTCOMES

PROCESSES

IDENTITY

2. The Processes

The **second**, middle layer, is about processes — this boils down to what system and action steps you put in place to allow your outcomes to come to fruition. These are things like:

"I will do a full-body stretch for 20 minutes every morning."

This is synonymous with strategies and tactics. These can be very useful, especially when you find one that clicks, and you'll see a number for you to experiment with, sprinkled throughout the journal.

These processes are likely to change over time as you test them out. See what works best for you and switch things up when you get bored / desensitized to them. For example, if you find that you're not stretching as consistently as you'd like in the morning, try setting it for a different time of the day, etc.

3a. Your Identity

This one's the **big kahuna**. This is the inner-most layer, identifying what your internal belief is of yourself as a person. The biggest mistake people make in enacting behavior change is placing way too much focus on the first two parts of this puzzle, while entirely forgetting about the third and the most impactful — how you view yourself.

By properly emphasizing WHO you want to grow into, you will maximize your self-respect, satisfaction, and ability to control your actions — more than any motivation or strategy can give you. Use this to guide you over time.

An example of setting your identity is:

"I'm someone who takes care of my body and maximizes mobility through stretching every day. I do what's right, not what's easy in taking the time to perform a daily stretching routine and staying consistent with my flexibility and mobility goals."

*After defining the identity you want to grow into for yourself, chances are this will **not change much**, but rather, only **strengthen over time** based on your actions.*

3b. Your Identity on Your Off-Days

As much as this plays a role in building towards your goals, *it's equally as important in regard to times when you fall off the wagon*.

Most people subconsciously forget about what their self-identity looks like when this happens, allowing a massive negative self-view to kick in.

This leads to a major emotional factor, *guilt*, kicking in, and as many studies have shown, *guilt is a willpower destroyer*.

Instead, mindfully set your identity in these situations... Grow into the person who uses every opportunity of falling off-track to further strengthen your ability to *switch from your off-days back to getting on track.*

Chances are, you won't have perfect consistency with fitness and stretching every single day, for the rest of your life, right? Life is about knowing which habits to employ, at the right time, to help you get the most fulfillment out of life.

This involves testing different things and seeing how they serve your life's purpose. In order to really do this, you must master the ability to switch back and forth and discover how to quickly rebuild the momentum you had with your habits, without any guilt that you 'lost your mojo.'

Be the type of person who can forgive themselves for mistakes, who will love themselves unconditionally, and who can be their own best friend (because if you can't, who will?).

We know these are big emphases on emotional states that can come off as 'fluffy', but the truth is, our fulfillment in life directly ties to our emotional states. Learning how to master them is the true feat of this journal, not just building up a specific habit.

Establishing Your Identity

Write your identity statement here.

What kind of person do you want to grow into through this process?

....
....
....
....
....
....
....

What kind of person do you want to be when you fall off the wagon of your habits? What do you want to remember about who you are, and how can you repurpose these days to serve your life?

....
....
....
....
....
....
....

Understanding Your Why

Who you want to grow into through this process is critical. Equally important is WHY.

The thing is, when we forget (and we forget quite often) the reason we're struggling to improve our lives, we tend to retreat to our habitual selves – to the person we were before we made the decision to change.

Having a clear understanding of your 'why' (what you want to change and why you want to change it) is what pulls you through the tough times you will inevitably face when altering your habits.

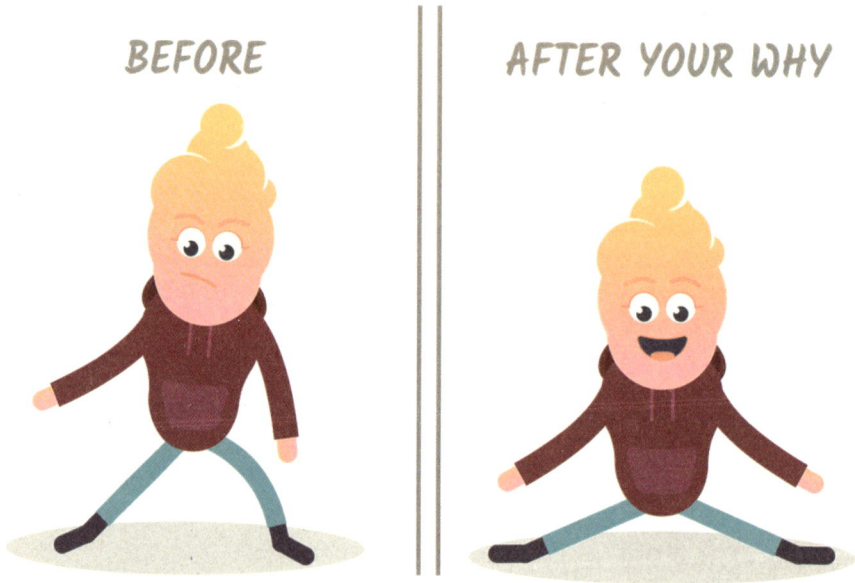

BEFORE

AFTER YOUR WHY

*On the next page are a few simple questions that **you should take your time to answer sincerely before moving on.** These questions are aimed at getting to the root of what drives you, why you bought this journal, and what you expect to gain from using it.*

1. What do I imagine my life would look like if I devoted time to stretching every day?

....

....

....

....

....

....

2. What sort of ripple effect would taking care of my body through stretching every day have on other areas of my life? On the lives of those around me?

....

....

....

....

....

....

3. What would I be missing out on if I didn't do this? How would missing those make me feel?

....

....

....

....

....

....

....

Bonus Question: What obstacles, if any, do I anticipate running into?
How might I overcome them?

....

....

....

....

....

....

....

....

....

Bookmark this section and flip back here the next time you're
struggling to stay consistent with this habit.

This section is your SOS Lifeline.

How This Journal Works

What To Expect

This journal is extremely simple and easy to use.

Every day for the next 66 days, you'll get a specific routine to follow, laid out roughly as follows:

1. You'll begin with a **dynamic warmup** that consists of 3 exercises to get your entire body warmed up and ready for the stretch.

2. You'll then get **6-10 upper body stretches to perform**, focused on the neck muscles, spine, abdomen, shoulders, chest, and arms.

3. The upper body stretches will be followed by **8-12 lower body stretches** focused on the lower back, hips, quadriceps, hamstrings, glutes, and calves.

4. Each day's routine will end with tracking the benefits you're experiencing, along with a blank space to write any notes about your body.

Now that you have the outline, we'll quickly run through why we structured the routines in this way by explaining the type of stretching we'll focus on and the importance of the dynamic warmup.

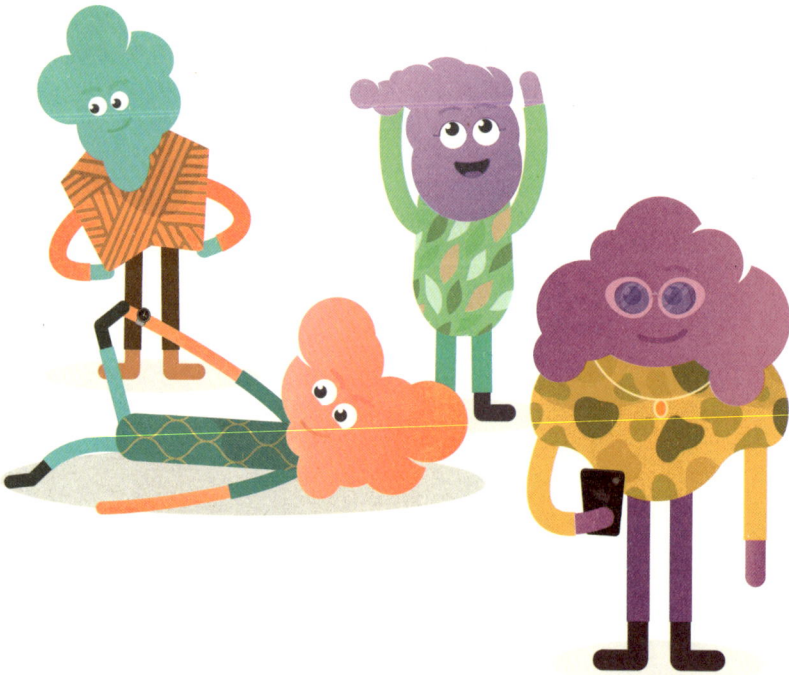

The Type of Stretching We'll Focus On

This journey will focus on traditional static stretching, while incorporating elements of dynamic stretching and PNF.

We chose static stretching as the primary type for the daily stretches in this journal because we believe that stretching requires relaxation, patience, and consistency, and muscles shouldn't be forced to do what they're not ready for.

In static stretching, you're holding a position for a prolonged period of time while trying to deepen the stretch and challenge the limit of your currently flexibility through relaxation. There is a concerted effort on relaxation in order to maximize flexibility, and the fact that you're not moving makes it easier to focus on the muscle being stretched.

That being said, dynamic stretching, static stretching, and PNF have all been found to improve flexibility and range of motion, with no one type significantly outperforming the others.

The truth is that there is only one type of stretching that really works when it comes to increasing flexibility, and range of motion...
CONSISTENT STRETCHING.

Every type of stretching works. They all make your body feel better to be in, and they all have a wide variety of health benefits associated with them.

One or another may be more effective in a unique circumstance, but they're all great at increasing flexibility and range of motion, and therefore mobility.

You begin improving flexibility by actually devoting time to stretching... Stretching only works if you do it consistently.

For 66 days, we're going to give you a complete routine every single day.

No thinking is required on your part. Your only job is to do the routines as consistently as possible.

The Importance of Warming Up

William Levine, orthopedic surgeon and director of sports medicine at *Columbia University Medical Center* in New York says:

> "To improve range of motion and avoid injury, you do need to stretch, but don't ever do it when muscles are cold... Always start with some mild aerobic warm-ups to get blood to the tissue before doing any stretching."

Warming up to stretching has been found to be **critical** to decreasing risk of injury and increasing the benefit of the time you spend stretching by increasing circulation and blood flow, and elevating the temperature of your muscle tissue.

That's why we'll provide a dynamic 2-3 minute full-body warm-up before each day's stretching routine to prepare your body for the stretch.

Getting Started:
Important Information

What Stretching Should Feel Like

Stretching is a relaxing activity that helps your body feel really good, immediately. But the process of stretching and increasing flexibility requires work and dedicated effort, and it won't always feel so pleasant to push the limit of your current flexibility.

For that reason, it's critical that you are able to differentiate between pain and the feeling of a stretch.

Discomfort vs. Pain

When you stretch a muscle, it's like forcing a rubber band to extend longer than it wants to, so naturally there is a resistance. Your body tells you what the limit is through the discomfort that comes when you've stretched a muscle to its current limit.

Your body speaks to you through the sensation of discomfort.

A sensation that wants to let go and relax because there is the experience of tension - that's the feeling of the stretch.

You should never feel agonizing **pain** when stretching, and if you are, there is something wrong. Your form could be off, or you could be stretching beyond a point that your body wants to allow for.

Fortunately, it isn't easy to injure yourself by over-stretching because your body doesn't really let you!

If you feel pain anywhere other than the area you're stretching, you should stop, and try to figure out what's causing that pain.

It's remarkably difficult to describe the difference in words, but remember that discomfort resulting from finding your current maximum limit during a stretch is not the same as pain.

Discomfort, even deep discomfort, is *probably* okay. Sharp sensations are definitely not okay.

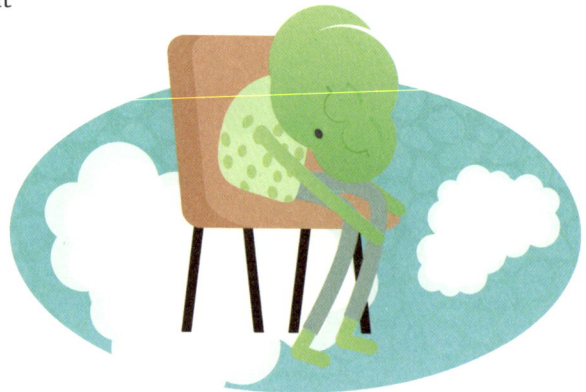

The Relationship Between Stretching & Breathing

As you begin this stretching journey, you'll quickly find that your breathing and your stretching have an intimate relationship.

That's because increasing flexibility through stretching is largely about relaxation.

If you can relax, not tense up in unnecessary places, and breathe through the discomfort you're experiencing as you stretch any given muscle, you'll find that the relaxation is the mechanism through which you can increase your flexibility.

When you breathe, you pull air into your lungs, causing the diaphragm to contract and press down on your internal organs. Then, when you exhale, refreshed blood moves throughout your entire body. The blood flow improves the elasticity of your muscles.

That's exactly why exhaling leads to feeling like you can increase the stretch.

You'll find the truth of this on Day 1.

When you exhale, you have an opportunity to take the stretch one notch further, and your body will tell you when the time comes.

When you're stretching, you'll almost always feel discomfort once you reach the current maximum flexibility for a given muscle. If you can hold through the discomfort for about 5-10 seconds, try to relax all unnecessary muscles, and simply breathe fully, you'll increase your flexibility instantly (at least for the moment).

Breathing is critical, but we don't recommend any sort of manipulation of the breath.

We recommend paying attention to your breathing as you stretch, trying to keep the whole body relaxed, and breathing fully so that you are aware of the moments where the discomfort starts to lessen and you can extend the length of the stretch. That's precisely how you increase flexibility.

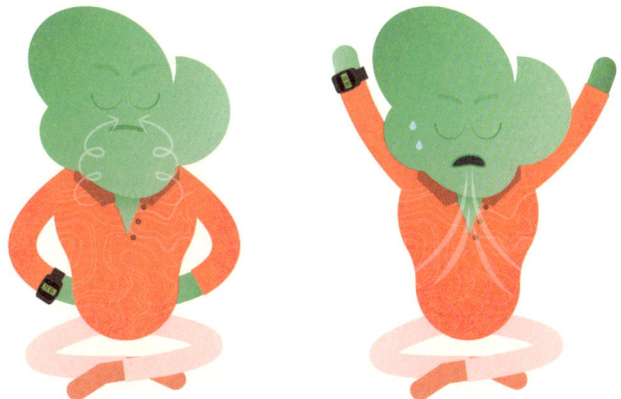

The <u>Extreme</u> Importance of Form

Before beginning any stretch, you have to be absolutely sure that you adequately understand how to perform the stretch without getting injured.

We provide explanations of each exercise, but if you're ever unclear, it only takes 30 seconds to look up any exercise or stretch online and see how others perform it to have a better understanding of what you need to do.

Our bodies are masters of compensation. Where the body can cheat, it will. There must be a conscious vigilance to retain proper form.

And let's be very clear: Form is **vitally** important.

<u>Without proper form:</u>

1. There is always a *risk of injury.*

2. You're most likely **missing the target muscle** because you're *compensating with body parts that don't need to be used.*

There is zero reason not to use proper form while performing any given stretch.

We will explain what proper form is in every stretch we provide, but if you're ever unclear, PLEASE search online for a video that delves further into how to perform the stretch properly until you're confident you can complete it without getting hurt.

Bonus tip: a commonly ignored yet incredibly useful strategy is to record yourself doing a specific stretch so you can actually SEE your form vs. tracking it mentally.

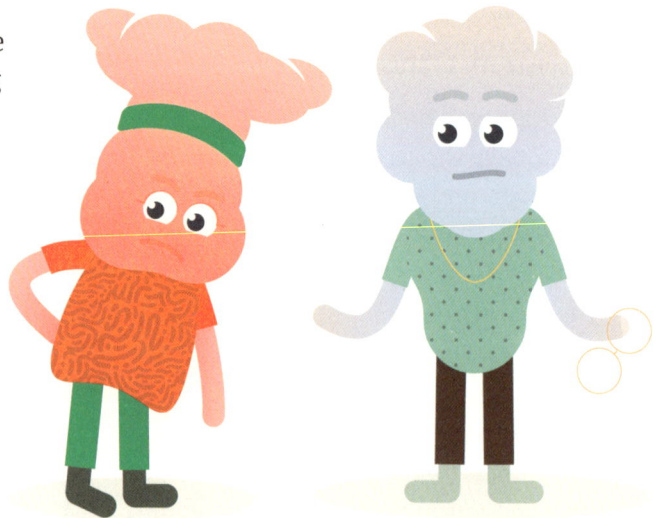

When Is the Best Time To Stretch?

Truthfully, the most important point we want to get across is that if you stretch consistently, you will have a better quality of life, regardless of when, or the type of stretching you perform.

But in order to actually build a new habit and find **consistency**, it's absolutely critical to have a plan for when and where you'll stretch, and to perform your stretching routine in the same place at the same time each day.

For the first few weeks, each routine will take about 10-15 minutes to complete, and afterwards, about 15-20 minutes.

That means that you need to dedicate a small portion of your day to it.

You don't want to be making decisions about where and when you'll stretch on a daily basis. You'll find that any day you do have to make those decisions without planning them beforehand, you're much less likely to actually perform the day's stretch.

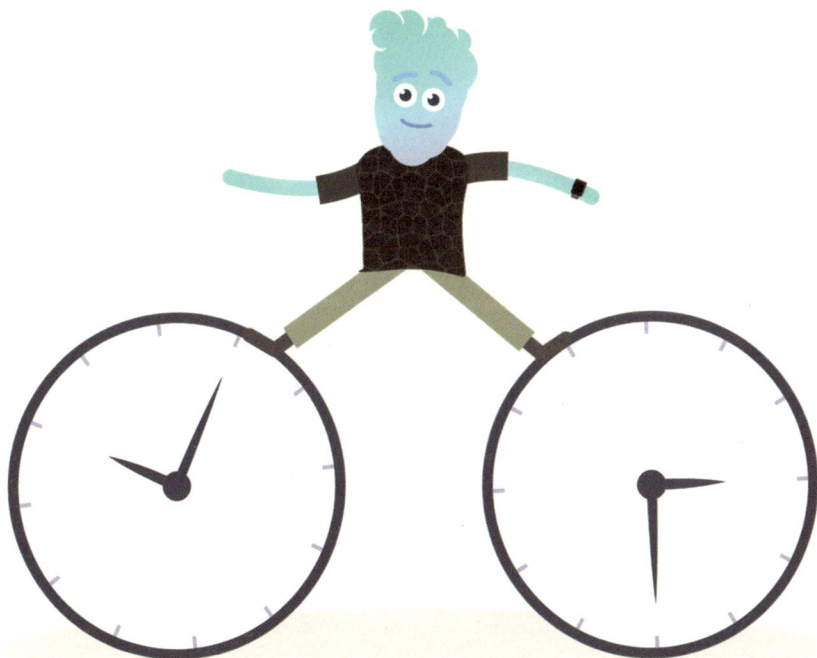

Here's what we recommend:

Give yourself time to stretch in the morning, and if your life circumstances don't allow for that, then in the evening before bed. That way, your routine is tied to a part of your day that takes place no matter what each day.

We more highly recommend doing your stretching in the morning because it helps prepare your body for the day ahead. It can play a role in relieving pain or tension from the night before, it helps increase blood flow, and movement will be more comfortable throughout the day.

If you can't stretch in the morning, stretching at night comes with its own benefits too. Devoting time to helping your body relax and relieve tension after a long day of moving around helps you get ready for bed, and there is research that supports a positive impact of stretching on sleep quality.

Either way, whether it's in the morning, at night, or a different time of the day, have a plan that you can perform with consistency each day, so that getting your routine started becomes a matter of habit.

Risks & Safety Tips

1. **Check with a health professional if you have ANY serious physical imitations, pre-existing injury or condition, or severe discomfort.** If your mobility and/or flexibility is severely limited and you are not comfortable performing any given stretch, or stretching at all causes significant discomfort, we recommend not doing any stretch provided in this journal before consulting a doctor, physical therapist, or other physical health professional.

2. **Do not skip the warmup exercises!** Like we explained before, we put them there because there has been actual research done that supports warming up in order to stretch. It's a simple 2-3 minute warmup that will activate your core and muscles all over your body so that you're ready for the stretch.

3. **Strive for symmetry.** Each of us has a slightly differently shaped body, different genetics, different moving habits, and a different lifestyle. Each of us has to go through the process of learning what our imbalances are, and although it'll take time, to find balance and symmetry. Simply keep in mind that you want to aim for symmetry in the body. When one side is more flexible, devote a little bit more time to the less flexible side, for example.

4. **Don't bounce.** The routines focus on static stretching - holding a position and maximizing the stretch through relaxation. Bouncing can cause injury. Only move as you feel more comfortable deepening a stretch. No sudden movements or bouncing!

5. **Try not to perform the routines immediately before exercise.** If you do want to connect the stretching to an exercise routine, we recommend performing the stretching routine after your workout. It's not a huge deal, but static stretching before exercise isn't ideal.

6. **Know when to exercise caution.** Stretching teaches you about your own body, and your body speaks to you as you stretch. It tells you what it likes, what it doesn't like but it may need, and what it absolutely can't handle. If something doesn't feel right, don't push it. Any time you have actual pain, stop immediately.

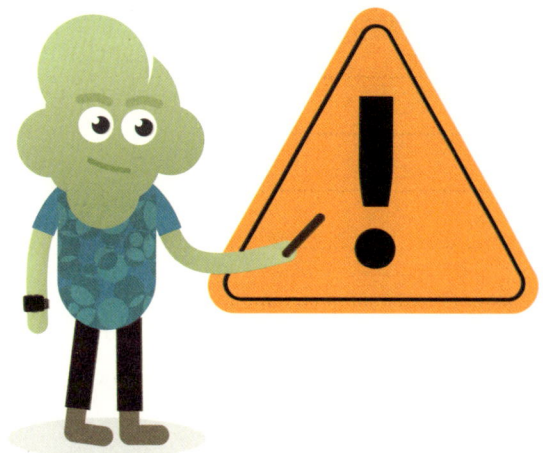

One Simple Idea

We hope that after reading the introductory pages, you're motivated and ready to tackle tomorrow with every ounce of energy you have.

We'll leave you to it with a breakdown of one simple idea...

1

Tomorrow, you will be exactly
who you are today.

2

The rest of your life is a future
projection of who you are today.

3

If you change today,
tomorrow will be different.

4

If you don't change today,
the rest of your life is predetermined.

Commit.

This week:
No matter what happens each day...

...whether I am exhausted
or have the __worst__ day of my life...

...whether I win the lottery
or have the __best__ day of my life...

<u>I **will** do my stretching routine.</u>

*My word is like **gold**.*

I will do whatever it takes to make this happen.

I will stretch at least this many times this week (circle one):

1   2   3   4   5   6   7

_____   _____
        Signature   Date

Phase 1:
Days
01 - 07

Hell Week

My main stretching goal for this phase:

Phase 1 Overview

Welcome to Day 1 of your stretching journey! Before you begin, we just want to quickly explain what to expect during this Phase so you're fully prepared.

<u>Each day, you'll get a 10-15 minute routine consisting of:</u>

• A dynamic warmup that includes 3 exercises to activate your muscles and get your blood pumping.

• 6 upper body stretches.

• 8 lower body stretches.

Days 1-7 are relatively light in terms of the amount of stretching compared to the rest of the journey. Use these 7 days to find the perfect time and place for you to stretch each day, and to get used to the discomfort that comes from stretching tense muscles.

Remember - your body speaks to you. It tells you what it needs, and it tells you what it can't handle, so focus on listening to what your body is telling you in each individual stretch.

Take mental note of what you're experiencing in each part of the body, how flexible you are in different areas,

whether your flexibility is symmetrical on different sides of the body, etc. Every bit of information you learn about yourself through what your body communicates is incredibly helpful.

If any stretch simply doesn't feel right, don't perform it. Find another stretch for the same muscle group that feels alright. You can find alternate exercises in the index, and they'll be listed out for you in the daily routines.

Remember, stretching is largely about learning to relax in order to deepen the stretch and push the limit of your current flexibility. Pay attention to your breathing, and when your body allows for it, deepen each stretch.

Lastly, enjoy the process and the many rewards it comes with!

We promise your body will thank you almost immediately. Good luck!

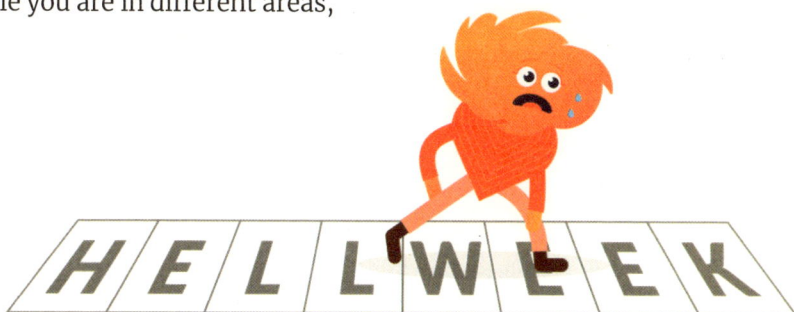

Day 1: Dynamic Warm-Up

Full Session Exercise Guide:
habitnest.com/pages/stretching-day-1

1. Walking Jacks (or Jumping Jacks)

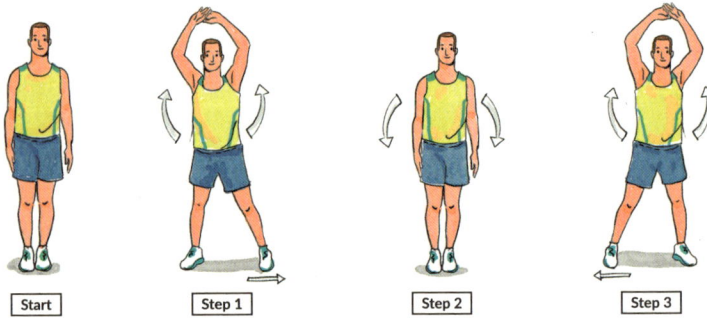

| Start | Step 1 | Step 2 | Step 3 |

Reps: .... *(Goal: 20-30)*

2. Bird-Dog

| Start | Step 1 | Step 2 | Step 3 |

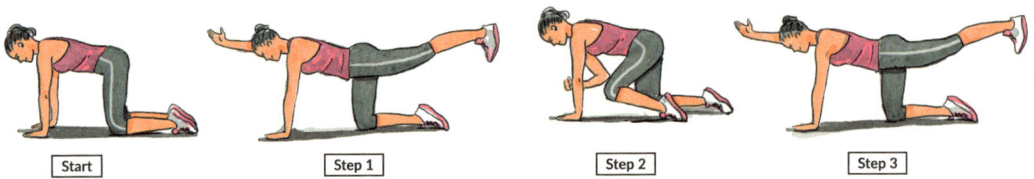

Reps: .... *(Goal: 10-15 each side)*

3. Air Squat to Calf Raise

(Don't let your knees pass your toes when you squat. Reach up towards the sky at the top as high as possible.)

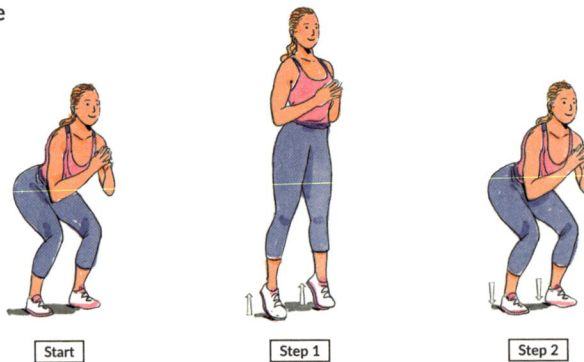

| Start | Step 1 | Step 2 |

Reps: .... *(Goal: 20-30)*

Day 1: Upper Body

DATE

1. Child's Pose

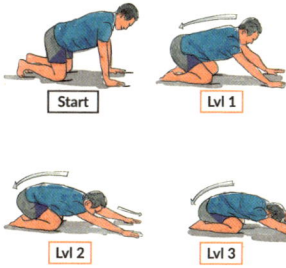

Start

Lvl 1

Lvl 2

Lvl 3

Focus on elongating the spine in both directions. Pull the top of the spine forward with the help of your fingertips, and pull the lower spine downward towards your feet, both physically and mentally.

Level:

Duration: (*Goal: 60 sec*)

2. Cat-Cow

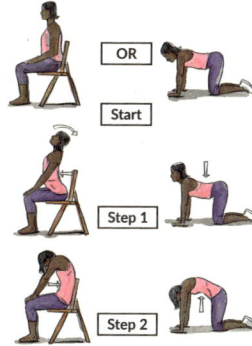

OR

Start

Step 1

Step 2

Try not to sway your entire body. Focus on the spine movement.

Duration: (*Goal: 30 sec*)

3. Lying Full Body Extension

Elongate the spine in both directions.

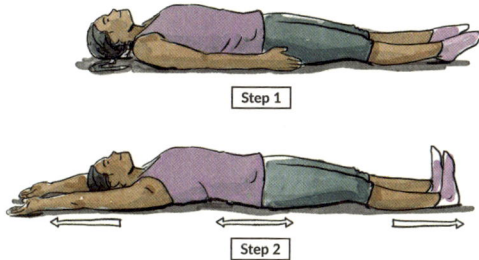

Step 1

Step 2

Duration: (*Goal: 30 sec*)

4. Up & Down Neck Tilt

Don't let any other part of your body tense up as you do this. Shoulders don't need to move!

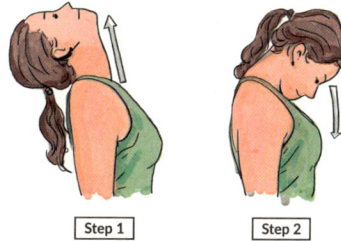

Step 1

Step 2

Duration: (*Goal: 30 sec, alternating*)

5. Lateral Side to Side Neck Rotation

Don't let any other part of your body tense up as you do this. Shoulders don't need to move!

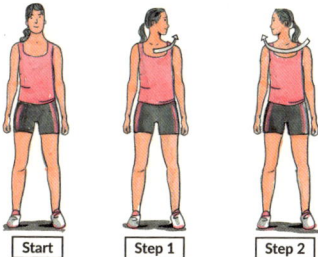

Start

Step 1

Step 2

Duration:

(*Goal: 30 sec, alternating*)

6. Elbow Opener

Don't move your torso at all during this stretch. It's only for your shoulders, chest, and neck.

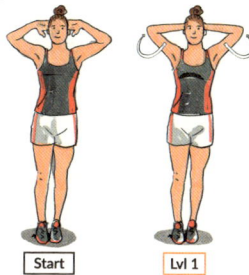

Start

Lvl 1

Duration:

(*Goal: 30 sec*)

7. Standing Oblique Stretch

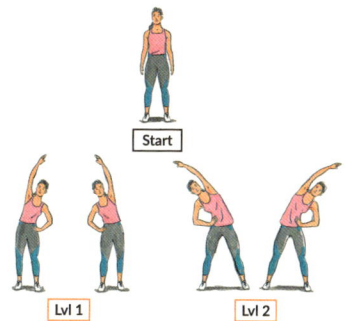

Start

Lvl 1

Lvl 2

Duration:

(*Goal: 15 sec each side*)

Level:

43

Day 1: Lower Body

1. Frog Pose

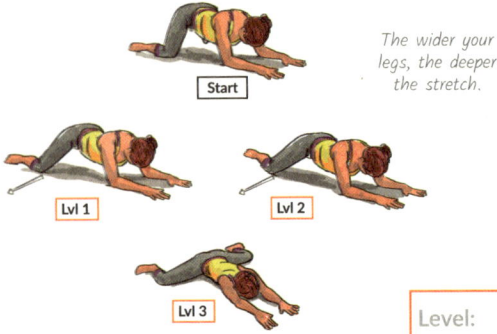

The wider your legs, the deeper the stretch.

Start

Lvl 1   Lvl 2

Lvl 3

Level: _____

Duration: _____

(Goal: 60 sec)

2. Butterfly

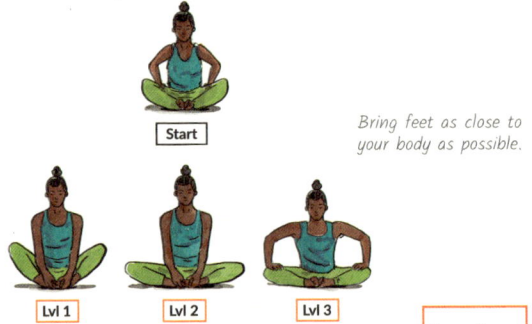

Start

Bring feet as close to your body as possible.

Lvl 1   Lvl 2   Lvl 3

Level: _____

Duration: _____

(Goal: 30 sec)

3. Knee to Chest stretch

Try not to arch your back. Entire spine on the floor!

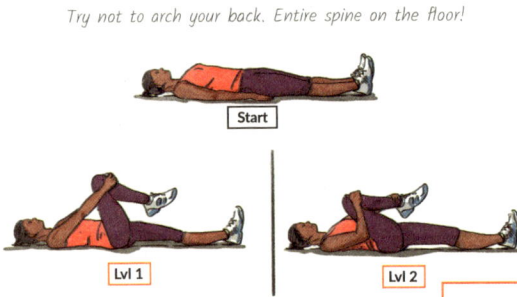

Start

Lvl 1   Lvl 2

Level: _____

Duration: _____

(Goal: 30 sec each side)

4. Runner's Lunge

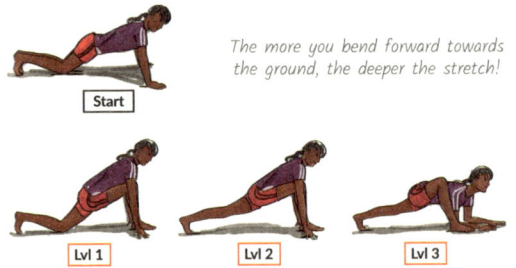

Start

The more you bend forward towards the ground, the deeper the stretch!

Lvl 1   Lvl 2   Lvl 3

Level: _____

Duration: _____

(Goal: 30 sec each side)

5. Lateral Squat

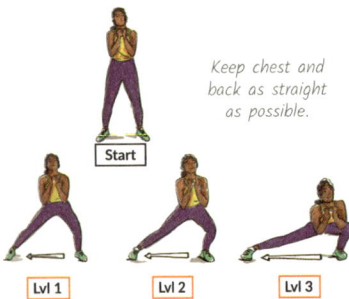

Keep chest and back as straight as possible.

Start

Lvl 1   Lvl 2   Lvl 3

Duration: _____

(Goal: 30 sec each side)   Level: _____

6. Lateral Squat w/ Toe Raise

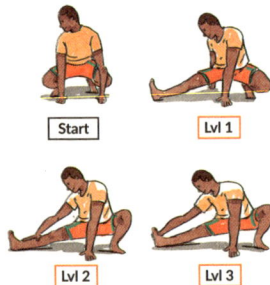

Start   Lvl 1

Lvl 2   Lvl 3

Duration: _____

(Goal: 30 sec each side)   Level: _____

7. Standing Wall Calf Stretch

Wear shoes if needed so you don't slide!

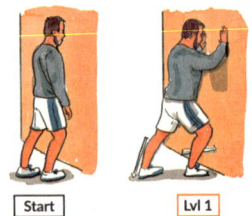

Start   Lvl 1

Duration: _____

(Goal: 15 sec each side)

Daily Reflection

Note: This section is completely optional!

Each day, you can log the benefits you're experiencing as a result of stretching. Stretching has an almost immediate impact on your quality of life, and you'll quickly begin to feel a lot of the physical benefits that come with the practice. Some benefits are a little less obvious, like the impact on your mental wellbeing.

Benefits I'm Experiencing:

Feel
Lighter

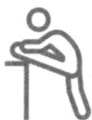

More Freedom
of Movement

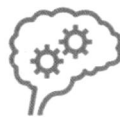

Improved
Mental Clarity

Less
Pain

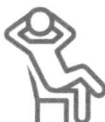

Less
Stressed

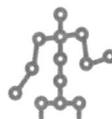

Improved
Posture

Notes On My Body:

....

....

....

....

....

....

Note: This section is completely optional! This space is meant for absolutely any thoughts that you have about your stretching habit, or your body in general.

You can write things like:
- How you're feeling today
- What you notice about how you move throughout the day
- What stretches have been feeling amazing
You get the idea!

Day 2: Dynamic Warm-Up

Full Session Exercise Guide:
habitnest.com/pages/stretching-day-2

1. Inch Worm Walk Out

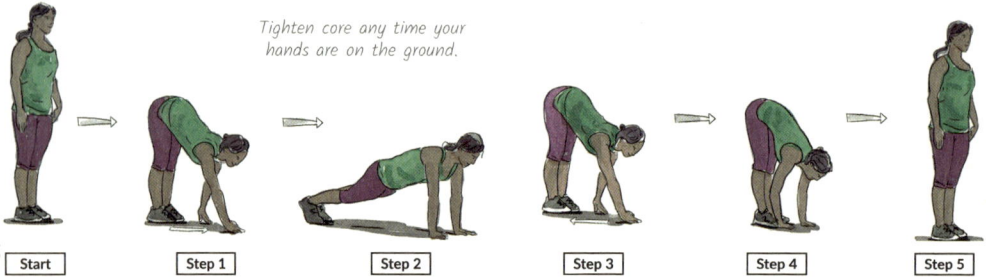

Tighten core any time your hands are on the ground.

| Start | Step 1 | Step 2 | Step 3 | Step 4 | Step 5 |

Reps: .... *(Goal: 10-15)*

2. Clam Opener w/ Side plank

Nothing wrong with taking a rest as you're completing your repetitions for each side!

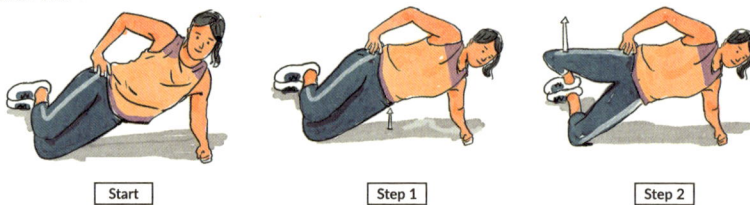

| Start | Step 1 | Step 2 |

Reps: .... *(Goal: 10-15 each side)*

3. Low Lunge w/ Elbow Twist

Here, you'll feel the stretch in the hip/groin area on your straight leg, and in your back on the same side. It feels good, so you can pause for a moment when you're reaching your elbow down!

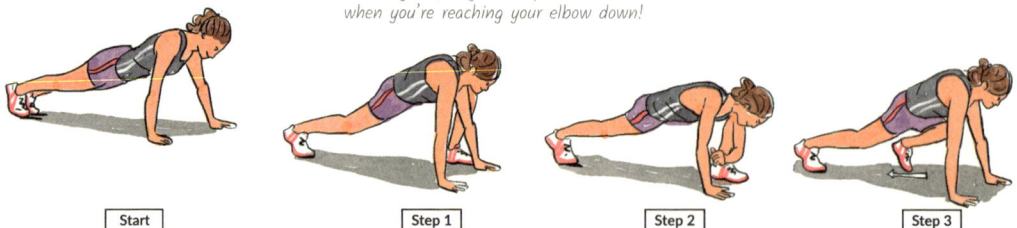

| Start | Step 1 | Step 2 | Step 3 |

Reps: .... *(Goal: 10-15 each side)*

Day 2: Upper Body

1. Child's Pose

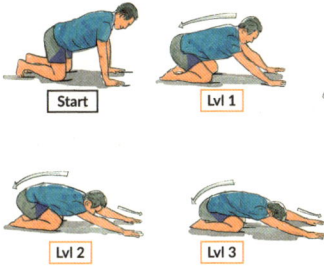

Extend hands to left and right for a deeper stretch on each side.

Start

Lvl 1

Lvl 2

Lvl 3

Level:

Duration:

(Goal: 60 sec)

2. Levator Scap Neck Stretch

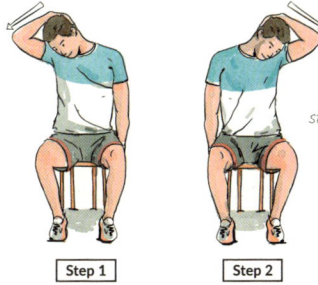

Remember: Pull only to the extent that the stretch feels comfortable.

Step 1

Step 2

Duration:

(Goal: 15 sec each side)

3. Side Neck Tilt

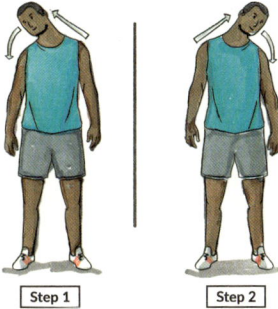

Ear to shoulder, chin up to the sky!

Step 1

Step 2

Duration:

(Goal: 15 sec each side)

4. Leaning Long Arm Shoulder Stretch

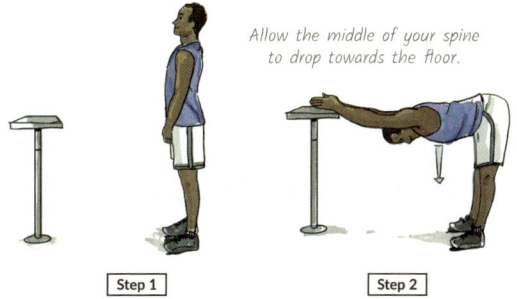

Allow the middle of your spine to drop towards the floor.

Step 1

Step 2

Duration:

(Goal: 30 sec)

5. Static Y Hold

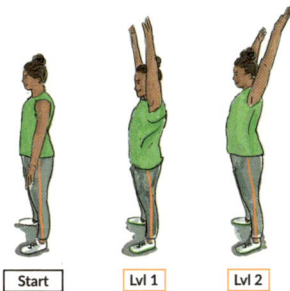

Start

Lvl 1

Lvl 2

Only the arms move. Torso shouldn't move at all!

Duration:

(Goal: 30 sec)

Level:

6. Open Book Chest Stretch

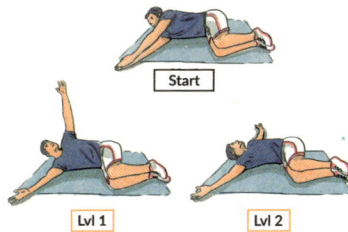

Start

Lvl 1

Lvl 2

Try to move your head and arm simultaneously.

Duration:

(Goal: 30 sec each side)

Level:

7. Seated Forward Curl

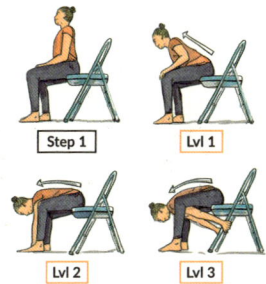

Step 1

Lvl 1

Lvl 2

Lvl 3

Think: Elongating the spine.

Duration:

(Goal: 30 sec)

Level:

47

Day 2: Lower Body

1. Seated Forward Fold Hamstring Stretch

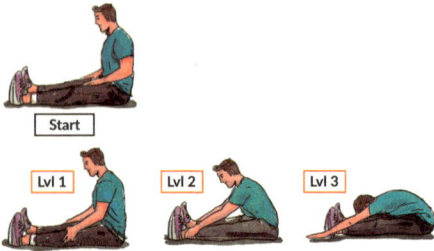

Start

Lvl 1   Lvl 2   Lvl 3

Level:

Duration: ....

(Goal: 30 sec)

2. Figure 4

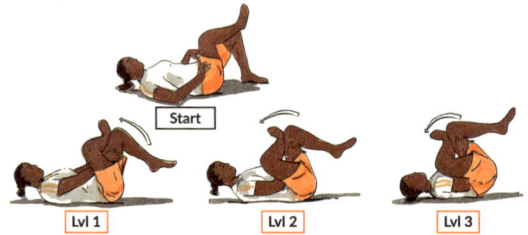

Start

Lvl 1   Lvl 2   Lvl 3

*Alternative: Sit in chair, cross one
leg over, and lean body forward.*

Level:

Duration: ....

(Goal: 30 sec each side)

3. Runner's Lunge

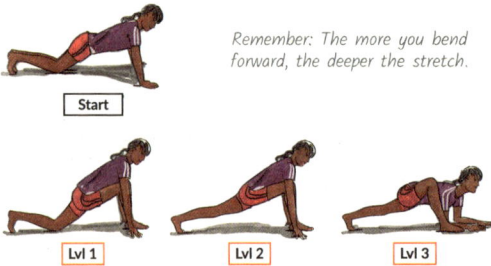

*Remember: The more you bend
forward, the deeper the stretch.*

Start

Lvl 1   Lvl 2   Lvl 3

Level:

Duration: ....

(Goal: 30 sec each side)

4. Standing Quad Stretch

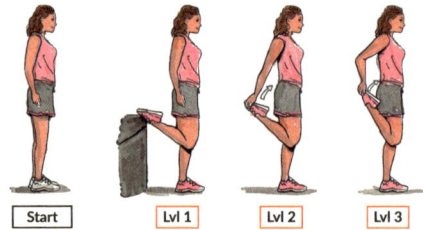

Start   Lvl 1   Lvl 2   Lvl 3

*Pull the leg straight up
behind you, not to the side.*

Level:

Duration: ....

(Goal: 30 sec each side)

5. Seated Single Leg Hamstring Stretch

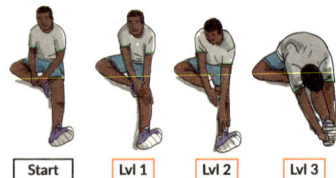

Start   Lvl 1   Lvl 2   Lvl 3

*Bend at the hip rather
than curving your spine.*

Duration: ....

(Goal: 30 sec each side)

Level:

6. Reclining Angle Bound Pose

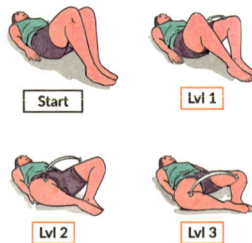

Start   Lvl 1

Lvl 2   Lvl 3

*The closer your feet to your butt,
the more you can open the hips.*

Duration: ....

(Goal: 30 sec)

Level:

7. Standing Wall Calf Stretch w/ Achilles Focus

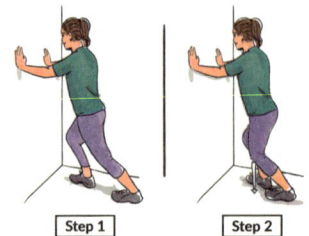

Step 1   Step 2

*The focus here is on the
Achilles of the front leg.*

Duration: ....

(Goal: 15 sec each side)

Daily Reflection

You may not feel the benefits of stretching every single day, and that's COMPLETELY okay. Never get discouraged by a lack of results. You're still putting money in the bank every time you stretch, and it comes with incredible returns as long as you find consistency.

Benefits I'm Experiencing:

Feel
Lighter

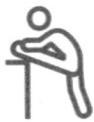

More Freedom
of Movement

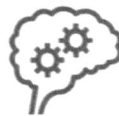

Improved
Mental Clarity

Less
Pain

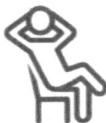

Less
Stressed

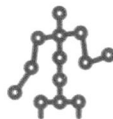

Improved
Posture

Notes On My Body:

....

....

....

....

....

....

One hugely important part of this process is beginning to pay attention to your movement throughout the day, and how the way you move impacts how your body feels.

For example, how's your posture in different times of the day? How do you walk? How do you sit? Our body is in constant use at every moment of our lives, and paying attention to the way we use it can show us what we need to improve.

Day 3: Dynamic Warm-Up

Full Session Exercise Guide:
habitnest.com/pages/stretching-day-3

1. World's Greatest Stretch

*You will learn to LOVE this movement.
Take it slowly the first few times
you do it.*

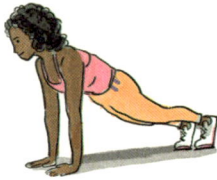 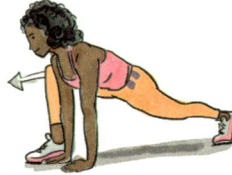 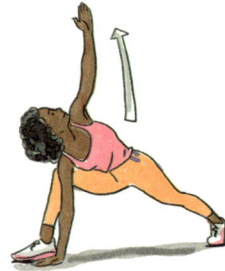

Start	Step 1	Step 2

Reps: .... *(Goal: 5-10 each side)*

2. Good Morning

*One of the best full body warmup exercises!
You're bending at the hip, and the knees.
Everything else maintains posture.*

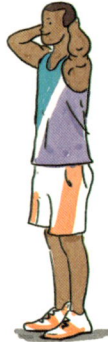 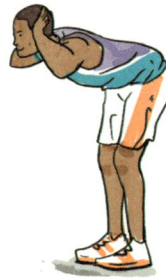

Start	Step 1

Reps: .... *(Goal: 15-20)*

3. Standing Hip Circles

*Open up as widely
as possible in back
and in front!*

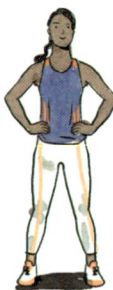 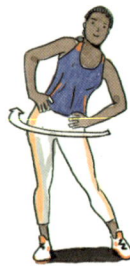 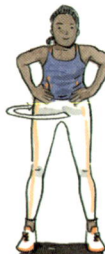 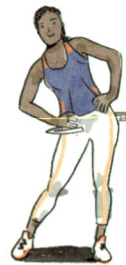

Start	Step 1	Step 2	Step 3

Reps: .... *(Goal: 10-15 each direction)*

Day 3: Upper Body

1. Side Neck Tilt

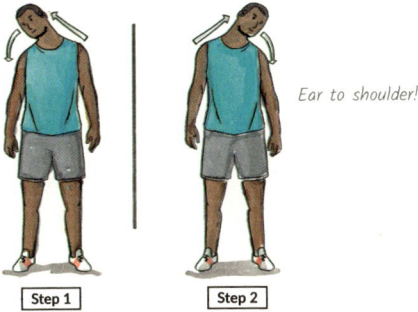

Step 1
Step 2

Ear to shoulder!

Duration: _____ *(Goal: 15 sec each side)*

2. Forward & Backward Neck Tilt

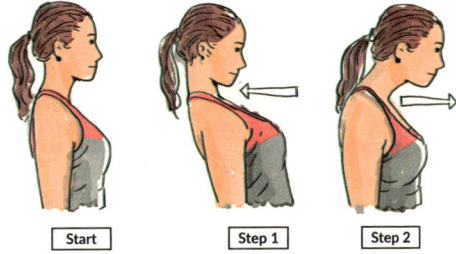

Start
Step 1
Step 2

Look straight ahead and move your head forward and backward.

Duration: _____ *(Goal: 30 sec, alternating)*

3. Forearm Stretch w/Hands on Surface

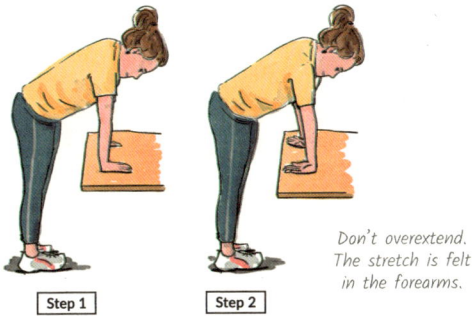

Step 1
Step 2

Don't overextend. The stretch is felt in the forearms.

Duration: _____ *(Goal: 15 sec each side of hand)*

4. Thread the Needle Shoulder Stretch

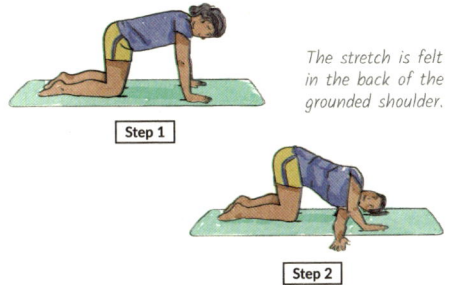

Step 1

The stretch is felt in the back of the grounded shoulder.

Step 2

Duration: _____ *(Goal: 30 sec each side)*

5. Floor Angel

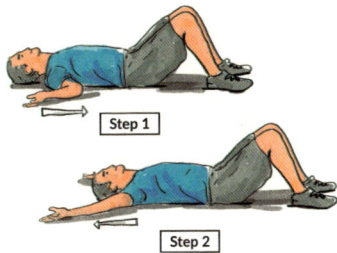

Step 1
Step 2

Duration: _____

(Goal: 30 sec, alternating)

6. Standing Oblique Stretch

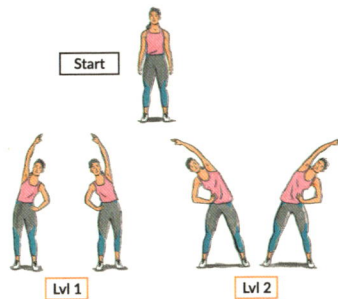

Start
Lvl 1
Lvl 2

Duration: _____

(Goal: 15 sec each side)

Level: _____

7. Behind the Back Tricep Extension

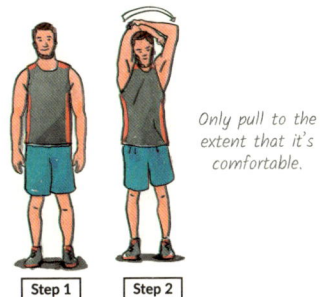

Only pull to the extent that it's comfortable.

Step 1
Step 2

Duration: _____

(Goal: 15 sec each side)

Day 3: Lower Body

1. Frog Pose

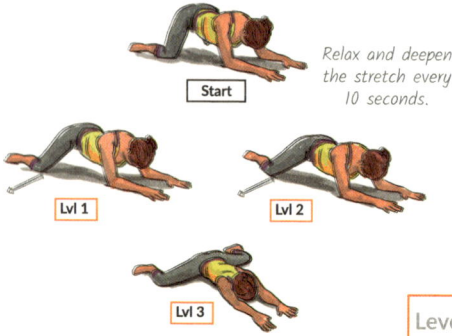

Relax and deepen the stretch every 10 seconds.

Start

Lvl 1   Lvl 2

Lvl 3

Level:

Duration: .... *(Goal: 60 sec)*

2. Seated Spinal Twist

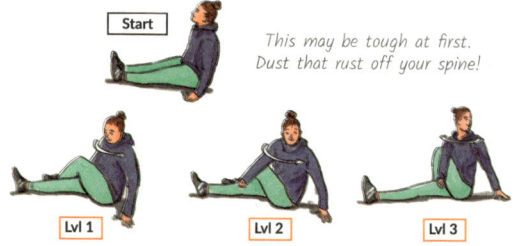

Start

This may be tough at first. Dust that rust off your spine!

Lvl 1   Lvl 2   Lvl 3

Level:

Duration: .... *(Goal: 30 sec each side)*

3. Sphinx/Cobra

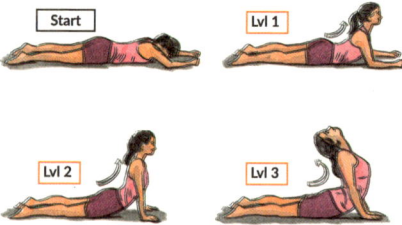

Start   Lvl 1

Lvl 2   Lvl 3

Listen to your body. If you feel the stretch deeply on your forearms, no need to do more.

Level:

Duration: .... *(Goal: 30 sec)*

4. Figure 4

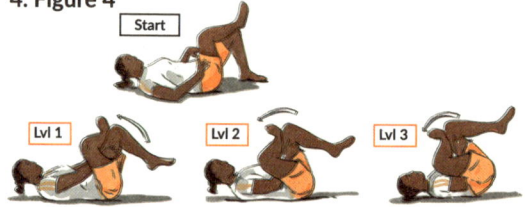

Start

Lvl 1   Lvl 2   Lvl 3

Eventually, you want your whole spine and head on the ground as you do this.

Level:

Duration: .... *(Goal: 30 sec each side)*

5. Lateral Squat

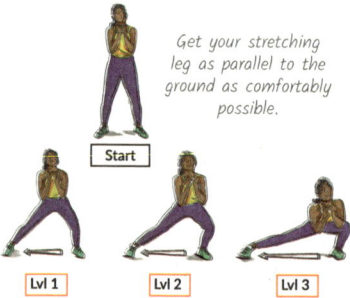

Get your stretching leg as parallel to the ground as comfortably possible.

Start

Lvl 1   Lvl 2   Lvl 3

Duration: ....

(Goal: 30 sec each side)   Level:

6. Lateral Squat w/ Toe Raise

Keep your chest and back as straight as possible without curling your spine.

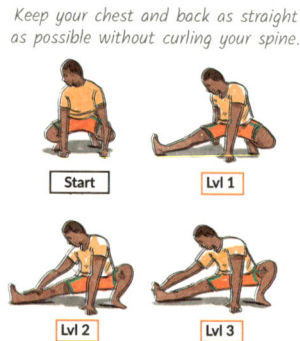

Start   Lvl 1

Lvl 2   Lvl 3

Duration: ....

(Goal: 30 sec each side)   Level:

7. Standing Quad Stretch

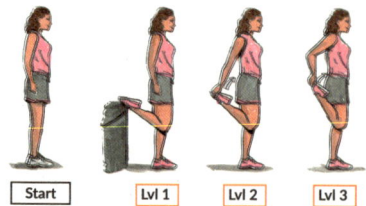

Start   Lvl 1   Lvl 2   Lvl 3

If you can't grab your shin, ankle, or foot, wear long pants and pull the bottom of your pants.

Duration: ....

(Goal: 30 sec each side)   Level:

Daily Reflection

Benefits I'm Experiencing:

Feel
Lighter

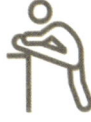

More Freedom
of Movement

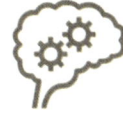

Improved
Mental Clarity

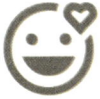

Less
Pain

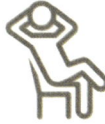

Less
Stressed

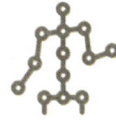

Improved
Posture

Notes On My Body:

....

....

....

....

....

....

....

Remember, this section is optional.

You may not have something new to write every day, but try not to ignore it completely.
When you do notice something new with regards to your body, whatever it is, write it down.

Writing helps solidify what you learn about yourself as opposed to simply having
a passing thought.

Day 4: Dynamic Warm-Up

Full Session Exercise Guide:
habitnest.com/pages/stretching-day-4

1. Standing Hamstring Scoop

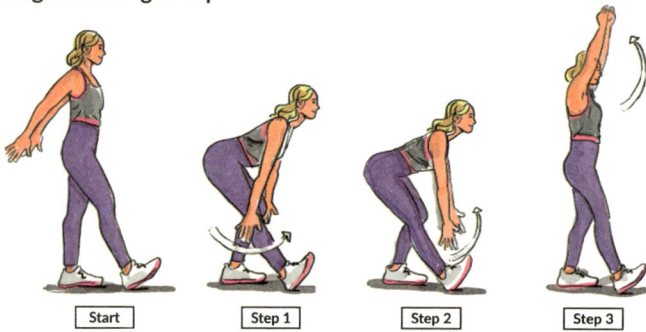

| Start | Step 1 | Step 2 | Step 3 |

Keep your spine straight.
Bend at the hip only.

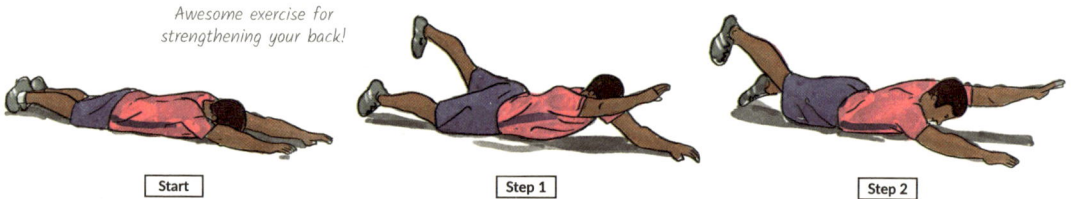

Reps: .... *(Goal: 10-15 each side)*

2. Aquaman

Awesome exercise for strengthening your back!

| Start | Step 1 | Step 2 |

Reps: .... *(Goal: 10-15)*

3. Towel Snatch

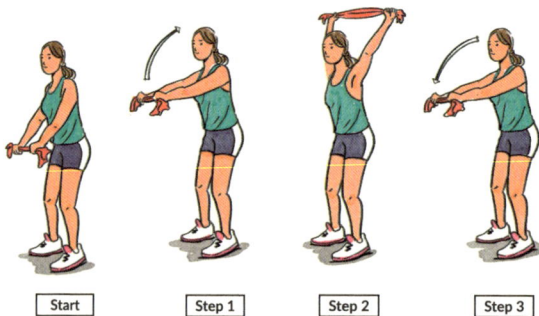

| Start | Step 1 | Step 2 | Step 3 |

Keep the tension high throughout the WHOLE exercise, on the way up & on the way down, by pulling on the towel as hard as you can. If you need a break, take it and then continue.

Reps: .... *(Goal: 15-20)*

Day 4: Upper Body

DATE

1. Child's Pose

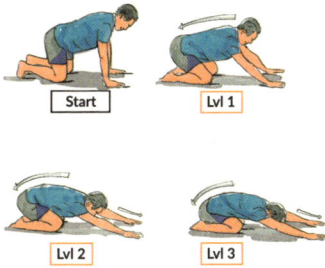

Start | Lvl 1

Lvl 2 | Lvl 3

Level:

Duration: _____ *(Goal: 60 sec)*

2. Up & Down Neck Tilt

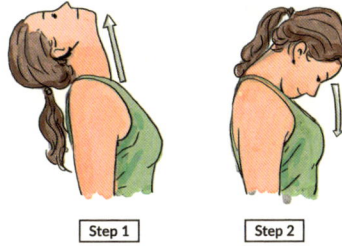

Step 1 | Step 2

The entire body should be relaxed. The only movement is in the neck.

Duration: _____ *(Goal: 30 sec, alternating)*

3. Levator Scap Neck Stretch

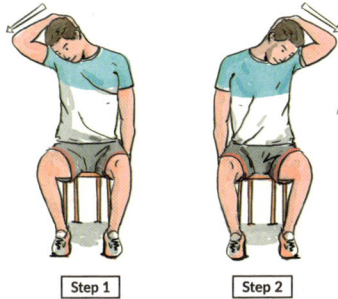

Step 1 | Step 2

Remember: Pull only to the extent that the stretch feels comfortable.

Duration: _____ *(Goal: 15 sec each side)*

4. Cross Arm Shoulder Stretch

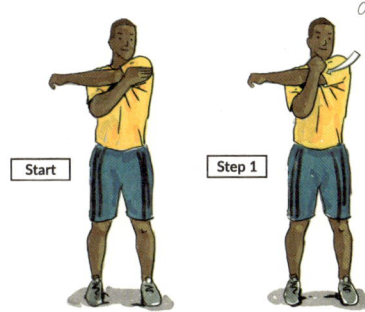

Only the arms move, not the torso!

Start | Step 1

Duration: _____ *(Goal: 15 sec each side)*

5. Locust Pose

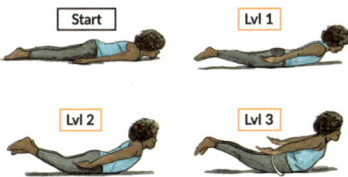

Start | Lvl 1

Lvl 2 | Lvl 3

If this is difficult, leave your legs on the ground for support.

Duration: _____

(Goal: 30 sec)

6. Doorway Pectoral Stretch

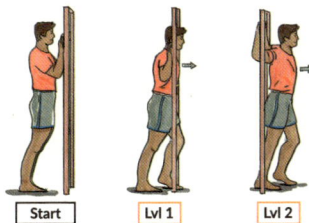

Start | Lvl 1 | Lvl 2

Duration: _____

(Goal: 30 sec)

Level:

7. Standing Oblique Stretch

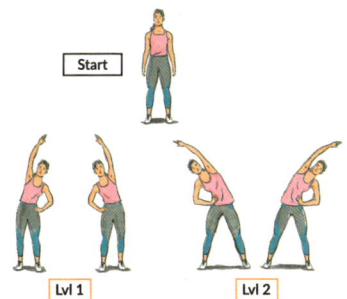

Start

Lvl 1 | Lvl 2

Duration: _____

(Goal: 15 sec each side)

Level:

Level:

Day 4: Lower Body

1. Frog Pose

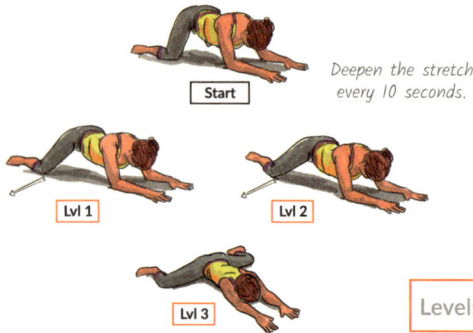

Start

Deepen the stretch every 10 seconds.

Lvl 1 Lvl 2

Lvl 3

Level:

Duration: ....

(Goal: 60 sec)

2. Butterfly

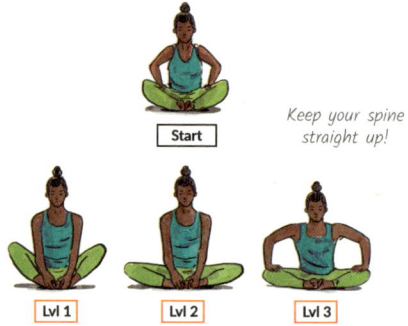

Start

Keep your spine straight up!

Lvl 1   Lvl 2   Lvl 3

Level:

Duration: ....

(Goal: 30 sec)

3. Seated Spinal Twist

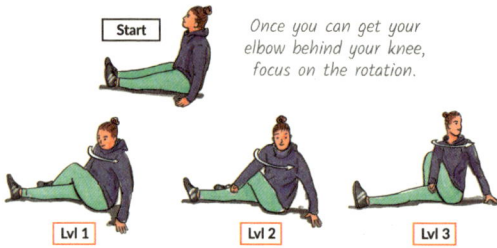

Start

Once you can get your elbow behind your knee, focus on the rotation.

Lvl 1   Lvl 2   Lvl 3

Level:

Duration: ....

(Goal: 30 sec each side)

4. Runner's Lunge

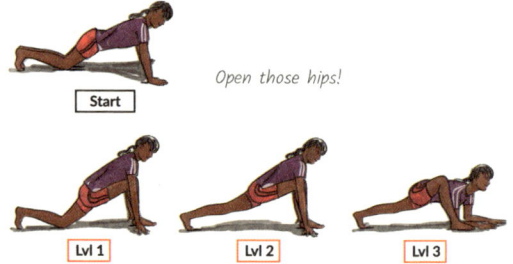

Start

Open those hips!

Lvl 1   Lvl 2   Lvl 3

Level:

Duration: ....

(Goal: 30 sec each side)

5. Pigeon Stretch

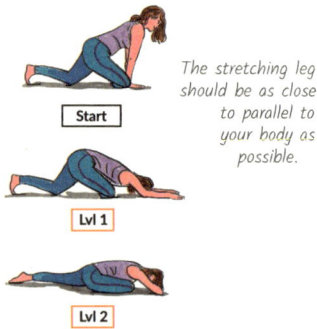

Start

The stretching leg should be as close to parallel to your body as possible.

Lvl 1

Lvl 2

Duration: ....

(Goal: 30 sec each side)

Level:

6. Pry Squat

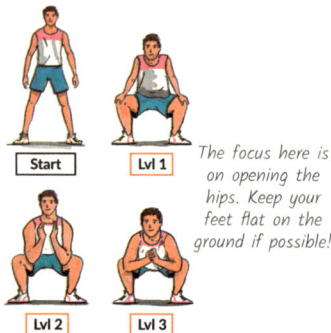

Start   Lvl 1

Lvl 2   Lvl 3

The focus here is on opening the hips. Keep your feet flat on the ground if possible!

Duration: ....

(Goal: 30 sec)

Level:

7. Downward Dog

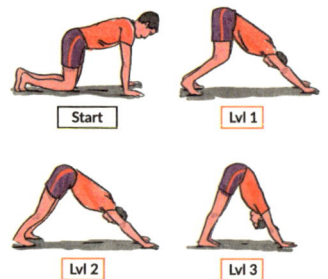

Start   Lvl 1

Lvl 2   Lvl 3

Remember to relax and only stretch to the extent it's comfortable.

Duration: ....

(Goal: 30 sec)

Level:

Daily Reflection

Benefits I'm Experiencing:

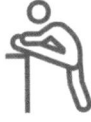

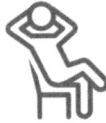

Feel Lighter	More Freedom of Movement	Improved Mental Clarity
Less Pain	Less Stressed	Improved Posture

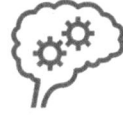

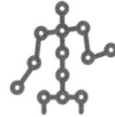

Notes On My Body:

....

....

....

....

....

....

....

What do you find is 'in the way' of actually completing your stretching routine on a daily basis? How can you combat these obstacles?

Day 5: Dynamic Warm-Up

Full Session Exercise Guide:
habitnest.com/pages/stretching-day-5

1. World's Greatest Stretch

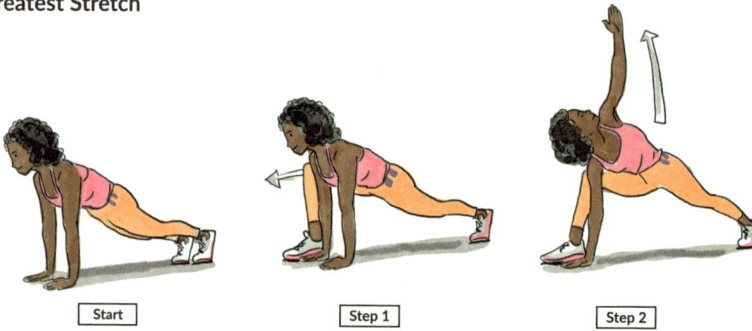

Start

Step 1

Step 2

Reps: .... *(Goal: 10-15)*

2. Mountain Climber

Keep your core tight throughout.
At first, slowly bring each knee up,
and speed up as you get comfortable.

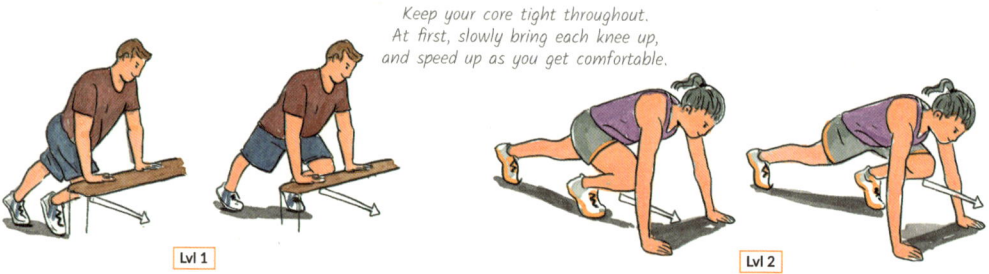

Lvl 1

Lvl 2

Level:

Reps: .... *(Goal: 30-50)*

3. Clam Opener w/ Side Plank

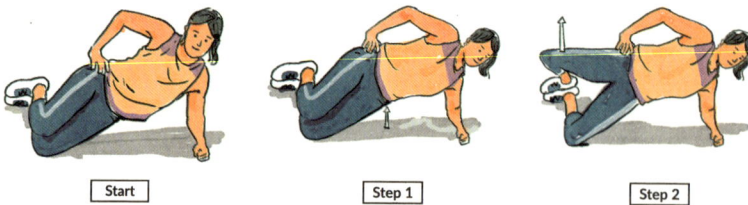

Start

Step 1

Step 2

Reps: .... *(Goal: 10-15 each side)*

Day 5: Upper Body

1. Child's Pose

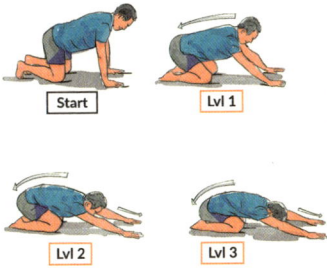

Start

Lvl 1

Imagine your spine elongating in each direction.

Lvl 2

Lvl 3

Level:

Duration: ....

(Goal: 60 sec)

2. Cat-Cow

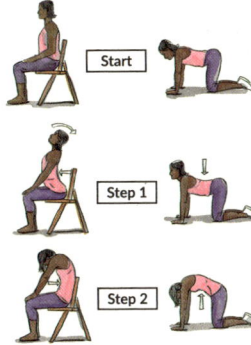

Start

Step 1

Step 2

Duration: ....

(Goal: 30 sec)

3. Side Neck Tilt

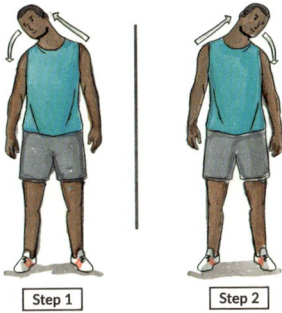

Step 1

Step 2

Duration: ....

(Goal: 15 sec each side)

4. Lareral Side to Side Neck Rotation

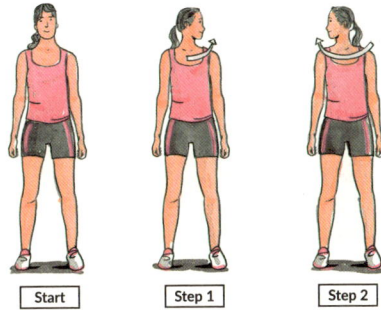

Start

Step 1

Step 2

Duration: ....

(Goal: 30 sec, alternating)

5. Static Y Hold

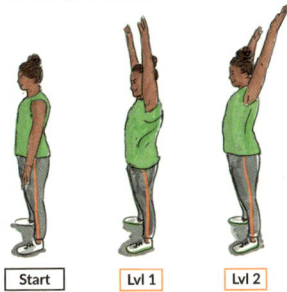

Start

Lvl 1

Lvl 2

Duration: ....

(Goal: 30 sec)

Level:

6. Elbow Opener

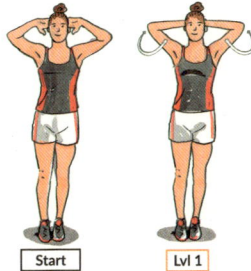

Start

Lvl 1

If it feels okay, stretch your head back slightly as you do this.

Duration: ....

(Goal: 30 sec)

7. Locust Pose

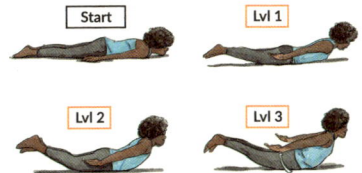

Start

Lvl 1

Lvl 2

Lvl 3

Duration: ....

(Goal: 30 sec)

Level:

Day 5: Lower Body

1. Frog Pose

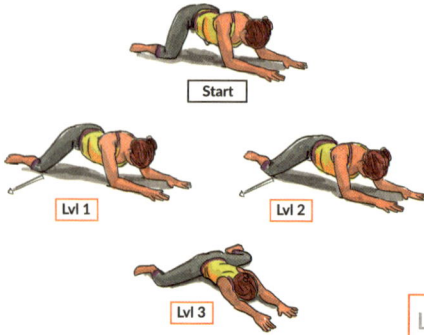

Start

Lvl 1   Lvl 2

Lvl 3

Level:

Duration: _____   (Goal: 60 sec)

2. Runner's Lunge

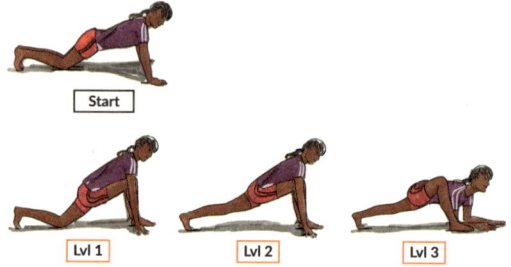

Start

Lvl 1   Lvl 2   Lvl 3

Level:

Duration: _____   (Goal: 30 sec each side)

3. Butterfly

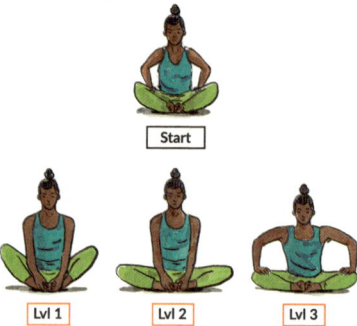

Start

Lvl 1   Lvl 2   Lvl 3

Level:

Duration: _____   (Goal: 30 sec)

4. Sphinx/Cobra

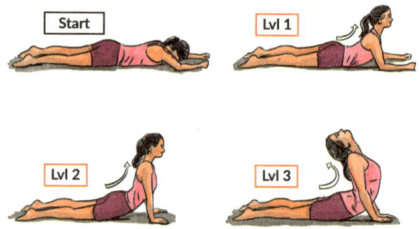

Start   Lvl 1

Lvl 2   Lvl 3

*You're not pulling your spine backwards.
You're stretching it UP and back.*

Level:

Duration: _____   (Goal: 30 sec)

5. Lateral Squat

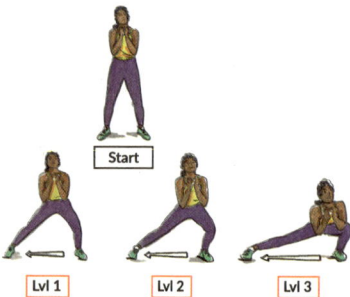

Start

Lvl 1   Lvl 2   Lvl 3

Duration: _____

(Goal: 30 sec each side)   Level:

6. Kneeling Quad Stretch

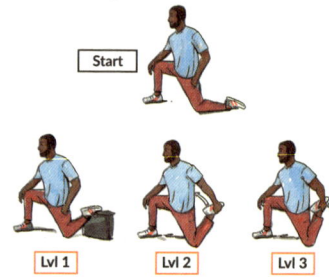

Start

Lvl 1   Lvl 2   Lvl 3

*You want the leg to remain directly
behind you, not to the side.*

Duration: _____

(Goal: 30 sec each side)   Level:

7. Hanging Calf Stretch

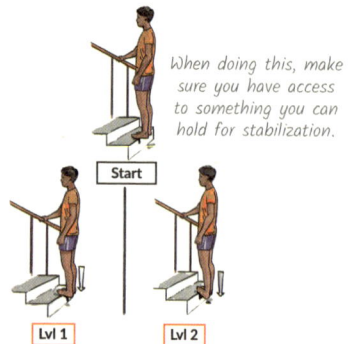

*When doing this, make
sure you have access
to something you can
hold for stabilization.*

Start

Lvl 1   Lvl 2

Duration: _____

(Goal: 30 sec)   Level:

Daily Reflection

Benefits I'm Experiencing:

Feel
Lighter

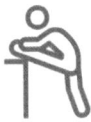

More Freedom
of Movement

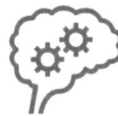

Improved
Mental Clarity

Less
Pain

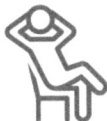

Less
Stressed

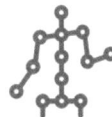

Improved
Posture

Notes On My Body:

....

....

....

....

....

....

....

*Which parts of your body seem to be unbalanced or asymmetrical
when it comes to flexibility? How can you devote a little extra time
to resolving the asymmetry?*

Day 6: Dynamic Warm-Up

Full Session Exercise Guide:
habitnest.com/pages/stretching-day-6

1. Rocking Feet w/ Arm Raise

*It may take a second to find the right sense
of stability as you perform this movement,
but you'll get used to it. Arms back as far
as possible in both directions!*

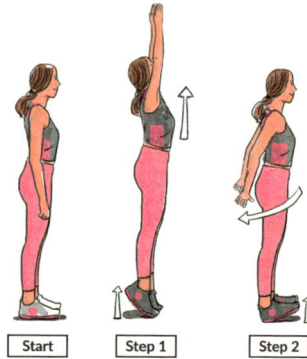

Start   Step 1   Step 2

Reps: *(Goal: 10-15)*

2. Plank w/ Shoulder Tap

*You can also do this on your knees if you're having difficulty
holding your body up. Do your best not to let your body
sway from left to right. As much as you can, hold your body
stable when you lift each arm to tap the opposite shoulder.*

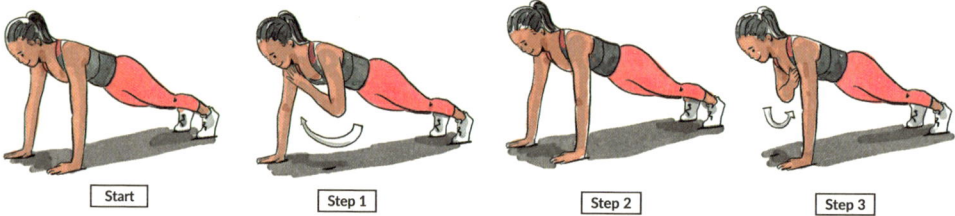

Start   Step 1   Step 2   Step 3

Reps: *(Goal: 10-15 each side)*

3. Split Squat

*Here, you perform the total number of reps
on one side before switching to the other side.
Will help you get in a little groove as you squat!*

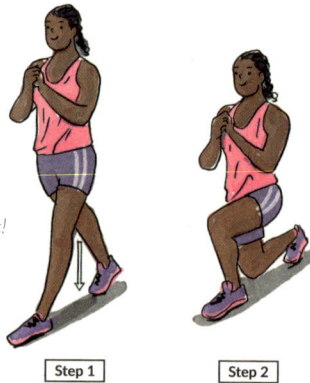

Step 1   Step 2

Reps: *(Goal: 10-15 each side)*

62

Day 6: Upper Body

DATE

1. Side Neck Tilt

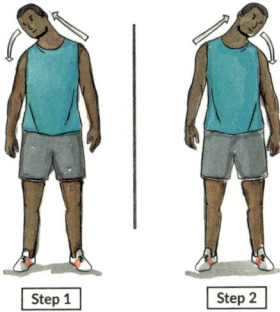

Step 1   Step 2

Duration: _____ *(Goal: 15 sec each side)*

2. Forward & Backward Neck Tilt

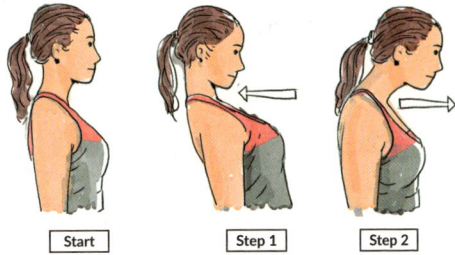

Start   Step 1   Step 2

Duration: _____ *(Goal: 30 sec, alternating)*

3. Child's Pose

Start   Lvl 1

Lvl 2   Lvl 3

Level: _____

Duration: _____ *(Goal: 60 sec)*

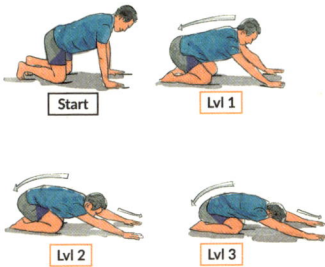

4. Sphinx/Cobra

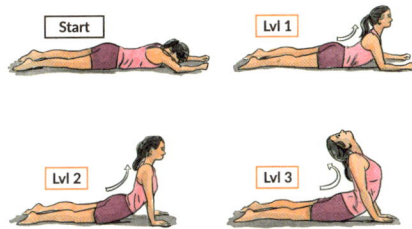

Start   Lvl 1

Lvl 2   Lvl 3

Level: _____

Duration: _____ *(Goal: 30 sec)*

5. Corner Chest Stretch

Find the right distance you need to be away from the wall for the stretch to feel good.

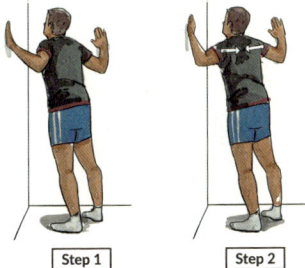

Step 1   Step 2

Duration: _____

(Goal: 30 sec)

6. Leaning Long Arm Shoulder Stretch

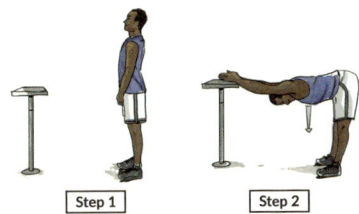

Step 1   Step 2

Duration: _____

(Goal: 30 sec)

7. Standing Oblique Stretch

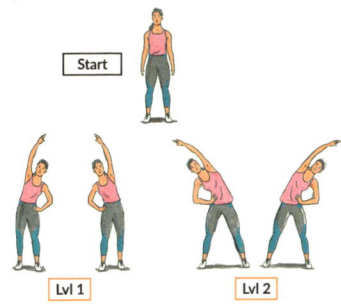

Start

Lvl 1   Lvl 2

Duration: _____

(Goal: 15 sec each side)   Level: _____

Day 6: Lower Body

1. Frog Pose

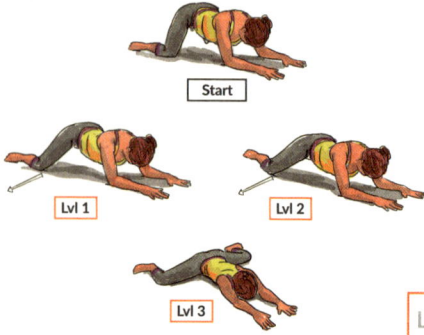

Start

Lvl 1   Lvl 2

Lvl 3

Duration: .... *(Goal: 60 sec)*

Level: [ ]

2. Pigeon Stretch

This is a super important stretch for loosening your glute muscles.

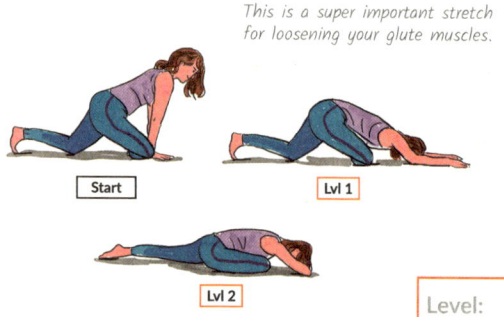

Start   Lvl 1

Lvl 2

Level: [ ]

Duration: .... *(Goal: 30 sec each side)*

3. Downward Dog

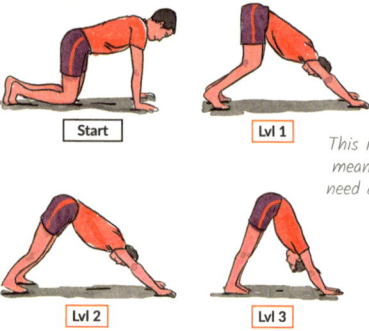

Start   Lvl 1

This is hard, and it's meant to be. If you need a break, take it.

Lvl 2   Lvl 3

Level: [ ]

Duration: .... *(Goal: 30 sec)*

4. Wig-Wag

Try to keep your back as parallel with the floor as possible while performing the stretch.

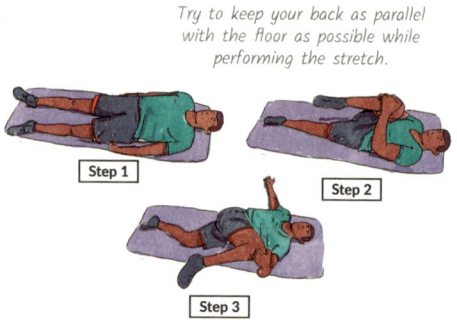

Step 1   Step 2

Step 3

Duration: .... *(Goal: 30 sec each side)*

5. Warrior II Pose

This is felt most in the hip of the straight leg.

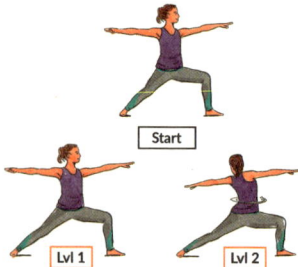

Start

Lvl 1   Lvl 2

Duration: ....

(Goal: 30 sec each side)   Level: [ ]

6. Pry Squat

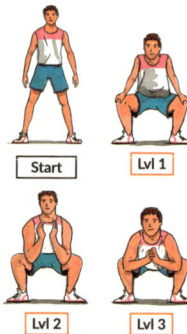

Start   Lvl 1

As low to the ground as possible with your feet flat.

Lvl 2   Lvl 3

Duration: ....

(Goal: 30 sec)   Level: [ ]

7. Standing Quad Stretch

Remember, try to keep your body nice and upright so you're not leaning forward.

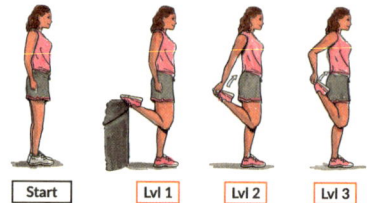

Start   Lvl 1   Lvl 2   Lvl 3

Duration: ....

(Goal: 30 sec each side)   Level: [ ]

Daily Reflection

Benefits I'm Experiencing:

Feel
Lighter

More Freedom
of Movement

Improved
Mental Clarity

Less
Pain

Less
Stressed

Improved
Posture

Notes On My Body:

....
....
....
....
....
....
....
....
....

Day 7: Dynamic Warm-Up

1. Inch Worm Walk Out

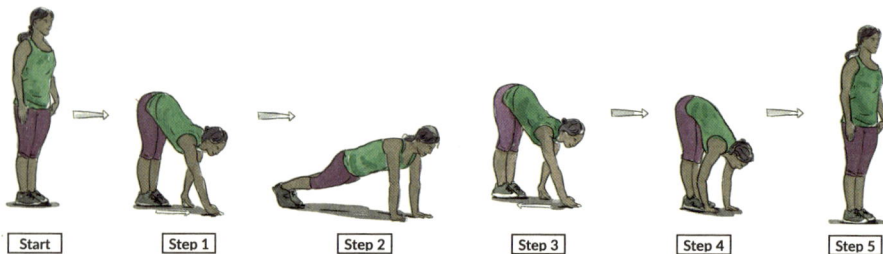

| Start | Step 1 | Step 2 | Step 3 | Step 4 | Step 5 |

Reps: .... *(Goal: 10-15)*

2. Good Morning

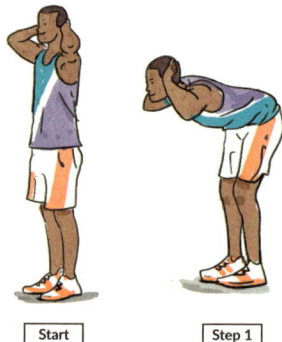

| Start | Step 1 |

Reps: .... *(Goal: 15-20)*

3. Knee Hug

Keep your body stable, without swaying, as you slowly lift each leg as high as possible.

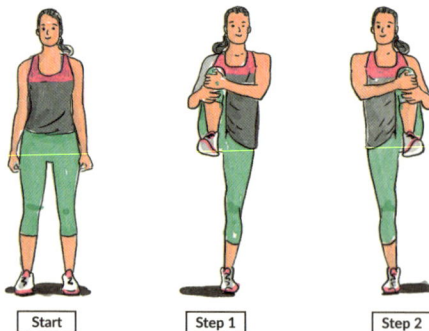

| Start | Step 1 | Step 2 |

Reps: .... *(Goal: 10-15 each side)*

Day 7: Upper Body

1. Child's Pose

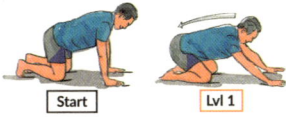

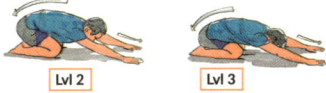

Extend to left and right for deeper lat stretches.

Level:

Duration: *(Goal: 60 sec)*

2. Up & Down Neck Tilt

Neck stretches often feel tedious, but they're important.

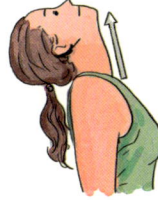 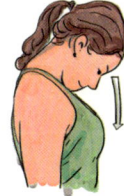

Step 1   Step 2

Duration: *(Goal: 30 sec, alternating)*

3. Lateral Side to Side Neck Rotation

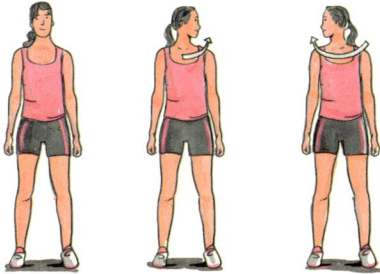

Start   Step 1   Step 2

Duration: *(Goal: 30 sec, alternating)*

4. Static Y Hold

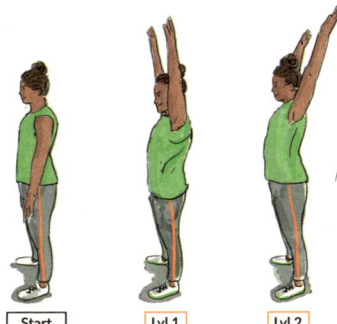

Arms back as FAR as possible without moving your torso.

Start   Lvl 1   Lvl 2

Level:

Duration: *(Goal: 30 sec)*

5. Open Book Chest Stretch

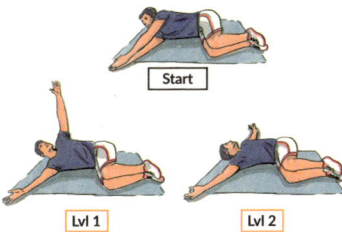

Start

Lvl 1   Lvl 2

Try to move your head and arm simultaneously while opening the arms and performing the stretch.

Duration:

(Goal: 30 sec each side)   Level:

6. Thread the Needle Shoulder Stretch

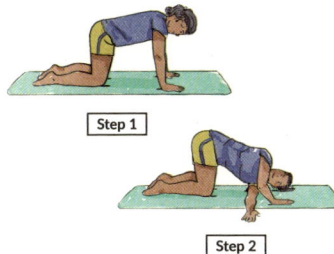

Step 1

Step 2

Duration:

(Goal: 30 sec each side)

7. Standing Oblique Stretch

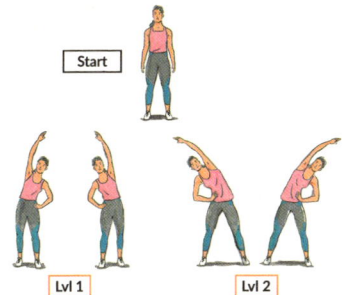

Start

Lvl 1   Lvl 2

Duration:

(Goal: 15 sec each side)   Level:

Day 7: Lower Body

1. Pigeon Stretch

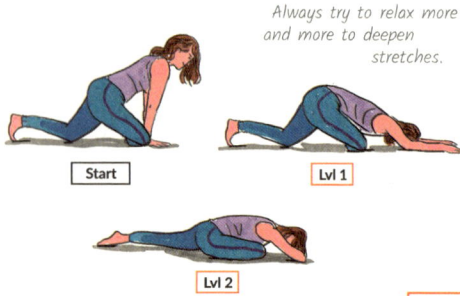

Always try to relax more and more to deepen stretches.

Start

Lvl 1

Lvl 2

Level: ___

Duration: ___   *(Goal: 30 sec each side)*

2. Butterfly

Start

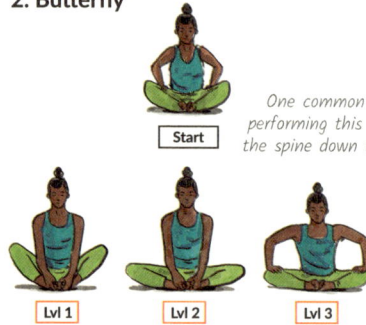

One common mistake while performing this stress is tensing the spine down towards the floor.

Lvl 1

Lvl 2

Lvl 3

Level: ___

Duration: ___   *(Goal: 30 sec)*

3. Runner's Lunge

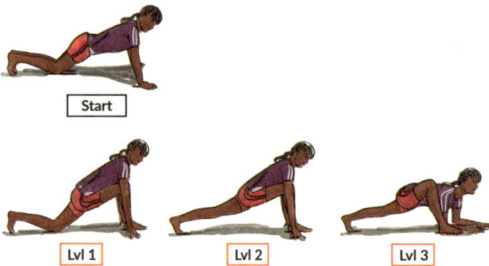

Start

Lvl 1

Lvl 2

Lvl 3

Level: ___

Duration: ___   *(Goal: 30 sec each side)*

4. Lateral Squat

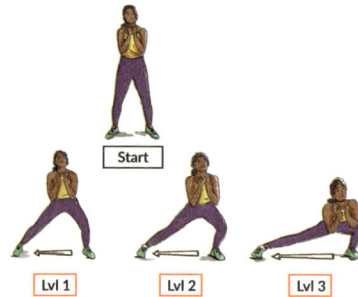

Start

Lvl 1

Lvl 2

Lvl 3

Level: ___

Duration: ___   *(Goal: 30 sec each side)*

5. Lateral Squat w/ Toe Raise

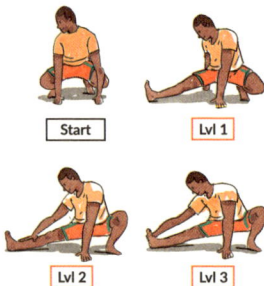

Start

Lvl 1

Lvl 2

Lvl 3

Duration: ___

(Goal: 30 sec each side)   Level: ___

6. Lying Quad Stretch

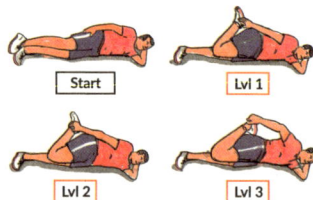

Start

Lvl 1

Lvl 2

Lvl 3

Duration: ___

(Goal: 30 sec each side)   Level: ___

7. Standing Wall Calf Stretch w/ Achilles Focus

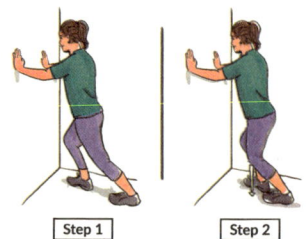

Step 1

Step 2

The stretch comes from lowering the knee on the lower calf of the stretching leg.

Duration: ___

(Goal: 15 sec each side)

Daily Reflection

There are A LOT of benefits to stretching, and of course only 6 of them are listed out here. Feel free to write any other benefits you're experiencing in your notes below.

For example, does increased freedom of movement impact your relationships in any way? Thinking about and writing actual examples of how you're benefitting from the practice will ALWAYS help motivate you to continue.

Benefits I'm Experiencing:

Feel
Lighter

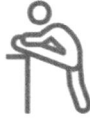

More Freedom
of Movement

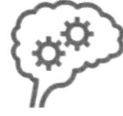

Improved
Mental Clarity

Less
Pain

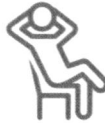

Less
Stressed

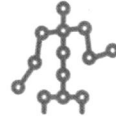

Improved
Posture

Notes On My Body:

....

....

....

....

....

....

....

How is your body feeling after 7 stretching sessions? Do you feel better, worse, or equal to what you expected at the beginning of the journey?

Recap Questions

1. In which parts of my body do I experience the most discomfort, pain, and/or tension?

    ....

    ....

    ....

2. What movements do I make in my life that don't feel seamless, or without any unnecessary discomfort or pain?

    ....

    ....

    ....

3. What stretches do I find help alleviate these symptoms that I need to spend more time on?

    ....

    ....

    ....

4. Which side of my body is generally more flexible? Are there any specific muscles I find have largely varying degrees of flexibility?

    ....

    ....

    ....

5. What stretches do I want to swap out completely because they just don't feel right? What can I replace those stretches with that target the same muscle(s)?

    ....

    ....

    ....

6. What physical habits do I have that I notice lead to tension or discomfort in the body?

....

....

....

....

7. What discomfort, pain, and/or tension do I experience that I don't know the cause of and want to pay attention to, with the goal of learning about my own physical habits?

....

....

....

....

Phase 1
Done.

Phase 2:
Days
08 - 21

Digging Deep & Staying Consistent

My main stretching goal for this phase:

Phase 2 Overview

You made it through Phase 1!

At this point, you've hopefully found the right place and time of day to dedicate to your stretching routine.

You've likely felt the immediate impact stretching has on the way your body feels throughout the day, and you're probably even a little more flexible than when you started.

It's time to kick it up a notch.

For the next few weeks, each day's routine will still include a dynamic warmup with 3 exercises, but now you'll perform 8 upper body stretches and 10 lower body stretches for a slightly longer routine.

During Phase 2, consistency is absolutely crucial. This is the time when it's critical to do your best to force yourself to stretch daily, especially when you don't feel like it.

Building a habit requires consistency, and the more often you stretch and see the clear positive impact it has on your daily life, the more likely you are to continue with it.

Remember, stretching regularly and activating the muscles in the body is a vital aspect of self-care.

The time you dedicate to relaxing and making your body happy is time that is extremely well spent. Your body carries you through life, and devoting at least 15-20 minutes a day to making it feel good shouldn't be thought of as a luxury. It's a necessity for living a physically comfortable, pain-free life.

Good luck in Phase 2!

Day 8: Dynamic Warm-Up

Full Session Exercise Guide:
habitnest.com/pages/stretching-day-8

1. Side Plank w/ Twist

Make sure your body is stable as you twist. You use each respective side of the core for this, and you'll definitely feel it afterwards!

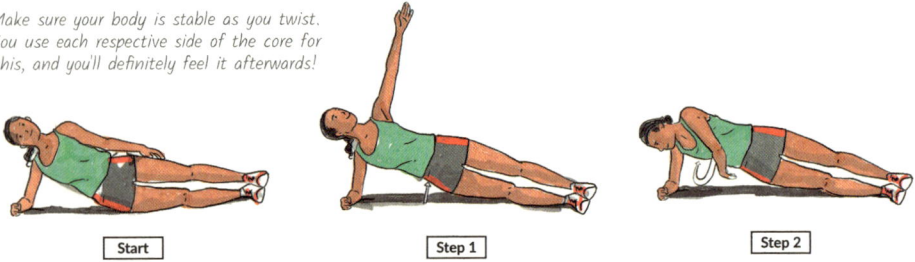

Start

Step 1

Step 2

Reps: .... *(Goal: 10-15 each side)*

2. Roundhouse Kick to Squat

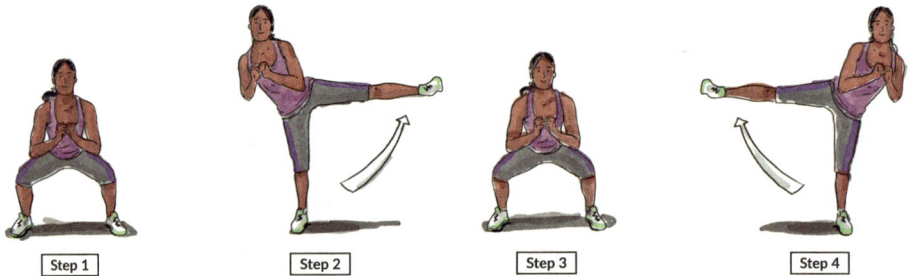

Step 1

Step 2

Step 3

Step 4

Reps: .... *(Goal: 10-20 each side)*

3. Glute Bridge

Keep your legs in a straight line as you push yourself up through your HEELS. Don't let your knees go outwards as you push up.

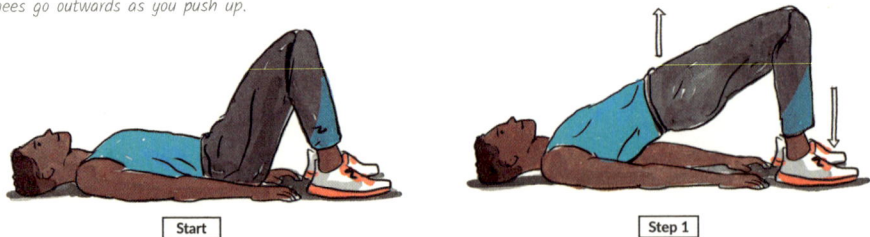

Start

Step 1

Reps: .... *(Goal: 20-30)*

Day 8: Upper Body

1. Up & Down Neck Tilt

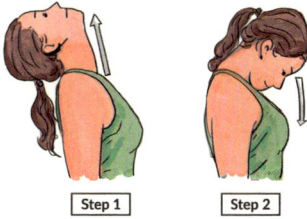

Step 1   Step 2

Duration: _____   (Goal: 30 sec, alternating)

2. Side Neck Stretch w/ Upside Down Palm on Wall

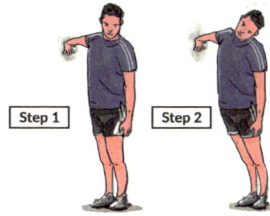

Step 1   Step 2

Reps: _____   (Goal: 30 sec each side)

3. Levator Scap Neck Stretch

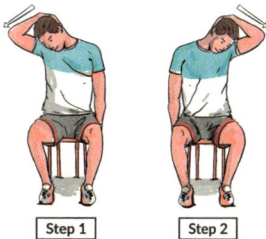

Step 1   Step 2

Duration: _____   (Goal: 15 sec each side)

4. Cross Arm Shoulder Stretch

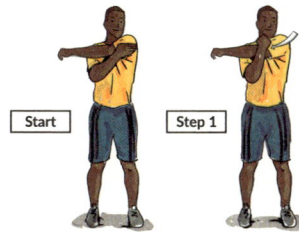

Start   Step 1

Duration: _____   (Goal: 15 sec each side)

5. Static Y Hold

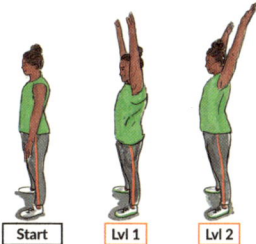

Start   Lvl 1   Lvl 2

Level: _____

Duration: _____   (Goal: 30 sec)

6. Reverse Prayer

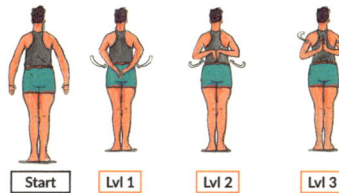

Start   Lvl 1   Lvl 2   Lvl 3

This is extremely difficult. Open your chest as wide as possible.

Level: _____

Duration: _____   (Goal: 30 sec)

7. Wall Lat Stretch

Keep your legs straight for a bonus hamstring stretch!

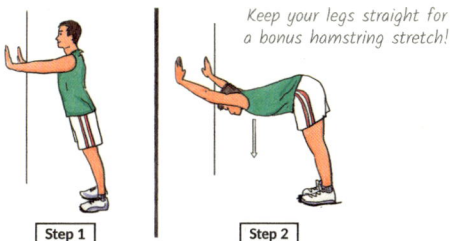

Step 1   Step 2

Duration: _____   (Goal: 30 sec)

8. Behind the Back Tricep Extension

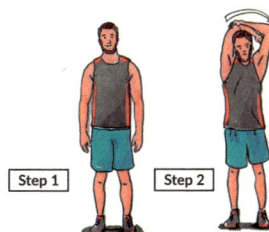

Step 1   Step 2

Duration: _____   (Goal: 15 sec each side)

Day 8: Lower Body

1. Frog Pose

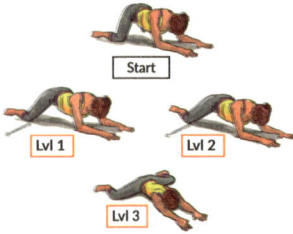
Start
Lvl 1   Lvl 2
Lvl 3

Duration:

(Goal: 60 sec)   Level:

2. Seated Forward Fold Hamstring Stretch

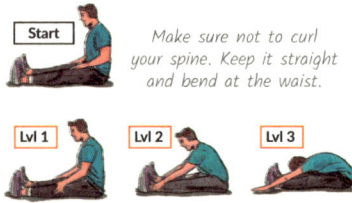
Start

Make sure not to curl your spine. Keep it straight and bend at the waist.

Lvl 1   Lvl 2   Lvl 3

Duration:

(Goal: 30 sec)   Level:

3. Lateral Squat

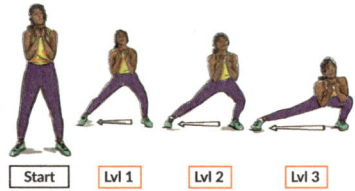
Start   Lvl 1   Lvl 2   Lvl 3

Duration:

(Goal: 30 sec each side)   Level:

4. Lateral Squat w/ Toe Raise

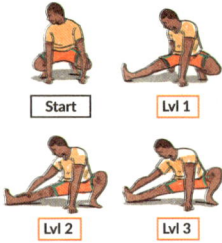
Start   Lvl 1
Lvl 2   Lvl 3

Duration:

(Goal: 30 sec each side)   Level:

5. Pigeon Stretch

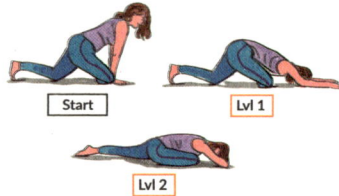
Start   Lvl 1
Lvl 2

Duration:

(Goal: 30 sec each side)   Level:

6. Downward Dog

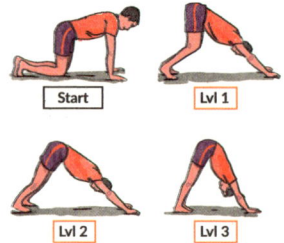
Start   Lvl 1
Lvl 2   Lvl 3

Duration:

(Goal: 30 sec)   Level:

7. Kneeling Quad Stretch

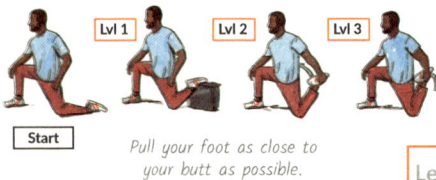
Lvl 1   Lvl 2   Lvl 3
Start

Pull your foot as close to your butt as possible.

Level:

Duration:

(Goal: 30 each side)

8. Runner's Lunge

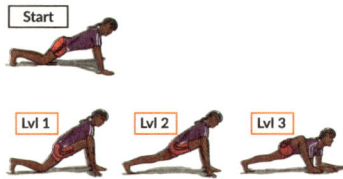
Start

Lvl 1   Lvl 2   Lvl 3

Level:

Duration:

(Goal: 30 each side)

9. Lying Hip Extension

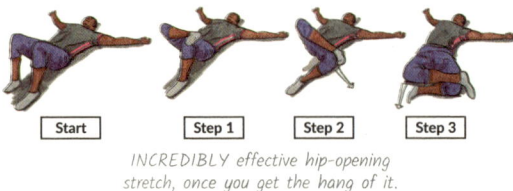
Start   Step 1   Step 2   Step 3

INCREDIBLY effective hip-opening stretch, once you get the hang of it.

Duration:

(Goal: 30 sec each side)

10. Hanging Calf Stretch

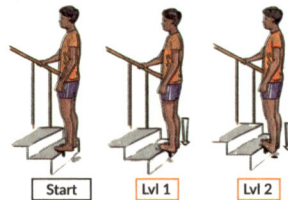

The more your foot is off the stair, the more you can deepen the stretch.

Start   Lvl 1   Lvl 2

Level:

Duration:

(Goal: 30 sec)

Daily Reflection

Benefits I'm Experiencing:

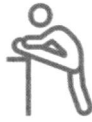

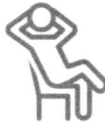

Feel Lighter	More Freedom of Movement	Improved Mental Clarity
Less Pain	Less Stressed	Improved Posture

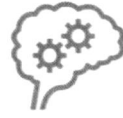

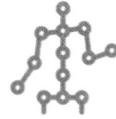

Notes On My Body:

Day 9: Dynamic Warm-Up

Full Session Exercise Guide:
habitnest.com/pages/stretching-day-9

1. Walking Jacks (or Jumping Jacks)

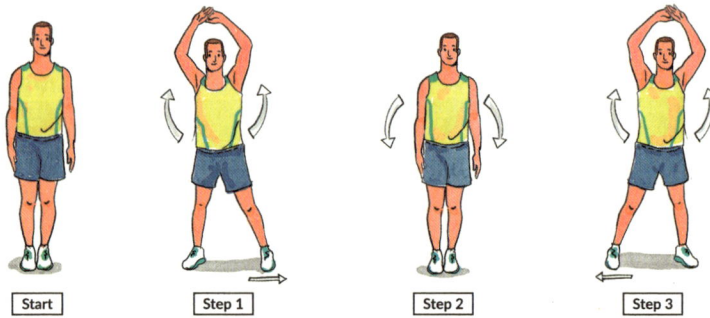

| Start | Step 1 | Step 2 | Step 3 |

Reps: .... *(Goal: 20-30)*

2. Bird-Dog   *(Goal: 20-30)*

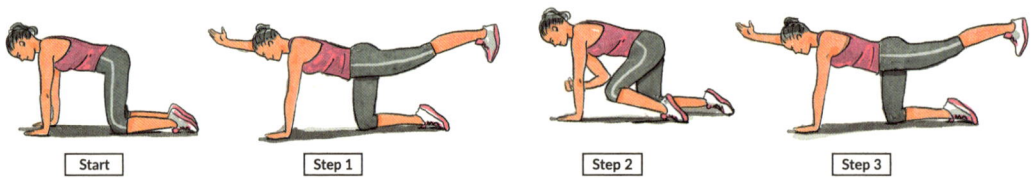

| Start | Step 1 | Step 2 | Step 3 |

Reps: .... *(Goal: 10-15 each side)*

3. Speed-Skater Arms

Simply get into a slight squat and twist all the way around, in a controlled manner, with your arms up!

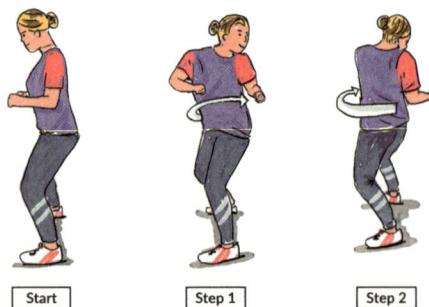

| Start | Step 1 | Step 2 |

Reps: .... *(Goal: 15-20)*

Day 9: Upper Body

1. Side Neck Tilt

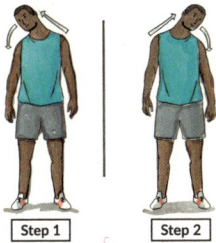

Step 1   Step 2

Duration: _____   *(Goal: 15 sec each side)*

2. Forward & Backward Neck Tilt

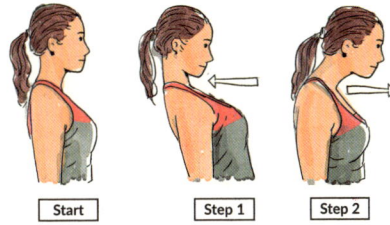

Start   Step 1   Step 2

Duration: _____   *(Goal: 30 sec, alternating)*

3. Forearm Stretch w/ Hands on Surface

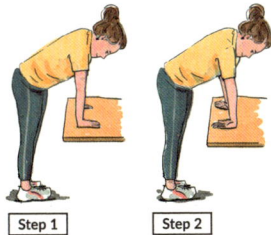

Step 1   Step 2

Duration: _____   *(Goal: 15 sec each side)*

4. Child's Pose

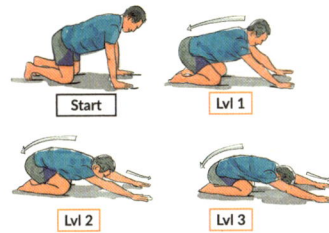

Start   Lvl 1

Lvl 2   Lvl 3

Level: _____

Duration: _____   *(Goal: 60 sec)*

5. Doorway Pectoral Stretch

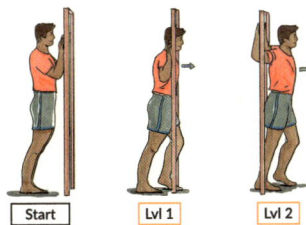

Remember to step forward to deepen the stretch, don't simply lean forward.

Start   Lvl 1   Lvl 2

Level: _____

Duration: _____   *(Goal: 30 sec)*

6. Static Y Hold

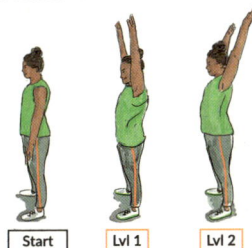

Start   Lvl 1   Lvl 2

Level: _____

Duration: _____   *(Goal: 30 sec)*

7. Standing Oblique Stretch

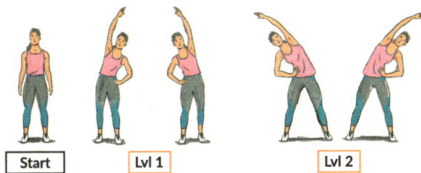

Start   Lvl 1   Lvl 2

Sometimes pointing your fingers in the direction you want your arm to move in helps you stretch farther.

Level: _____

Duration: _____   *(Goal: 15 sec each side)*

8. Sphinx/Cobra

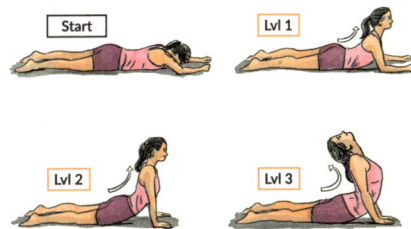

Start   Lvl 1

Lvl 2   Lvl 3

Level: _____

Duration: _____   *(Goal: 30 sec)*

Day 9: Lower Body

1. Butterfly

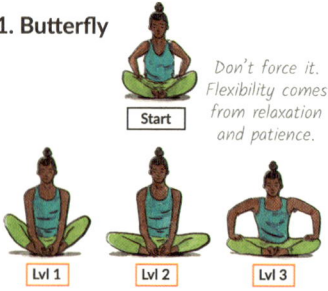

Don't force it. Flexibility comes from relaxation and patience.

Duration: ....

(Goal: 30 sec)

Level:

2. Pry Squat

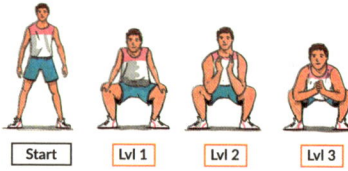

Duration: ....

(Goal: 30 sec)

Level:

3. Figure 4

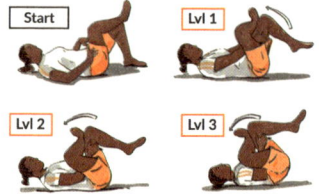

Push up with your free leg first, and THEN pull with your arms.

Duration: ....

(Goal: 30 sec each side)

Level:

4. Seated Forward Fold Hamstring Stretch

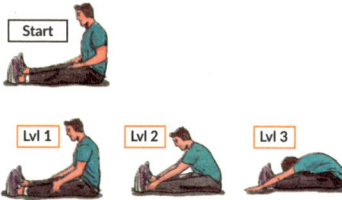

Duration: ....

(Goal: 30 sec)

Level:

5. Lateral Squat

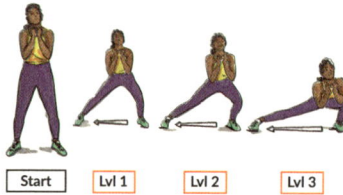

Duration: ....

(Goal: 30 sec each side)

Level:

6. Pigeon Stretch

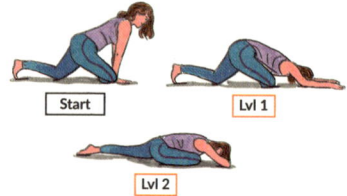

Duration: ....

(Goal: 30 sec each side)

Level:

7. Lying Quad Stretch

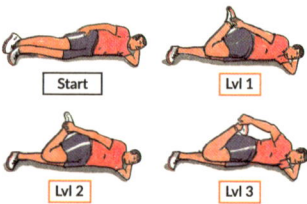

Level:

Duration: ....

(Goal: 30 sec each side)

8. Downward Dog

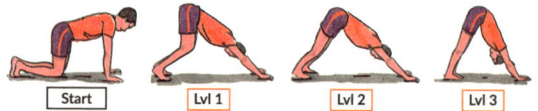

Level:

Duration: ....

(Goal: 30 sec)

9. Reverse Tabletop

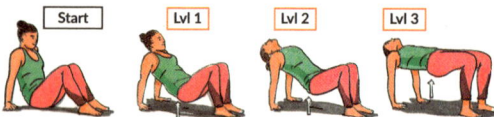

This is TOUGH to do, but it'll be worth it.

Level:

Duration: ....

(Goal: 30 sec)

10. Standing Wall Calf Stretch

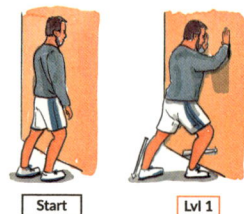

Duration: ....

(Goal: 15 sec each side)

Daily Reflection

Benefits I'm Experiencing:

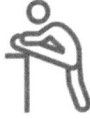

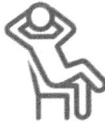

Feel Lighter	More Freedom of Movement	Improved Mental Clarity
Less Pain	Less Stressed	Improved Posture

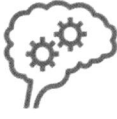

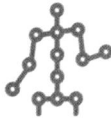

Notes On My Body:

....

....

....

....

....

....

....

....

....

1. Low Lunge w/ Elbow Twist

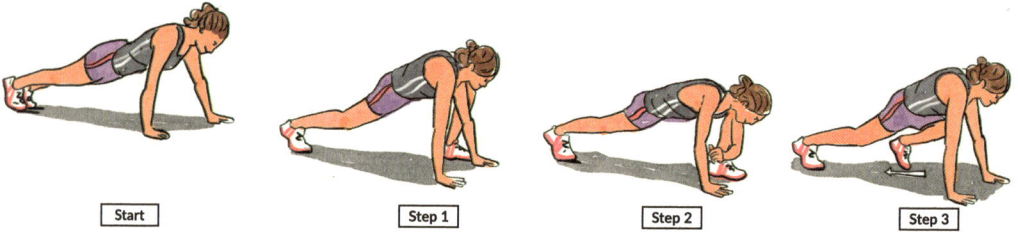

Start | Step 1 | Step 2 | Step 3

Reps: .... (*Goal: 10-15 each side*)

2. Plank w/ Shoulder Tap

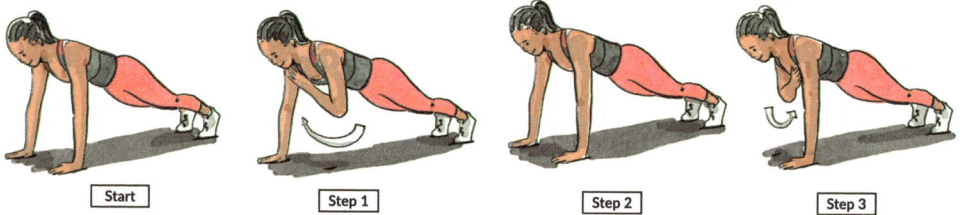

Start | Step 1 | Step 2 | Step 3

Reps: .... (*Goal: 10-15 each side*)

3. Mountain Climber

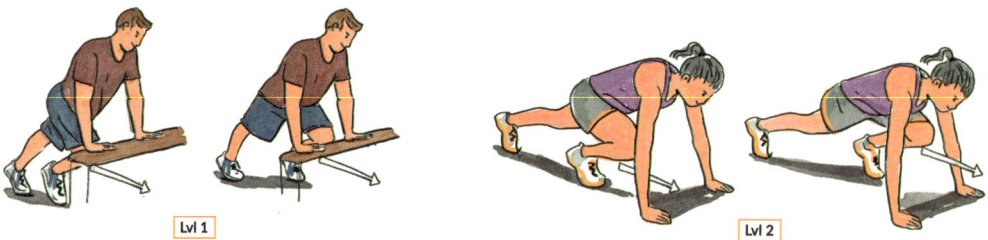

Lvl 1 | Lvl 2

Level:

Reps: .... (*Goal: 30-40*)

Day 10: Upper Body

1. Child's Pose

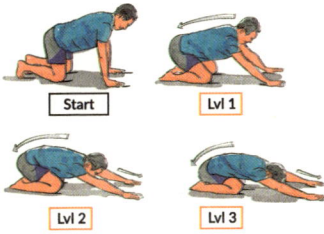

Start   Lvl 1

Lvl 2   Lvl 3

Level:

Duration:

(Goal: 60 sec)

2. Sphinx/Cobra

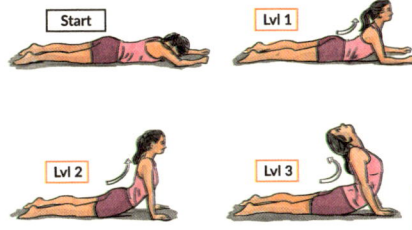

Start   Lvl 1

Lvl 2   Lvl 3

Level:

Duration:

(Goal: 30 sec)

3. Seated Spinal Twist

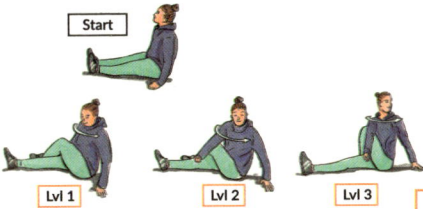

Start

Lvl 1   Lvl 2   Lvl 3

Level:

Duration:

(Goal: 15 sec each side)

4. Open Book Chest Stretch

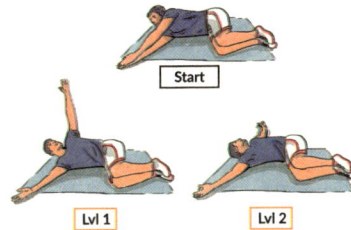

Start

Lvl 1   Lvl 2

Level:

Duration:

(Goal: 15 sec each side)

5. Leaning Long Arm Shoulder Stretch

Step back further and let your torso drop. Let gravity do its thing.

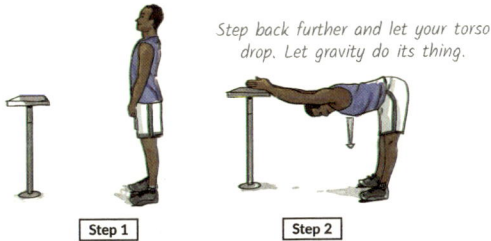

Step 1   Step 2

Duration:

(Goal: 30 sec)

6. Locust Pose

If needed, leave your legs on the ground and use them as leverage to lift your upper body.

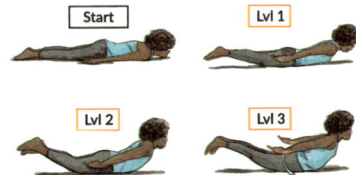

Start   Lvl 1

Lvl 2   Lvl 3

Level:

Duration:

(Goal: 30 sec)

7. Corner Chest Stretch

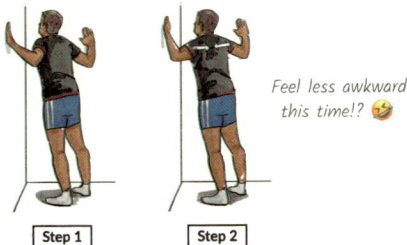

Feel less awkward this time!? 🤣

Step 1   Step 2

Duration:

(Goal: 30 sec)

8. Surface Tricep Stretch

Place your elbow on the wall and lean forward if it feels comfortable.

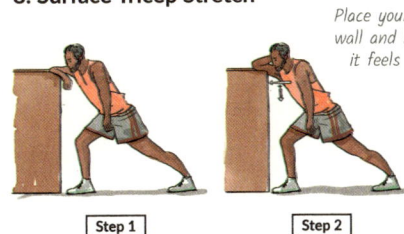

Step 1   Step 2

Duration:

(Goal: 15 sec each side)

Day 10: Lower Body

1. Frog Pose

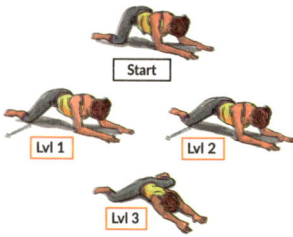

Start

Lvl 1

Lvl 2

Lvl 3

Duration:
....

(Goal: 60 sec)

Level:

2. Scorpion Pose

You'll feel it in the hip of the stretching leg. Keep your torso on the ground.

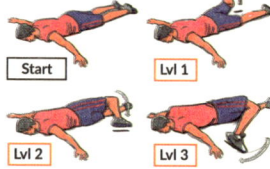

Start

Lvl 1

Lvl 2

Lvl 3

Duration:
....

(Goal: 30 sec each side)

Level:

3. Halfway Center Split

This is an inner thigh stretch, not the back of the hamstrings.

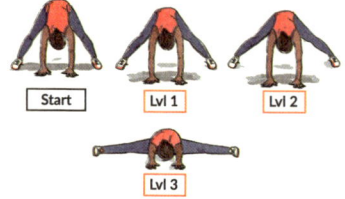

Start

Lvl 1

Lvl 2

Lvl 3

Duration:
....

(Goal: 30 sec)

Level:

4. Prone Quad Stretch

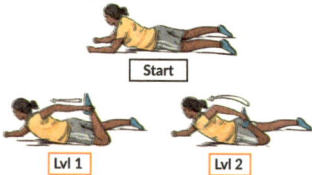

Start

Lvl 1

Lvl 2

Use the non-stretching forearm to support and balance this position by placing it on the ground under your head.

Duration:
....

(Goal: 30 sec each side)

Level:

5. Downward Dog

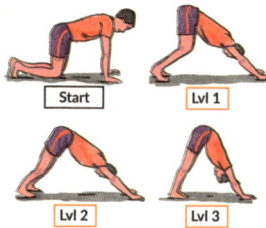

Start

Lvl 1

Lvl 2

Lvl 3

Duration:
....

(Goal: 30 sec)

Level:

6. Figure 4

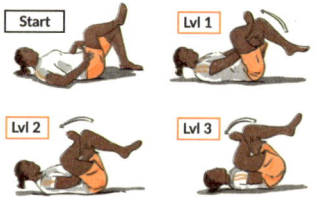

Start

Lvl 1

Lvl 2

Lvl 3

Duration:
....

(Goal: 30 sec each side)

Level:

7. Knee to Chest Stretch

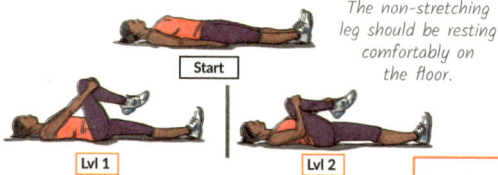

The non-stretching leg should be resting comfortably on the floor.

Start

Lvl 1

Lvl 2

Level:

Duration:
....

(Goal: 30 sec each side)

8. Lateral Squat

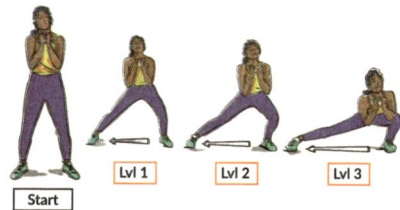

Lvl 1

Lvl 2

Lvl 3

Start

Level:

Duration:
....

(Goal: 30 sec each side)

9. Lateral Squat w/ Toe Raise

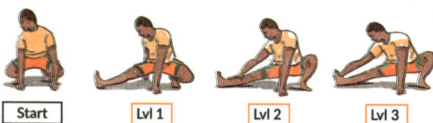

Start

Lvl 1

Lvl 2

Lvl 3

Level:

Duration:
....

(Goal: 30 sec each side)

10. Hanging Calf Stretch

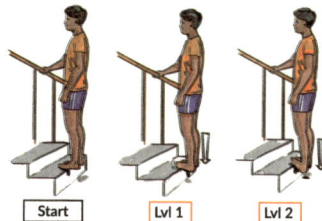

Start

Lvl 1

Lvl 2

Level:

Duration:
....

(Goal: 30 sec)

Daily Reflection

Benefits I'm Experiencing:

Feel
Lighter

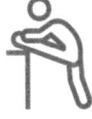

More Freedom
of Movement

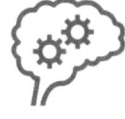

Improved
Mental Clarity

Less
Pain

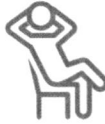

Less
Stressed

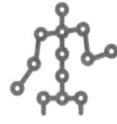

Improved
Posture

Notes On My Body:

....

....

....

....

....

....

....

....

Day 11: Dynamic Warm-Up

Full Session Exercise Guide:
habitnest.com/pages/stretching-day-11

1. Standing Hamstring Scoop

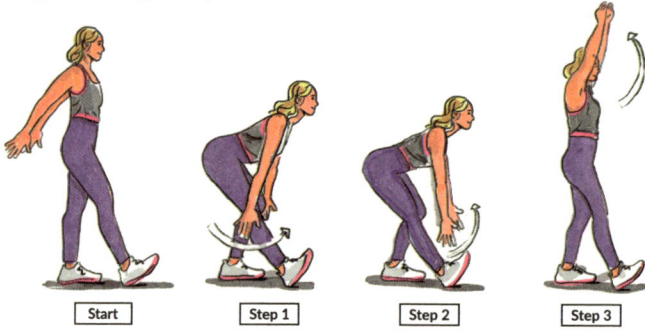

| Start | Step 1 | Step 2 | Step 3 |

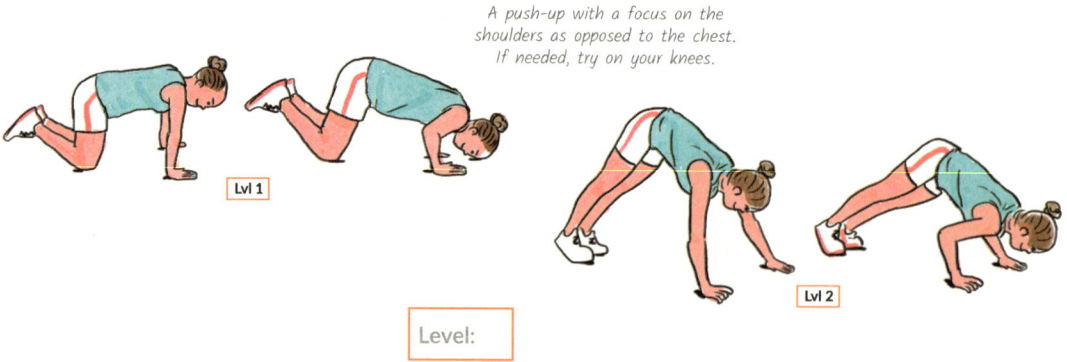

Reps: .... *(Goal: 15-20)*

2. Good Morning

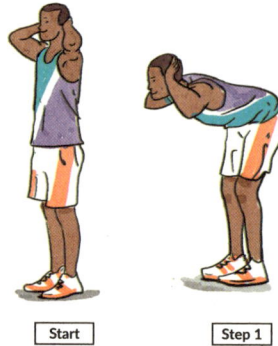

| Start | Step 1 |

Reps: .... *(Goal: 15-20)*

3. Pike Push-Up

A push-up with a focus on the shoulders as opposed to the chest. If needed, try on your knees.

Lvl 1

Lvl 2

Level:

Reps: .... *(Goal: 15-20)*

Day 11: Upper Body

1. Up & Down Neck Tilt

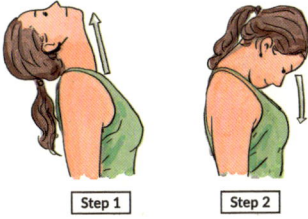

Step 1   Step 2

Duration: .... *(Goal: 30 sec, alternating)*

2. Side Neck Tilt

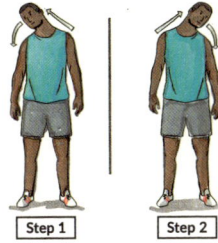

Step 1   Step 2

Duration: .... *(Goal: 15 sec each side)*

3. Levator Scap Neck Stretch

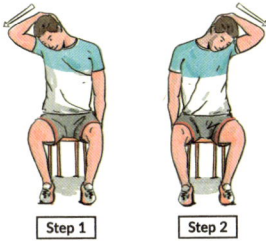

Step 1   Step 2

Duration: .... *(Goal: 15 sec each side)*

4. Child's Pose

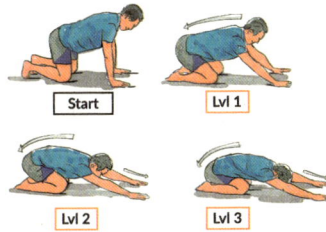

Start   Lvl 1
Lvl 2   Lvl 3

Level:

Duration: .... *(Goal: 60 sec)*

5. Cat-Cow

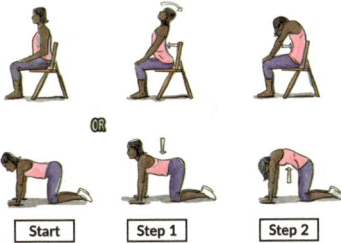

OR

Start   Step 1   Step 2

Duration: .... *(Goal: 30 sec, alternating)*

6. Behind the Back Elbow to Elbow Grip

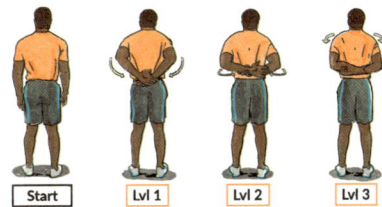

Start   Lvl 1   Lvl 2   Lvl 3

Focus on opening your chest and shoulders.

Level:

Duration: .... *(Goal: 30 sec)*

7. Thread the Needle Shoulder Stretch

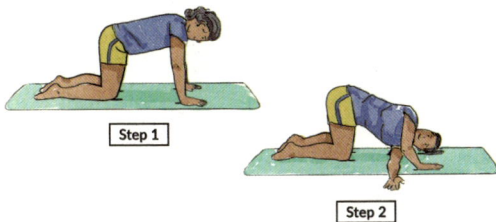

Step 1

Step 2

Duration: .... *(Goal: 30 sec each side)*

8. Doorway Pectoral Stretch

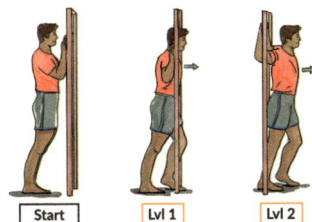

Start   Lvl 1   Lvl 2

Level:

Duration: .... *(Goal: 30 sec)*

Day 11: Lower Body

1. Frog Pose

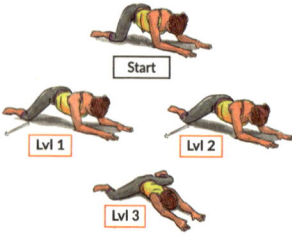

Start
Lvl 1
Lvl 2
Lvl 3

Duration:
....

(Goal: 60 sec)

Level:

2. Butterfly

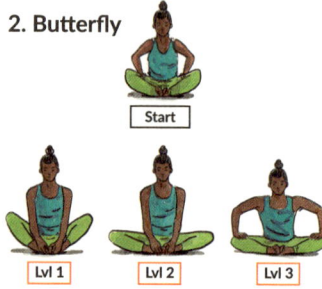

Start
Lvl 1
Lvl 2
Lvl 3

Duration:
....

(Goal: 30 sec)

Level:

3. Runner's Lunge

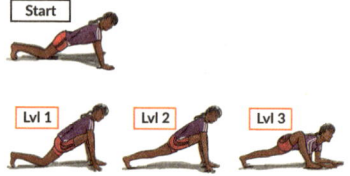

Start
Lvl 1
Lvl 2
Lvl 3

Duration:
....

(Goal: 30 sec each side)

Level:

4. Pigeon Stretch

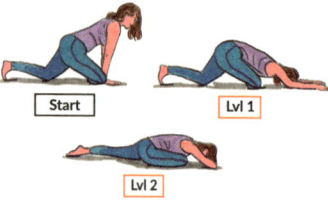

Start
Lvl 1
Lvl 2

Duration:
....

(Goal: 30 sec each side)

Level:

5. Halfway Center Split

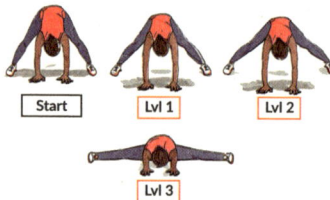

Start
Lvl 1
Lvl 2
Lvl 3

Duration:
....

(Goal: 30 sec)

Level:

6. Figure 4

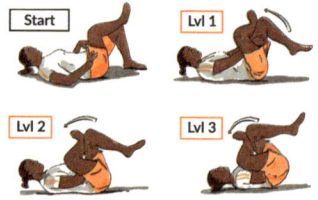

Start
Lvl 1
Lvl 2
Lvl 3

Duration:
....

(Goal: 30 sec each side)

Level:

7. Lying Hamstring Extension

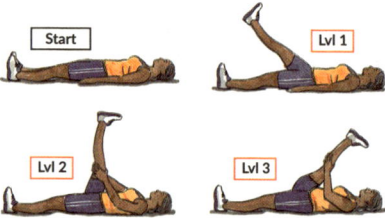

Start
Lvl 1
Lvl 2
Lvl 3

Keep your leg as straight as possible and lift.

Level:

Duration:
....

(Goal: 30 sec each side)

8. Kneeling Quad Stretch

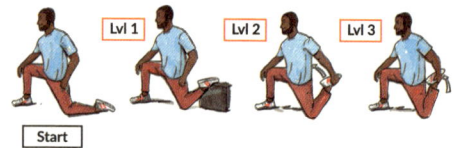

Lvl 1
Lvl 2
Lvl 3
Start

Level:

Duration:
....

(Goal: 30 sec each side)

9. Standing Wall Calf Stretch

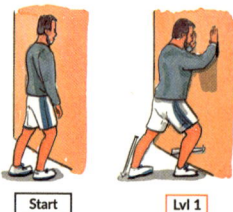

Start
Lvl 1

Duration:
....

(Goal: 15 sec each side)

10. Standing Wall Calf Stretch w/ Achilles Focus

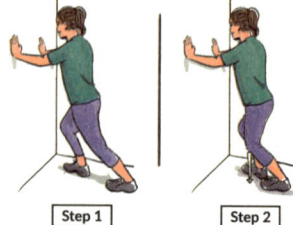

Step 1
Step 2

Duration:
....

(Goal: 15 sec each side)

Daily Reflection

You're circling the same icons every day, and it's easy to get desensitized to a process like this.

Remember, as you circle, try to really feel that there is a concrete difference in how you experience life when you stretch vs. when you don't.

The benefits you experience when you invest in your own well-being are easy to take for granted.

Benefits I'm Experiencing:

Feel
Lighter

More Freedom
of Movement

Improved
Mental Clarity

Less
Pain

Less
Stressed

Improved
Posture

Notes On My Body:

....
....
....
....
....
....
....
....
....

With reference to your body, what are you grateful for?

Day 12: Dynamic Warm-Up

Full Session Exercise Guide:
habitnest.com/pages/stretching-day-12

1. Knee Hug

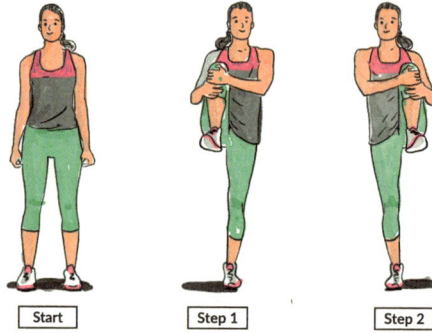

| Start | Step 1 | Step 2 |

Reps: _____ (Goal: 10-15 each side)

2. Low Lunge w/ Elbow Twist

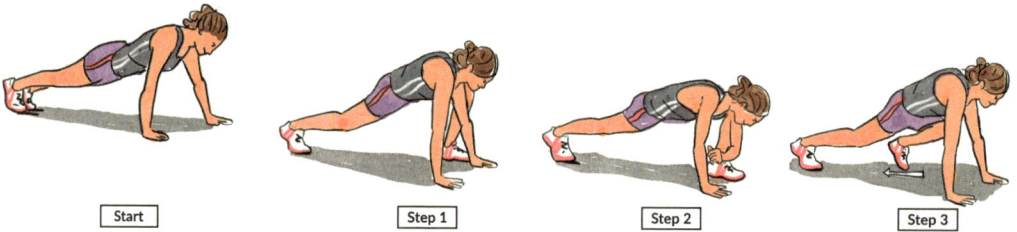

| Start | Step 1 | Step 2 | Step 3 |

Reps: _____ (Goal: 10-15 each side)

3. Y Raise

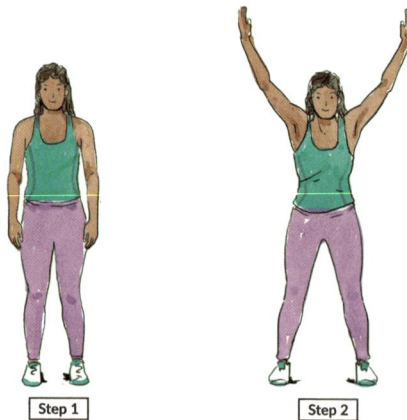

| Step 1 | Step 2 |

Reps: _____ (Goal: 15-20)

Day 12: Upper Body

1. Child's Pose

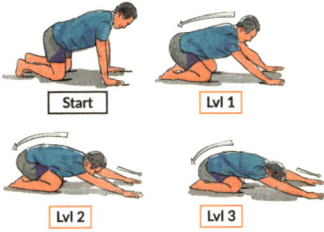

Start
Lvl 1
Lvl 2
Lvl 3

Level:

Duration: ....

(Goal: 60 sec)

2. Cat-Cow

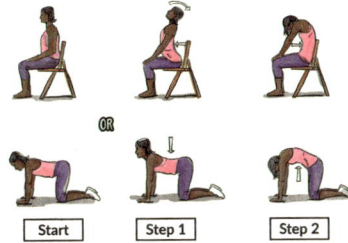

OR

Start
Step 1
Step 2

Duration: ....

(Goal: 30 sec, alternating)

3. Sphinx/Cobra

Remember, extend head and abdomen abdomen UPWARDS.

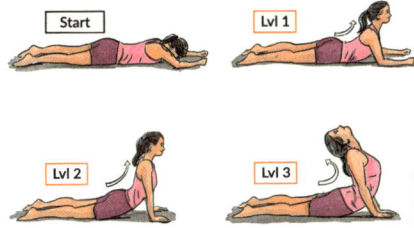

Start
Lvl 1
Lvl 2
Lvl 3

Level:

Duration: ....

(Goal: 30 sec)

4. Seated Spinal Twist

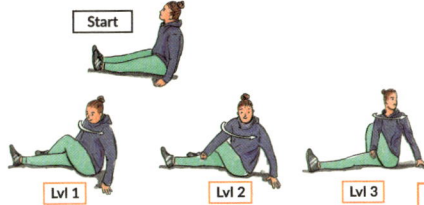

Start
Lvl 1
Lvl 2
Lvl 3

Level:

Duration: ....

(Goal: 15 sec each side)

5. Cross Arm Shoulder Stretch

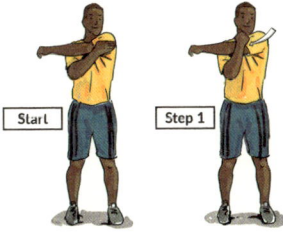

Start
Step 1

Duration: ....

(Goal: 15 sec each side)

6. Reverse Prayer

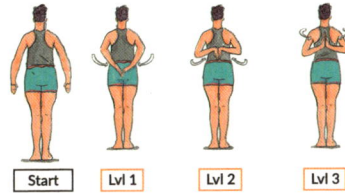

Start
Lvl 1
Lvl 2
Lvl 3

Level:

Duration: ....

(Goal: 30 sec)

7. Open Book Chest Stretch

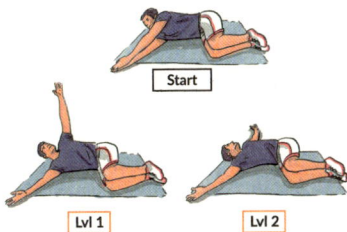

Start
Lvl 1
Lvl 2

Level:

Duration: ....

(Goal: 30 sec each side)

8. Floor Angel

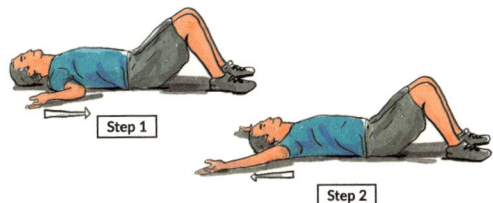

Step 1
Step 2

Duration: ....

(Goal: 30 sec, alternating)

Day 12: Lower Body

1. Reclining Angle Bound Pose

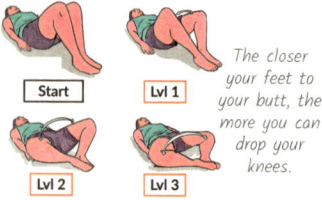

Start

Lvl 1

Lvl 2

Lvl 3

The closer your feet to your butt, the more you can drop your knees.

Duration:

(Goal: 30 sec)

Level:

2. Scorpion Pose

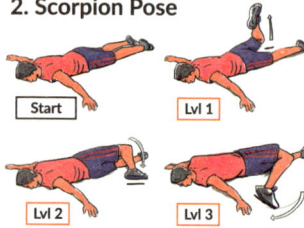

Start

Lvl 1

Lvl 2

Lvl 3

Duration:

(Goal: 30 sec each side)

Level:

3. Reverse Tabletop

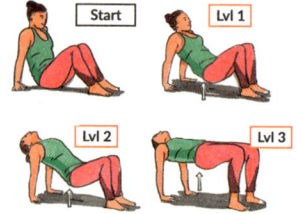

Push through your heels and hands to lift your torso up.

Start

Lvl 1

Lvl 2

Lvl 3

Duration:

(Goal: 30 sec)

Level:

4. Warrior II Pose

Twist away from the hip on your straight leg.

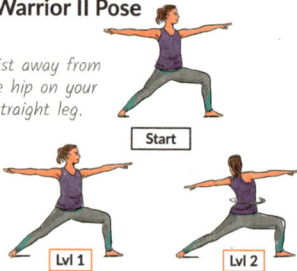

Start

Lvl 1

Lvl 2

Duration:

(Goal: 30 sec each side)

Level:

5. Seated Forward Fold Hamstring Stretch

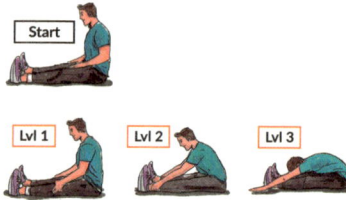

Start

Lvl 1

Lvl 2

Lvl 3

Duration:

(Goal: 30 sec)

Level:

6. Lateral Squat

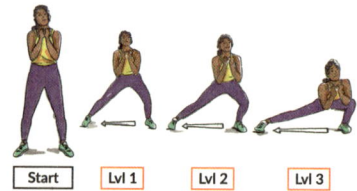

Start

Lvl 1

Lvl 2

Lvl 3

Duration:

(Goal: 30 sec each side)

Level:

7. Lateral Squat w/ Toe Raise

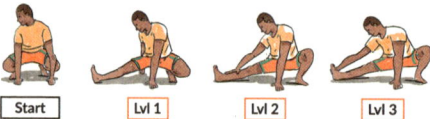

Start

Lvl 1

Lvl 2

Lvl 3

Level:

Duration:

(Goal: 30 sec each side)

8. Pigeon Stretch

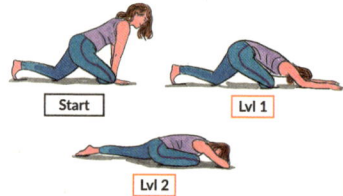

Start

Lvl 1

Lvl 2

Level:

Duration:

(Goal: 30 sec each side)

9. Prone Quad Stretch

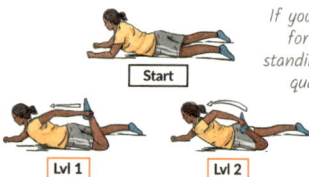

If you're not ready for this, try a standing or kneeling quad stretch.

Start

Lvl 1

Lvl 2

Level:

Duration:

(Goal: 30 sec each side)

10. Hanging Calf Stretch

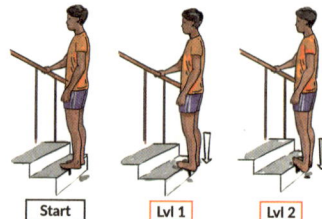

Start

Lvl 1

Lvl 2

Level:

Duration:

(Goal: 30 sec)

Daily Reflection

Benefits I'm Experiencing:

Feel
Lighter

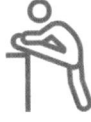

More Freedom
of Movement

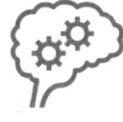

Improved
Mental Clarity

Less
Pain

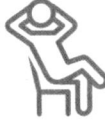

Less
Stressed

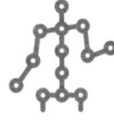

Improved
Posture

Notes On My Body:

Day 13: Dynamic Warm-Up

Full Session Exercise Guide:
habitnest.com/pages/stretching-day-13

1. World's Greatest Stretch

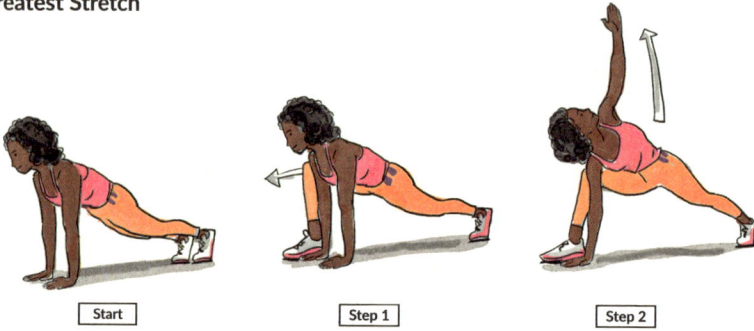

Start

Step 1

Step 2

Reps: *(Goal: 5-10 each side)*

2. Air Squat to Calf Raise

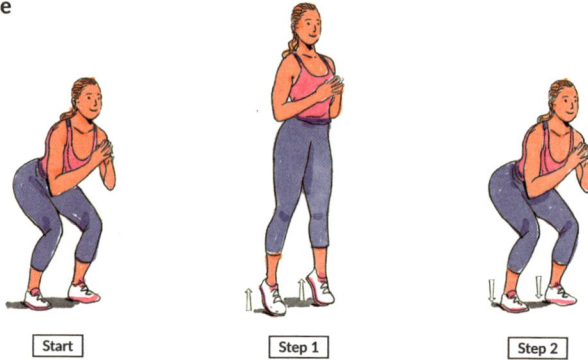

Start

Step 1

Step 2

Reps: *(Goal: 25-30)*

3. Aquaman

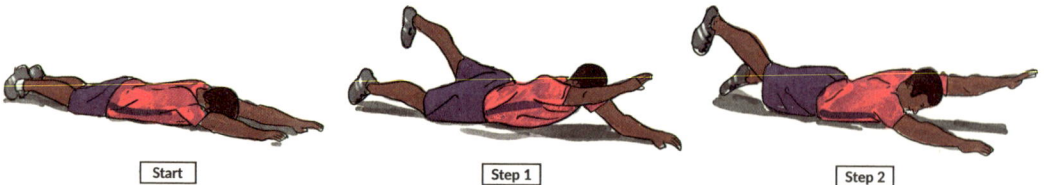

Start

Step 1

Step 2

Reps: *(Goal: 15-20)*

Day 13: Upper Body

1. Side Neck Stretch w/ Upside Down Palm On Wall

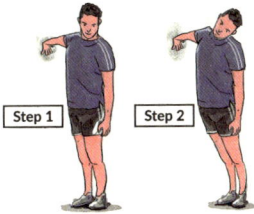

Step 1 Step 2

Let your head drop to your shoulder ONLY to the extent it feels comfortable.

Duration: _____

(Goal: 15 sec each side)

2. Levator Scap Neck Stretch

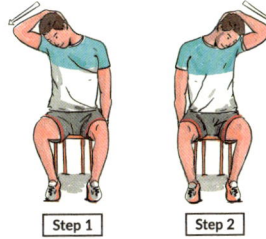

Step 1 Step 2

Duration: _____

(Goal: 15 sec each side)

3. Child's Pose

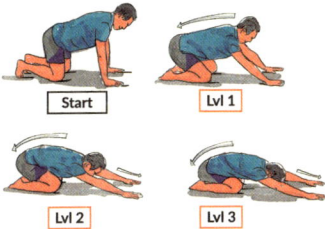

Start Lvl 1 Lvl 2 Lvl 3

Level: _____

Duration: _____

(Goal: 60 sec)

4. Standing Oblique Stretch

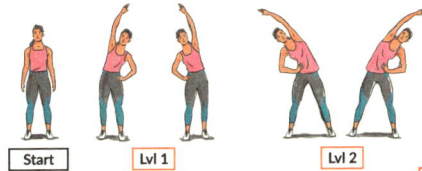

Start Lvl 1 Lvl 2

Level: _____

Duration: _____

(Goal: 15 sec each side)

5. Leaning Long Arm Shoulder Stretch

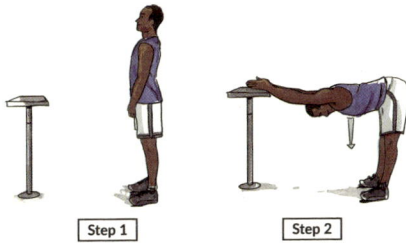

Step 1 Step 2

Duration: _____

(Goal: 30 sec)

6. Sphinx/Cobra

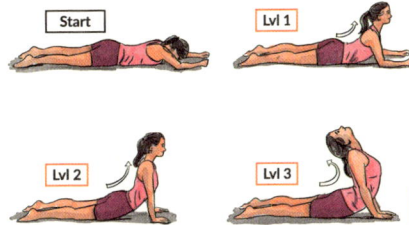

Start Lvl 1 Lvl 2 Lvl 3

Level: _____

Duration: _____

(Goal: 30 sec)

7. Elbow Opener

Open your chest as if you were trying to touch your elbows to each other behind your body.

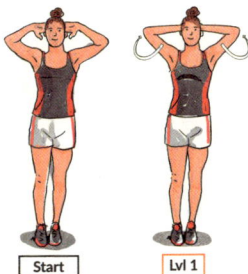

Start Lvl 1

Duration: _____

(Goal: 30 sec)

8. Corner Chest Stretch

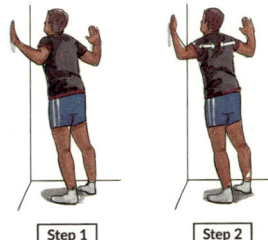

Step 1 Step 2

Duration: _____

(Goal: 30 sec)

Day 13: Lower Body

1. Frog Pose

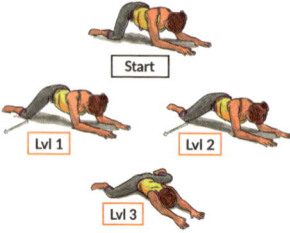

Start

Lvl 1   Lvl 2

Lvl 3

Duration:

(Goal: 60 sec)   Level:

2. Warrior II Pose

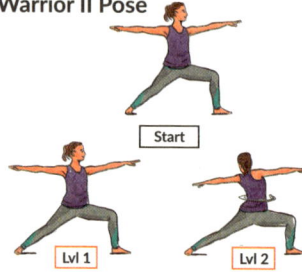

Start

Start

Lvl 1   Lvl 2

Duration:

(Goal: 30 sec each side)   Level:

3. Runner's Lunge

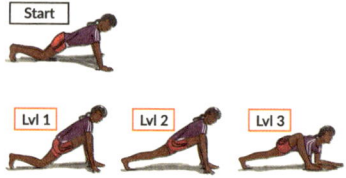

Start

Lvl 1   Lvl 2   Lvl 3

Duration:

(Goal: 30 sec each side)   Level:

4. Wig-Wag

This is felt primarily in the glute of the top leg.

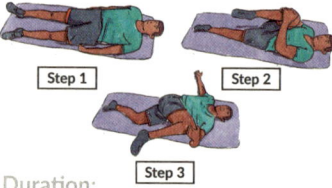

Step 1   Step 2

Step 3

Duration:

(Goal: 30 sec each side)

5. Figure 4

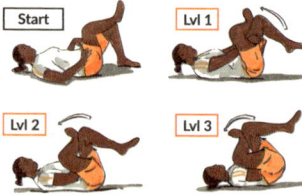

Start   Lvl 1

Lvl 2   Lvl 3

Duration:

(Goal: 30 sec each side)   Level:

6. Downward Dog

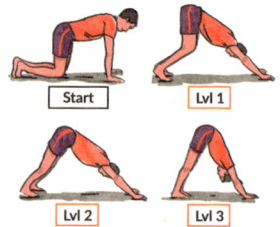

Start   Lvl 1

Lvl 2   Lvl 3

Duration:

(Goal: 30 sec)   Level:

7. Seated Forward Fold Hamstring Stretch

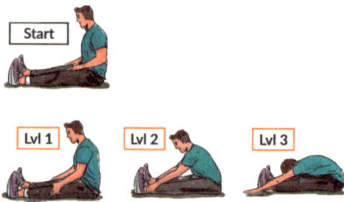

Start

Lvl 1   Lvl 2   Lvl 3

Level:

Duration:

(Goal: 30 sec)

8. Kneeling Quad Stretch

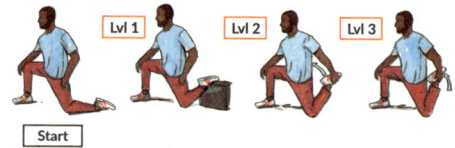

Lvl 1   Lvl 2   Lvl 3

Start

Level:

Duration:

(Goal: 30 sec each side)

9. Standing Wall Calf Stretch

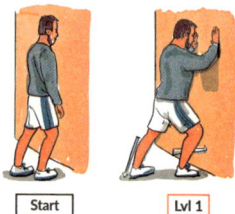

Start   Lvl 1

Duration:

(Goal: 15 sec each side)

10. Standing Wall Calf Stretch w/ Achilles Focus

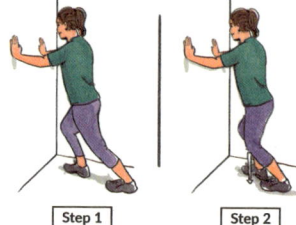

Step 1   Step 2

Duration:

(Goal: 15 sec each side)

Daily Reflection

Benefits I'm Experiencing:

Feel
Lighter

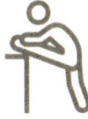

More Freedom
of Movement

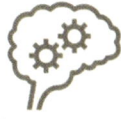

Improved
Mental Clarity

Less
Pain

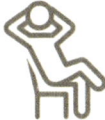

Less
Stressed

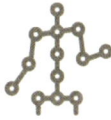

Improved
Posture

Notes On My Body:

Day 14: Dynamic Warm-Up

Full Session Exercise Guide:
habitnest.com/pages/stretching-day-14

1. Inch Worm Walk Out

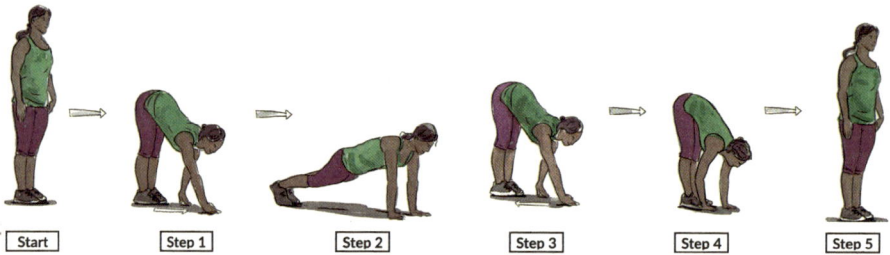

| Start | Step 1 | Step 2 | Step 3 | Step 4 | Step 5 |

Reps: _____ *(Goal: 15-20)*

2. Plank w/ Shoulder Tap

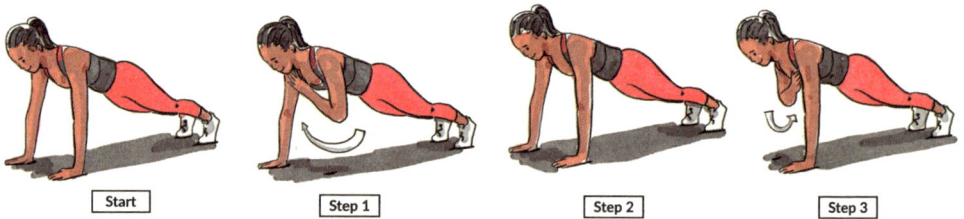

| Start | Step 1 | Step 2 | Step 3 |

Reps: _____ *(Goal: 10-15 each side)*

3. Rocking Feet w/ Arm Raise

Bring your arms as far back as possible in EACH direction.

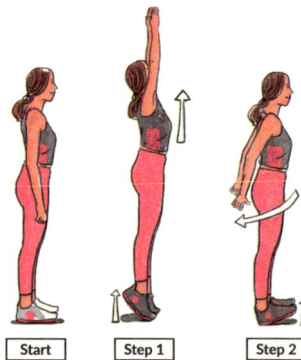

| Start | Step 1 | Step 2 |

Reps: _____ *(Goal: 10-15 in each direction)*

Day 14: Upper Body

1. Forearm Stretch w/ Hands On Surface

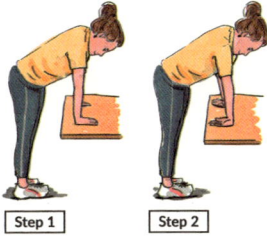

Step 1   Step 2

Duration: _____   (Goal: 15 sec each side)

2. Behind the Back Tricep Extension

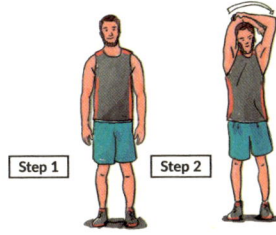

Step 1   Step 2

Duration: _____   (Goal: 15 sec each side)

3. Child's Pose

Start   Lvl 1
Lvl 2   Lvl 3

Level: _____

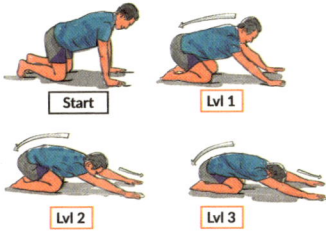

Duration: _____   (Goal: 60 sec)

4. Sphinx/Cobra

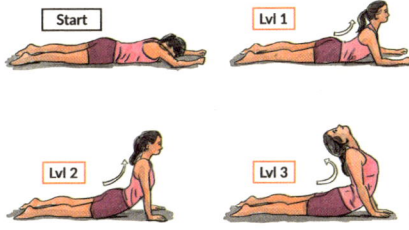

Start   Lvl 1
Lvl 2   Lvl 3

Level: _____

Duration: _____   (Goal: 30 sec)

5. Seated Spinal Twist

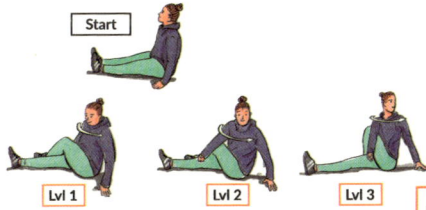

Start
Lvl 1   Lvl 2   Lvl 3

Level: _____

Duration: _____   (Goal: 15 sec each side)

6. Cross Arm Shoulder Stretch

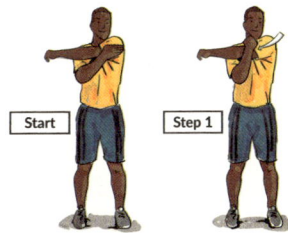

Start   Step 1

Duration: _____   (Goal: 15 sec each side)

7. Elbow Opener

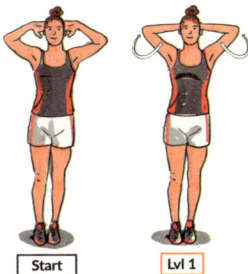

Start   Lvl 1

Duration: _____   (Goal: 30 sec)

8. Open Book Chest Stretch

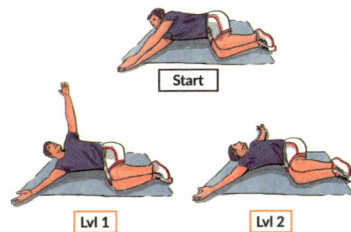

Start
Lvl 1   Lvl 2

Level: _____

Duration: _____   (Goal: 30 sec each side)

Day 14: Lower Body

1. Frog Pose

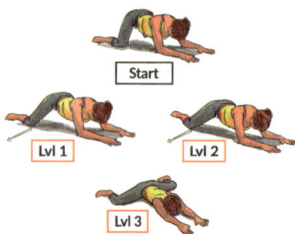

Duration:
....

(Goal: 60 sec)

Level:

2. Butterfly

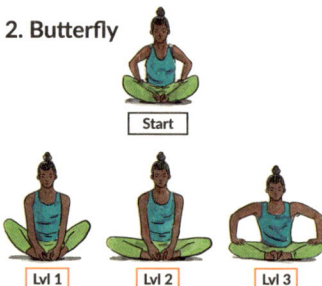

Duration:
....

(Goal: 30 sec)

Level:

3. Halfway Center Split

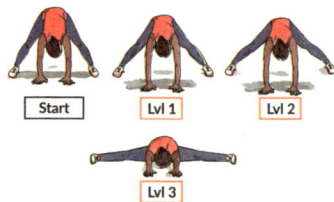

Duration:
....

(Goal: 30 sec)

Level:

4. Knee to Chest Stretch

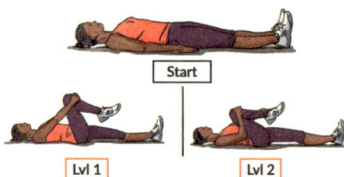

Duration:
....

(Goal: 30 sec each side)

Level:

5. Figure 4

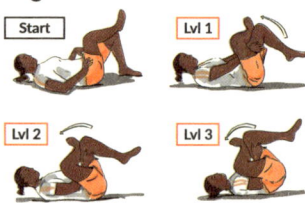

Duration:
....

(Goal: 30 sec each side)

Level:

6. Lying Hip Extension

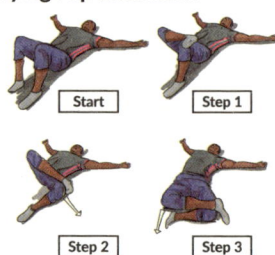

Duration:
....

(Goal: 30 sec each side)

7. Lateral Squat

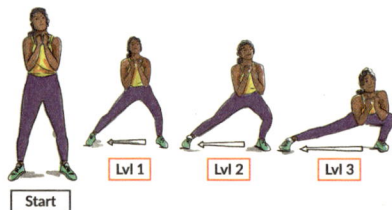

Level:

Duration:
....

(Goal: 30 sec each side)

8. Lateral Squat w/ Toe Raise

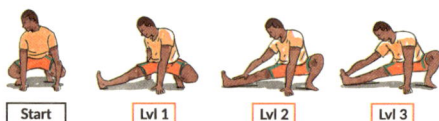

Level:

Duration:
....

(Goal: 30 sec each side)

9. Standing Quad Stretch

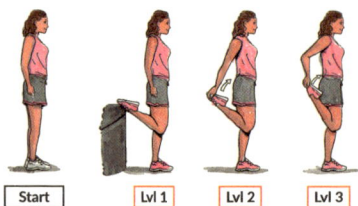

Level:

Duration:
....

(Goal: 30 sec each side)

10. Hanging Calf Stretch

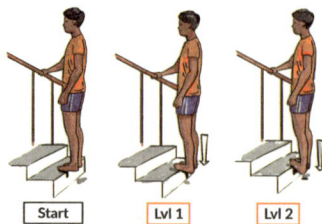

Level:

Duration:
....

(Goal: 30 sec)

Daily Reflection

Benefits I'm Experiencing:

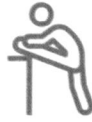

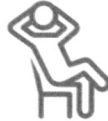

Feel Lighter	More Freedom of Movement	Improved Mental Clarity
Less Pain	Less Stressed	Improved Posture

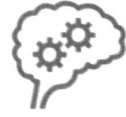

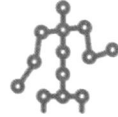

Notes On My Body:

....

....

....

....

....

....

....

....

....

Day 15: Dynamic Warm-Up

Full Session Exercise Guide:
habitnest.com/pages/stretching-day-15

1. Push-Up

Lvl 1

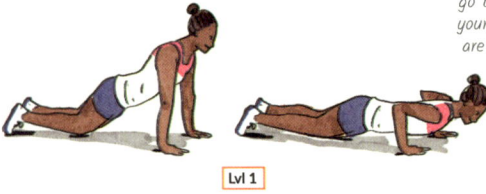

The whole body is in one straight line. Butt doesn't go up in the air, and hips don't fall to the floor. Use your core to keep the body in one line. If your knees are on the ground, then the straight line goes from the top of your head to your knees.

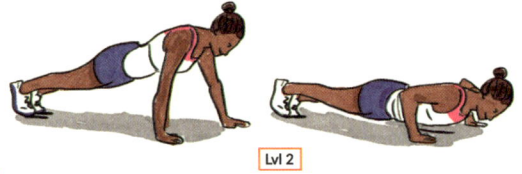

Lvl 2

Level:

Reps: *(Goal: 15-25)*

2. Good Morning

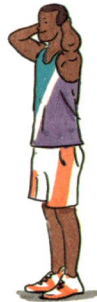

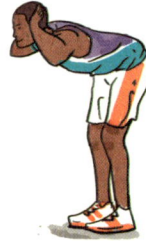

Start   Step 1

Reps: *(Goal: 15-20)*

3. Standing Hip Circles

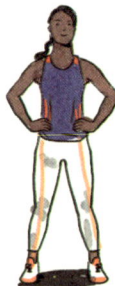

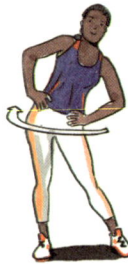

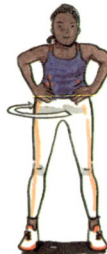

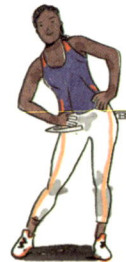

Start   Step 1   Step 2   Step 3

Reps: *(Goal: 10-15 in each direction)*

Day 15: Upper Body

1. Up & Down Neck Tilt

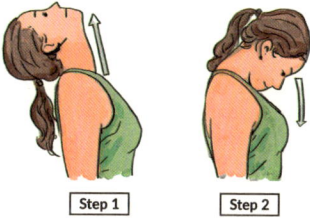

Step 1 | Step 2

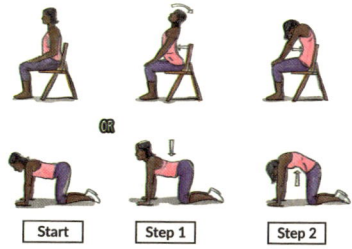

Duration: _____ (Goal: 30 sec, alternating)

2. Side Neck Tilt

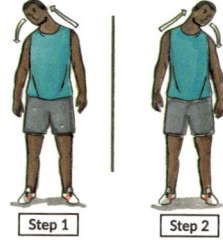

Step 1 | Step 2

Duration: _____ (Goal: 15 sec each side)

3. Forward & Backward Neck Tilt

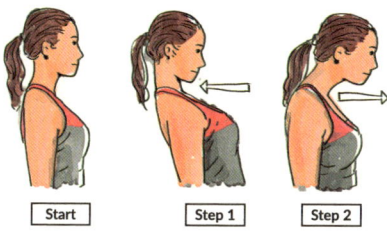

Start | Step 1 | Step 2

Duration: _____ (Goal: 30 sec, alternating)

4. Lateral Side to Side Neck Rotation

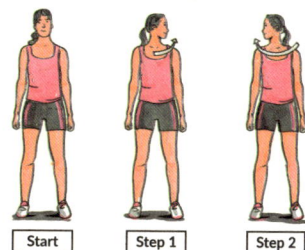

Start | Step 1 | Step 2

Duration: _____ (Goal: 30 sec, alternating)

5. Child's Pose

Start | Lvl 1
Lvl 2 | Lvl 3

Level: _____

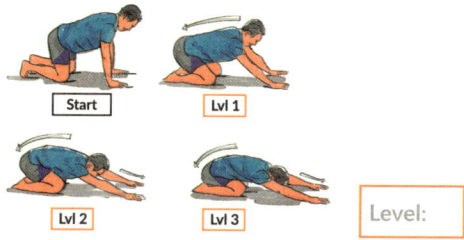

Duration: _____ (Goal: 60 sec)

6. Cat-Cow

OR

Start | Step 1 | Step 2

Duration: _____ (Goal: 30 sec, alternating)

7. Static Y Hold

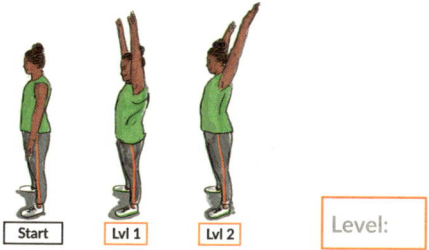

Start | Lvl 1 | Lvl 2

Level: _____

Duration: _____ (Goal: 30 sec)

8. Corner Chest Stretch

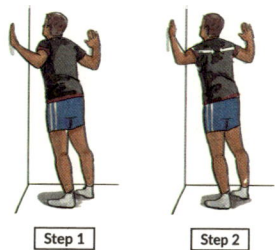

Step 1 | Step 2

Duration: _____ (Goal: 30 sec)

103

Day 15: Lower Body

1. Frog Pose

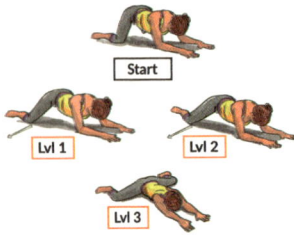

Duration:
....

(Goal: 60 sec)

Level:

2. Butterfly

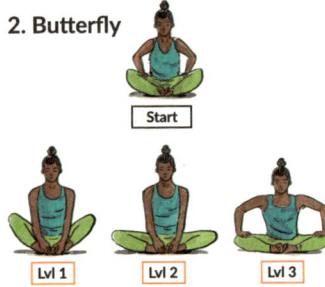

Duration:
....

(Goal: 30 sec)

Level:

3. Scorpion Pose

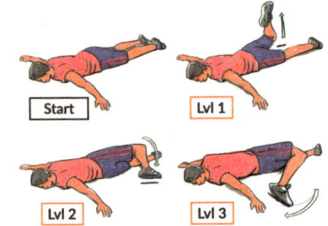

Duration:
....

(Goal: 30 sec each side)

Level:

4. Runner's Lunge

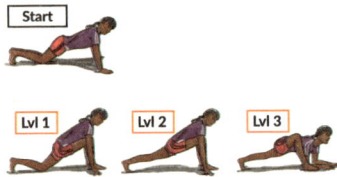

Duration:
....

(Goal: 30 sec each side)

Level:

5. Figure 4

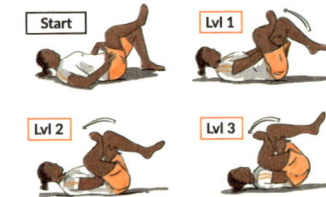

Duration:
....

(Goal: 30 sec each side)

Level:

6. Seated Single Leg Hamstring Stretch

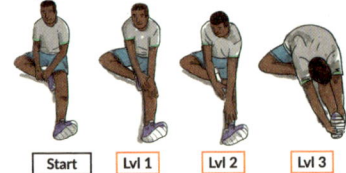

Remember not to curve the spine. You bend at the hip.

Duration:
....

(Goal: 30 sec each side)

Level:

7. Downward Dog

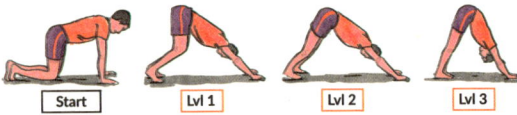

Level:

Duration:
....

(Goal: 30 sec)

8. Lateral Squat

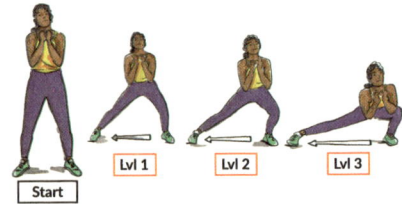

Level:

Duration:
....

(Goal: 30 sec each side)

9. Lateral Squat w/ Toe Raise

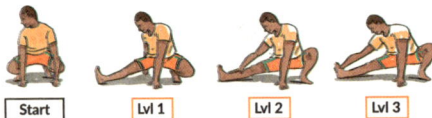

Level:

Duration:
....

(Goal: 30 sec each side)

10. Reverse Tabletop

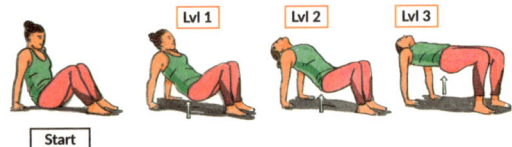

Level:

Duration:
....

(Goal: 30 sec)

Daily Reflection

Benefits I'm Experiencing:

Feel
Lighter

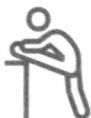

More Freedom
of Movement

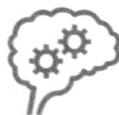

Improved
Mental Clarity

Less
Pain

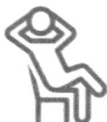

Less
Stressed

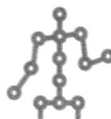

Improved
Posture

Notes On My Body:

....

....

....

....

....

....

....

....

What part of your body do you enjoy stretching least?
It's probably what you need to focus on most!

Day 16: Dynamic Warm-Up

1. World's Greatest Stretch

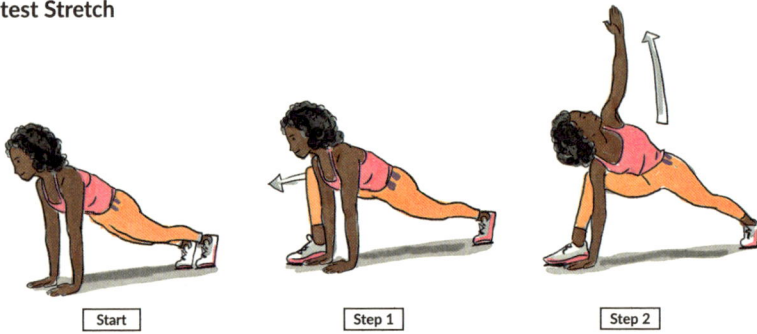

| Start | Step 1 | Step 2 |

Reps: .... *(Goal: 10-15 each side)*

2. Air Squat to Calf Raise

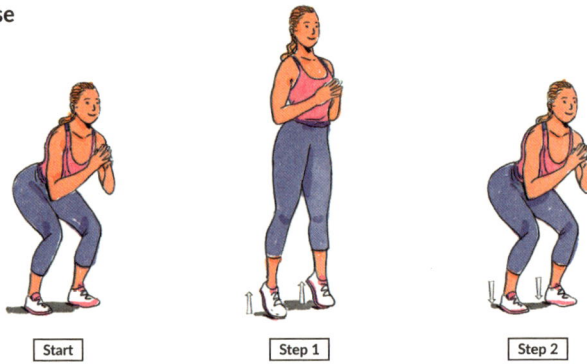

| Start | Step 1 | Step 2 |

Reps: .... *(Goal: 25-30)*

3. Pike Push-Up

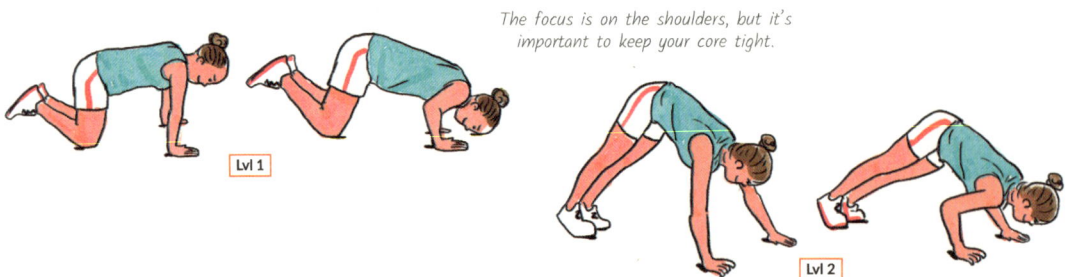

The focus is on the shoulders, but it's important to keep your core tight.

Lvl 1

Lvl 2

Level:

Reps: .... *(Goal: 15-25)*

Day 16: Upper Body

1. Seated Forward Curl

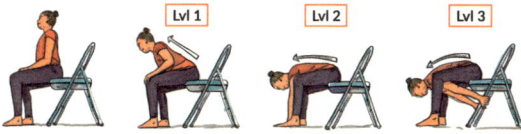

Start   **Lvl 1**   **Lvl 2**   **Lvl 3**

Imagine you're pulling your spine out through the top of your head without moving your lower body.

Level:

Duration: ....

(Goal: 30 sec)

2. Seated Spinal Twist

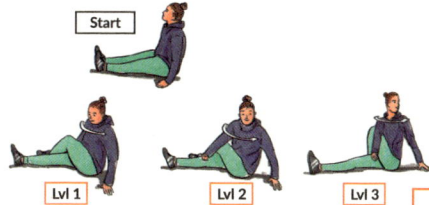

Start   **Lvl 1**   **Lvl 2**   **Lvl 3**

Level:

Duration: ....

(Goal: 15 sec each side)

3. Sphinx/Cobra

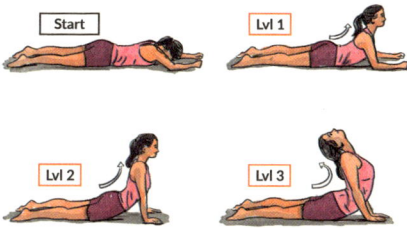

Start   **Lvl 1**   **Lvl 2**   **Lvl 3**

Level:

Duration: ....

(Goal: 30 sec)

4. Leaning Long Arm Shoulder Stretch

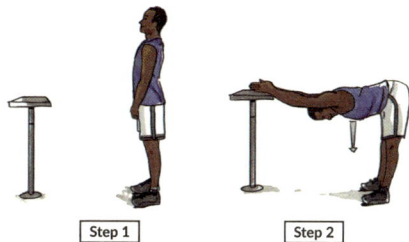

Step 1   **Step 2**

Duration: ....

(Goal: 30 sec)

5. Behind the Back Elbow to Elbow Grip

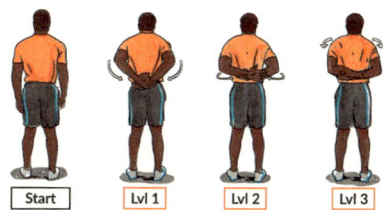

Start   **Lvl 1**   **Lvl 2**   **Lvl 3**

Level:

Duration: ....

(Goal: 30 sec)

6. Standing Oblique Stretch

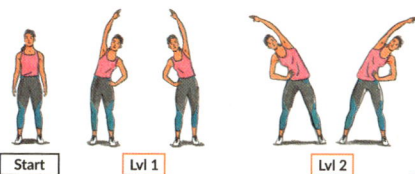

Start   **Lvl 1**   **Lvl 2**

Level:

Duration: ....

(Goal: 15 sec each side)

7. Locust Pose

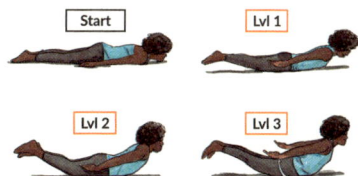

Start   **Lvl 1**   **Lvl 2**   **Lvl 3**

Level:

Duration: ....

(Goal: 30 sec)

8. Behind the Back Tricep Extension

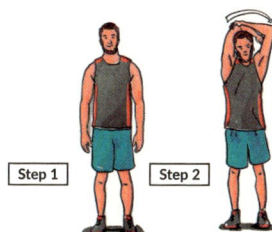

Step 1   **Step 2**

Duration: ....

(Goal: 15 sec each side)

Day 16: Lower Body

1. Frog Pose

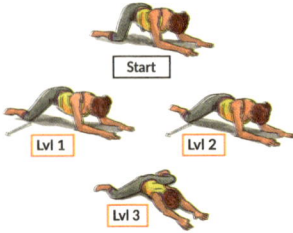

Start

Lvl 1   Lvl 2

Lvl 3

Duration:
....

(Goal: 60 sec)   Level: [ ]

2. Pry Squat

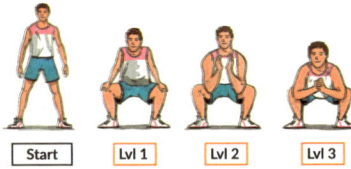

Start   Start   Lvl 1   Lvl 2   Lvl 3

Duration:
....

(Goal: 30 sec)   Level: [ ]

3. Happy Baby Pose

If you can't grab your feet, grab your shins. Gravity is on your side.

Start

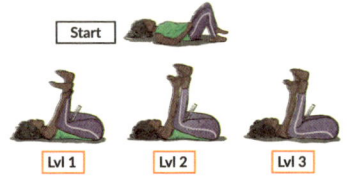

Lvl 1   Lvl 2   Lvl 3

Duration:
....

(Goal: 30 sec)   Level: [ ]

4. Pigeon Stretch

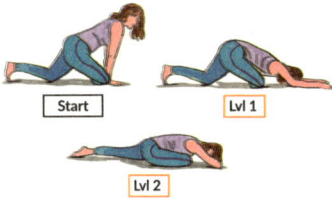

Start   Lvl 1

Lvl 2

Duration:
....

(Goal: 30 sec each side)   Level: [ ]

5. Reclining Angle Bound Pose

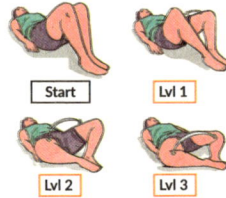

Start   Lvl 1

Lvl 2   Lvl 3

Duration:
....

(Goal: 30 sec)   Level: [ ]

6. Seated Forward Fold Hamstring Stretch

Start   *Always pay attention to whether you're even 1% more flexible than the last time.*

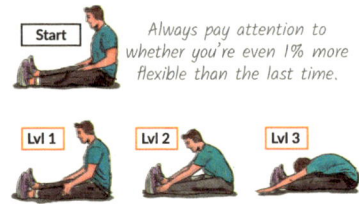

Lvl 1   Lvl 2   Lvl 3

Duration:
....

(Goal: 30 sec)   Level: [ ]

7. Kneeling Quad Stretch

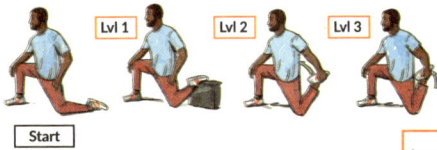

Lvl 1   Lvl 2   Lvl 3

Start

Level: [ ]

Duration:
....

(Goal: 30 sec each side)

8. Lateral Squat

The inner thighs are often neglected in strength and flexibility!

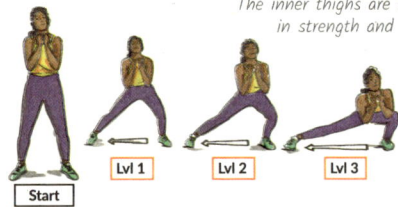

Lvl 1   Lvl 2   Lvl 3

Start

Level: [ ]

Duration:
....

(Goal: 30 sec each side)

9. Lateral Squat w/ Toe Raise

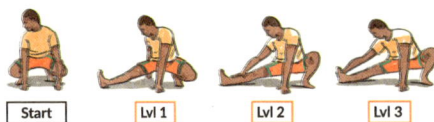

Start   Lvl 1   Lvl 2   Lvl 3

Level: [ ]

Duration:
....

(Goal: 30 sec each side)

10. Hanging Calf Stretch

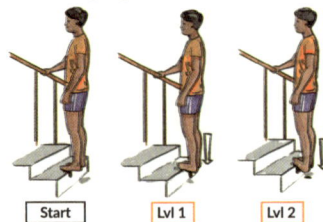

Start   Lvl 1   Lvl 2

Level: [ ]

Duration:
....

(Goal: 30 sec)

Daily Reflection

Benefits I'm Experiencing:

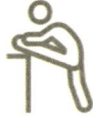

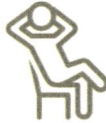

Feel Lighter	More Freedom of Movement	Improved Mental Clarity
Less Pain	Less Stressed	Improved Posture

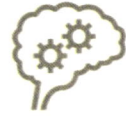

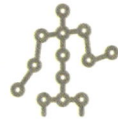

Notes On My Body:

Day 17: Dynamic Warm-Up

Full Session Exercise Guide:
habitnest.com/pages/stretching-day-17

1. Walking Jacks (or Jumping Jacks)

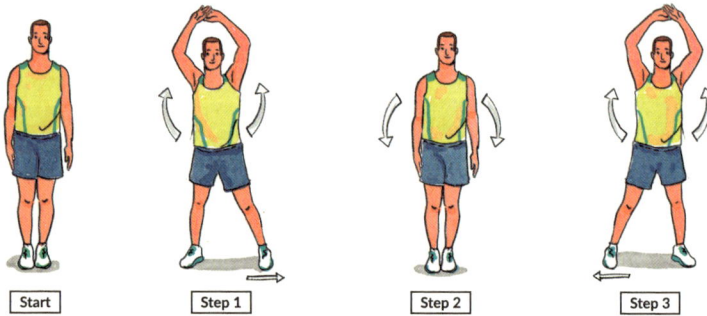

Start	Step 1	Step 2	Step 3

Reps: _____ *(Goal: 20-30)*

2. Clam Opener w/ Side Plank

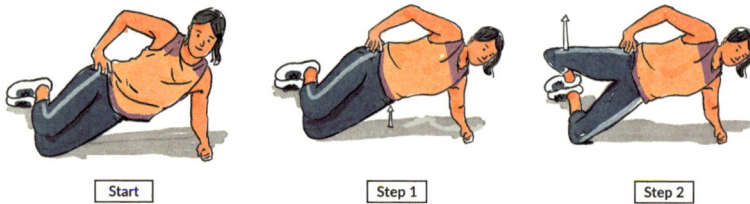

Start	Step 1	Step 2

Reps: _____ *(Goal: 10-15 each side)*

3. Towel Snatch

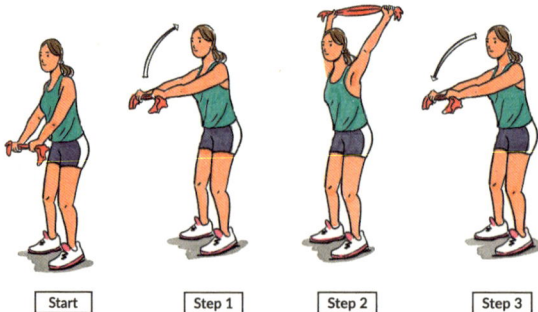

Start	Step 1	Step 2	Step 3

Only you know if you're really maintaining tension throughout the whole movement. Don't cheat yourself.

Reps: _____ *(Goal: 15-20)*

Day 17: Upper Body

1. Up & Down Neck Tilt

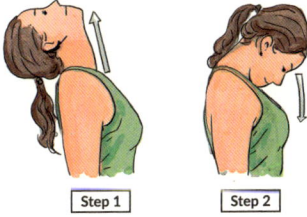

Step 1   Step 2

Duration: *(Goal: 30 sec, alternating)*

2. Lateral Side to Side Neck Rotation

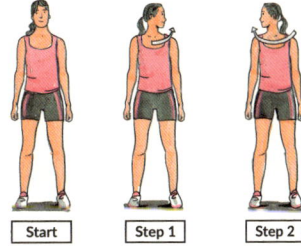

Start   Step 1   Step 2

Duration: *(Goal: 30 sec, alternating)*

3. Levator Scap Neck Stretch

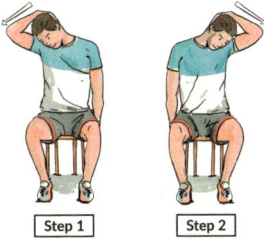

Step 1   Step 2

Duration: *(Goal: 15 sec each side)*

4. Cat-Cow

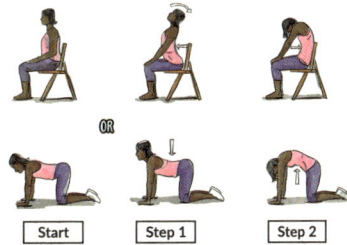

OR

Start   Step 1   Step 2

Duration: *(Goal: 30 sec, alternating)*

5. Standing Oblique Stretch

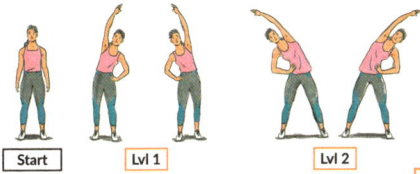

Start   Lvl 1   Lvl 2

Level:

Duration: *(Goal: 15 sec each side)*

6. Cross Arm Shoulder Stretch

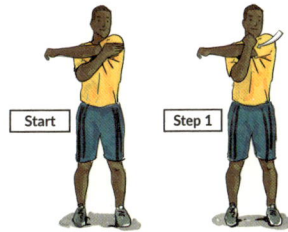

Start   Step 1

Duration: *(Goal: 15 sec each side)*

7. Doorway Pectoral Stretch

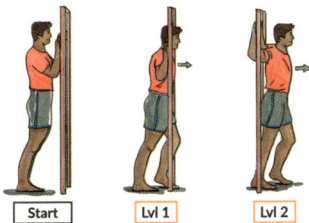

Start   Lvl 1   Lvl 2

Level:

Duration: *(Goal: 30 sec)*

8. Forearm Stretch w/ Hands on Surface

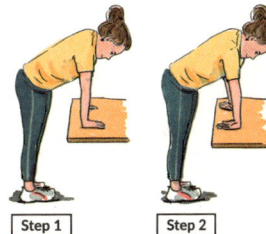

Step 1   Step 2

Level:

Duration: *(Goal: 15 sec each side)*

Day 17: Lower Body

1. Halfway Center Split

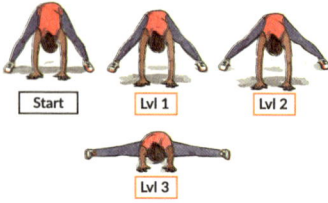

Start   Lvl 1   Lvl 2

Lvl 3

Duration: ....

(Goal: 30 sec)   Level:

2. Butterfly

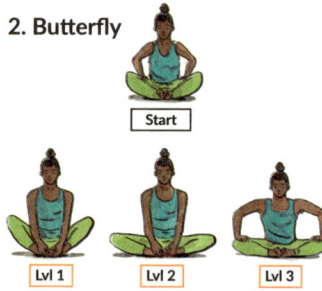

Start

Lvl 1   Lvl 2   Lvl 3

Duration: ....

(Goal: 30 sec)   Level:

3. Scorpion Pose

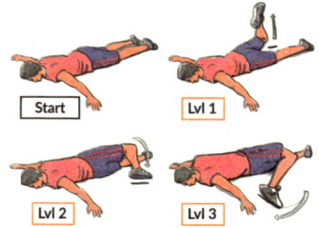

Start   Lvl 1

Lvl 2   Lvl 3

Duration: ....

(Goal: 30 sec each side)   Level:

4. Lying Hip Extension

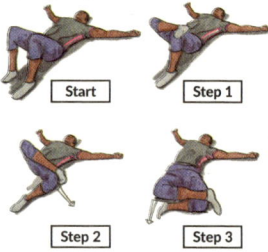

Start   Step 1

Step 2   Step 3

Duration: ....

(Goal: 30 sec each side)

5. Figure 4

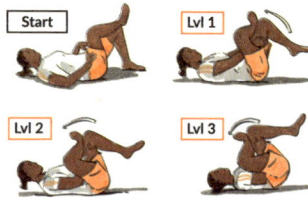

Start   Lvl 1

Lvl 2   Lvl 3

Duration: ....

(Goal: 30 sec each side)   Level:

6. Downward Dog

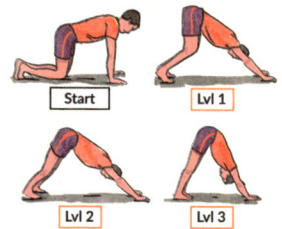

Start   Lvl 1

Lvl 2   Lvl 3

Duration: ....

(Goal: 30 sec)   Level:

7. Lying Quad Stretch

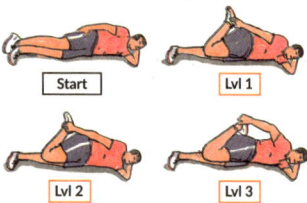

Start   Lvl 1

Lvl 2   Lvl 3

Level:

Duration: ....   *(Goal: 30 sec each side)*

8. Reclining Angle Bound Pose

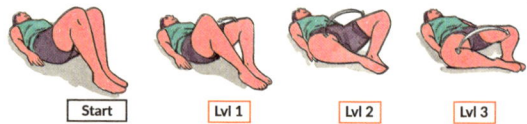

Start   Lvl 1   Lvl 2   Lvl 3

Try not to arch your back!   Level:

Duration: ....   *(Goal: 30 sec)*

9. Knee to Chest Stretch

If needed, keep non-stretching leg bent with your foot on the ground.

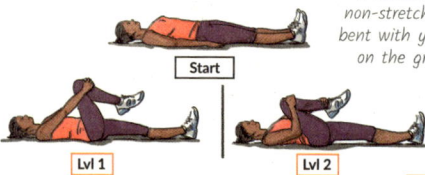

Start

Lvl 1   Lvl 2

Level:

Duration: ....   *(Goal: 30 sec each side)*

10. Standing Wall Calf Stretch

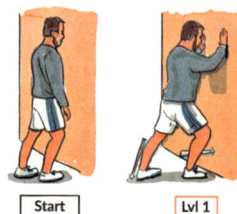

Start   Lvl 1

Duration: ....   *(Goal: 30 sec)*

Daily Reflection

Benefits I'm Experiencing:

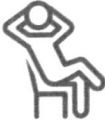

Feel Lighter	More Freedom of Movement	Improved Mental Clarity
Less Pain	Less Stressed	Improved Posture

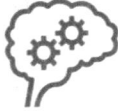

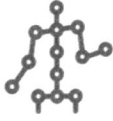

Notes On My Body:

....

....

....

....

....

....

....

....

Day 18: Dynamic Warm-Up

Full Session Exercise Guide:
habitnest.com/pages/stretching-day-18

1. World's Greatest Stretch

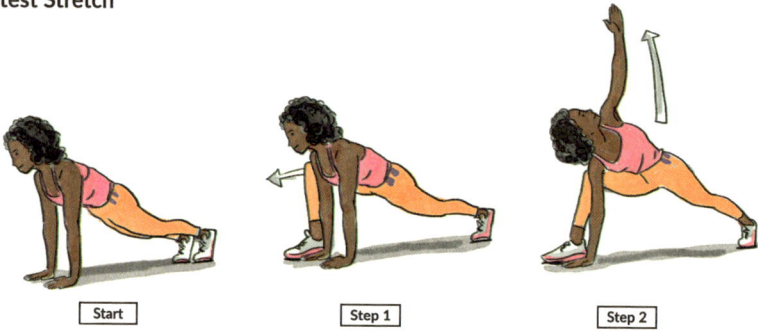

Start

Step 1

Step 2

Reps: _____ *(Goal: 10-15 each side)*

2. Split Squat

Step 1

Step 2

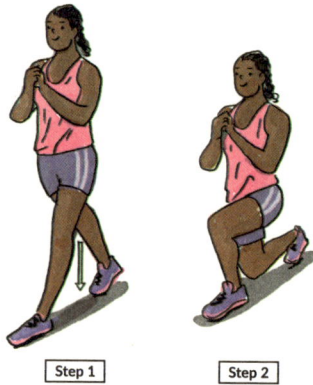

Reps: _____ *(Goal: 15-20 each side)*

3. Push-Up

Lvl 1

Lvl 2

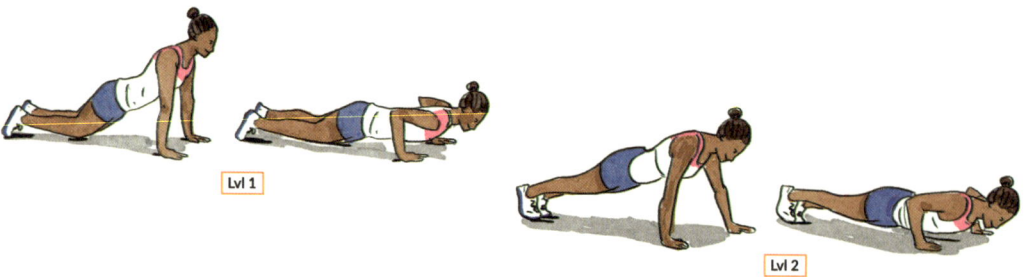

Reps: _____ *(Goal: 15-25)*

Day 18: Upper Body

1. Side Neck Tilt

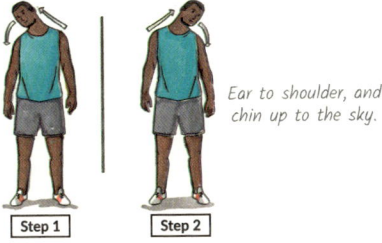

Ear to shoulder, and chin up to the sky.

Step 1   Step 2

Duration: _____   *(Goal: 15 sec each side)*

2. Child's Pose

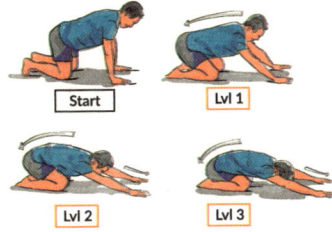

Start   Lvl 1   Lvl 2   Lvl 3

Level: _____

Duration: _____   *(Goal: 60 sec)*

3. Sphinx/Cobra

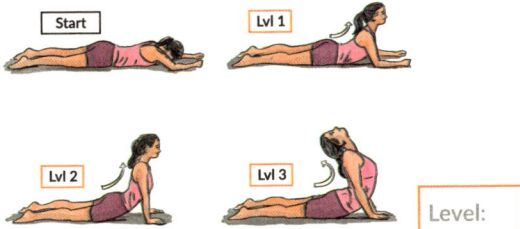

Start   Lvl 1   Lvl 2   Lvl 3

Level: _____

Duration: _____   *(Goal: 30 sec)*

4. Standing Oblique Stretch

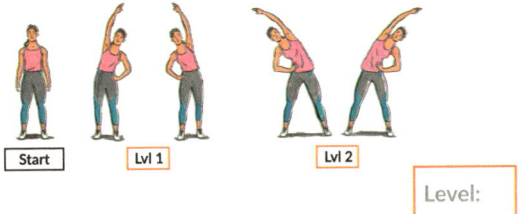

Start   Lvl 1   Lvl 2

Level: _____

Duration: _____   *(Goal: 15 sec each side)*

5. Thread the Needle Shoulder Stretch

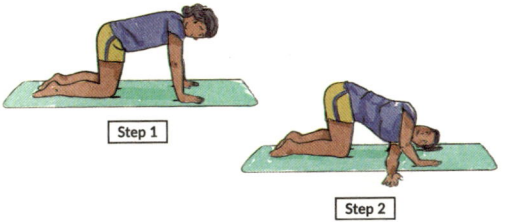

Step 1   Step 2

Duration: _____   *(Goal: 15 sec each side)*

6. Static Y Hold

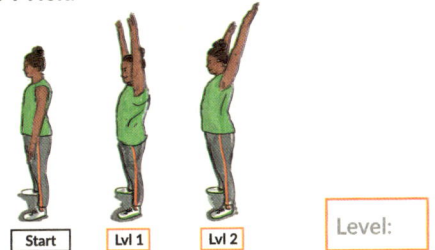

Start   Lvl 1   Lvl 2

Level: _____

Duration: _____   *(Goal: 30 sec)*

7. Reverse Prayer

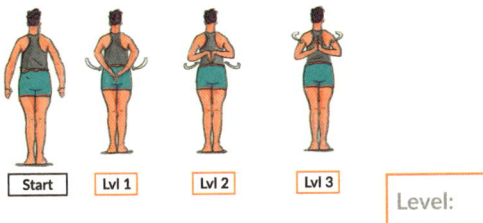

Start   Lvl 1   Lvl 2   Lvl 3

Level: _____

Duration: _____   *(Goal: 30 sec)*

8. Surface Tricep Stretch

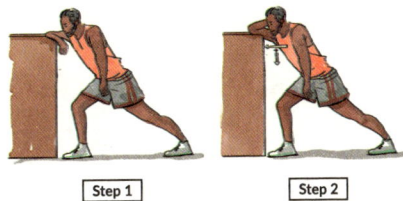

Step 1   Step 2

Duration: _____   *(Goal: 15 sec each side)*

Day 18: Lower Body

1. Warrior II Pose

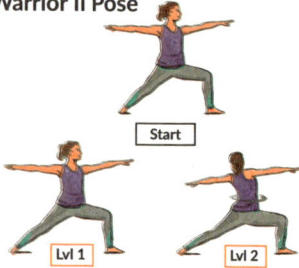

Start

Lvl 1   Lvl 2

Duration:
....

(Goal: 30 sec each side)   Level:

2. Halfway Center Split

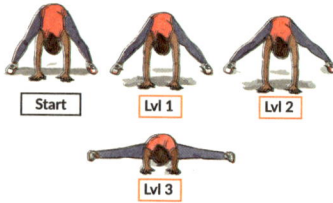

Start   Lvl 1   Lvl 2

Lvl 3

Duration:
....

(Goal: 30 sec)   Level:

3. Pigeon Stretch

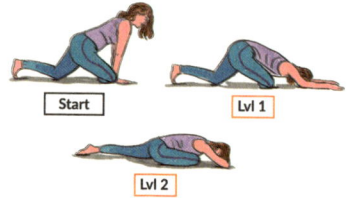

Start   Lvl 1

Lvl 2

Duration:
....

(Goal: 30 sec each side)   Level:

4. Runner's Lunge

Start

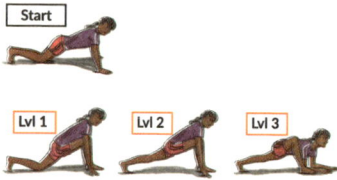

Lvl 1   Lvl 2   Lvl 3

Duration:
....

(Goal: 30 sec each side)   Level:

5. Figure 4

Start   Lvl 1

Lvl 2   Lvl 3

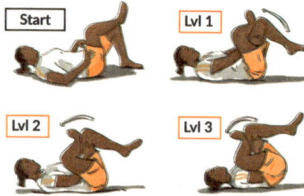

Duration:
....

(Goal: 30 sec each side)   Level:

6. Seated Single Leg Hamstring Stretch

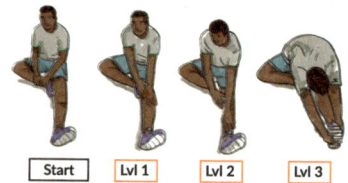

Start   Lvl 1   Lvl 2   Lvl 3

Duration:
....

(Goal: 30 sec each side)   Level:

7. Prone Quad Stretch

Start

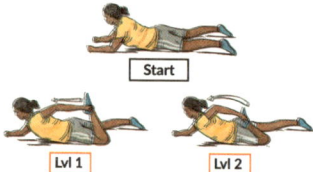

Lvl 1   Lvl 2

Level:

Duration:
....

(Goal: 30 sec each side)

8. Lateral Squat

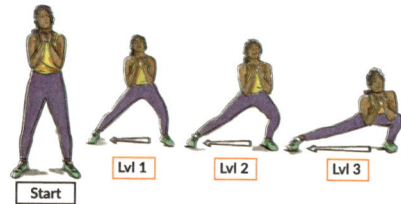

Lvl 1   Lvl 2   Lvl 3

Start

Level:

Duration:
....

(Goal: 30 sec each side)

9. Lying Hip Extension

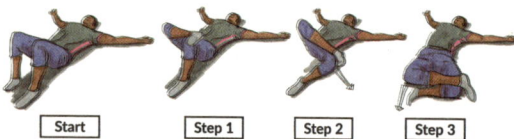

Start   Step 1   Step 2   Step 3

Duration:
....

(Goal: 30 sec each side)

10. Standing Wall Calf Stretch

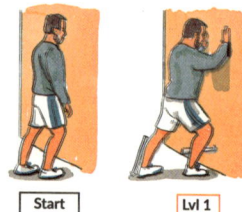

Start   Lvl 1

Level:

Duration:
....

(Goal: 30 sec)

116

Daily Reflection

Benefits I'm Experiencing:

Feel
Lighter

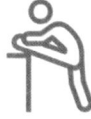

More Freedom
of Movement

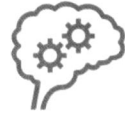

Improved
Mental Clarity

Less
Pain

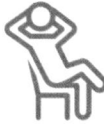

Less
Stressed

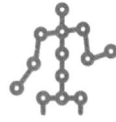

Improved
Posture

Notes On My Body:

Day 19: Dynamic Warm-Up

Full Session Exercise Guide:
habitnest.com/pages/stretching-day-19

1. Plank w/ Shoulder Tap

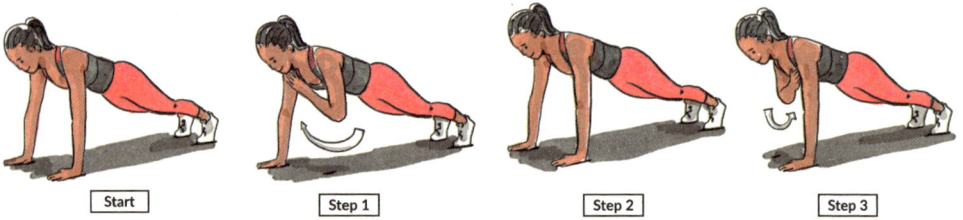

| Start | Step 1 | Step 2 | Step 3 |

Reps: .... *(Goal: 10-15 each side)*

2. Side Plank w/ Twist

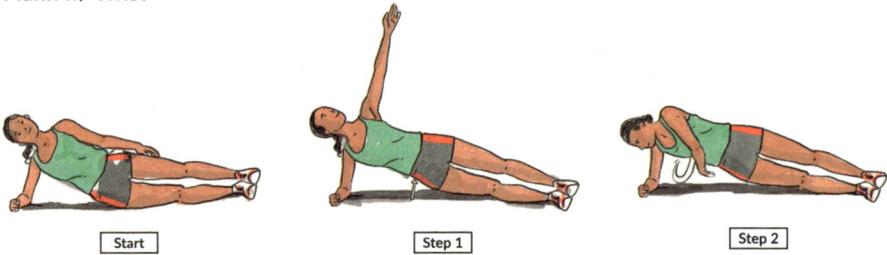

| Start | Step 1 | Step 2 |

Reps: .... *(Goal: 10-15 each side)*

3. Good Morning

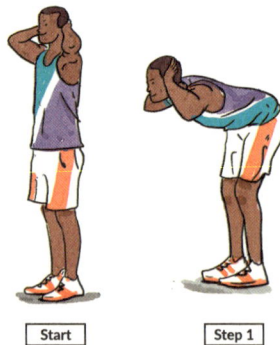

| Start | Step 1 |

Reps: .... *(Goal: 15-20)*

Day 19: Upper Body

1. Levator Scap Neck Stretch

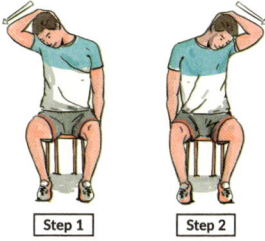

| Step 1 | Step 2 |

Duration: *(Goal: 15 sec each side)*

2. Side Neck Tilt

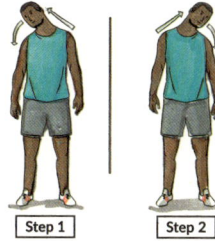

| Step 1 | Step 2 |

Duration: *(Goal: 15 sec each side)*

3. Forward & Backward Neck Tilt

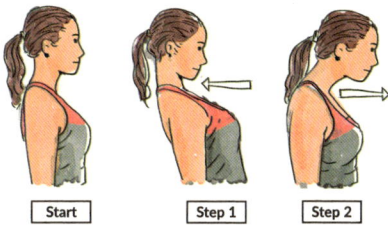

| Start | Step 1 | Step 2 |

Duration: *(Goal: 30 sec, alternating)*

4. Child's Pose

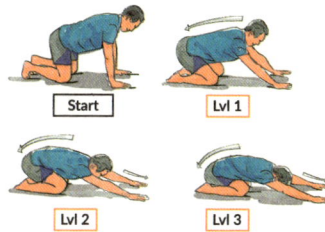

| Start | Lvl 1 |
| Lvl 2 | Lvl 3 |

Level:

Duration: *(Goal: 60 sec)*

5. Cat-Cow

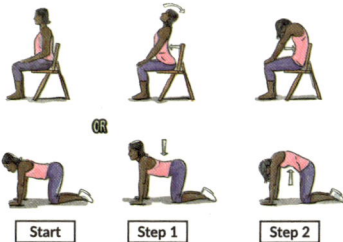

OR

| Start | Step 1 | Step 2 |

Duration: *(Goal: 30 sec, alternating)*

6. Elbow Opener

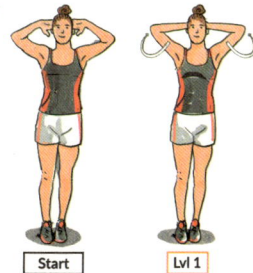

| Start | Lvl 1 |

Duration: *(Goal: 30 sec)*

7. Doorway Pectoral Stretch

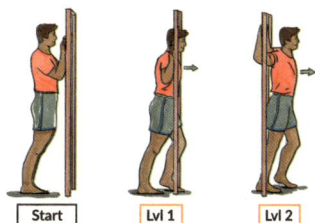

| Start | Lvl 1 | Lvl 2 |

Level:

Duration: *(Goal: 30 sec)*

8. Locust Pose

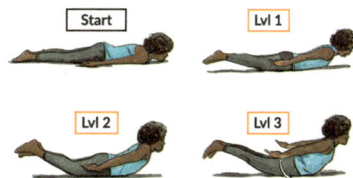

| Start | Lvl 1 |
| Lvl 2 | Lvl 3 |

Level:

Duration: *(Goal: 30 sec)*

Day 19: Lower Body

1. Frog Pose

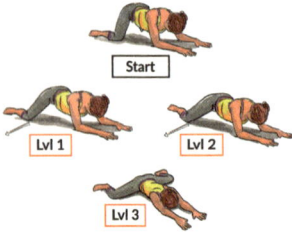

Start

Lvl 1   Lvl 2

Lvl 3

Duration:

(Goal: 60 sec)   Level:

2. Butterfly

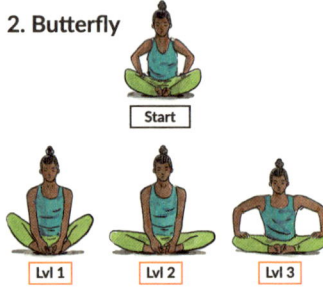

Start

Lvl 1   Lvl 2   Lvl 3

Duration:

(Goal: 30 sec)   Level:

3. Reverse Tabletop

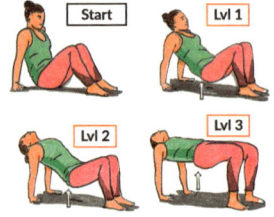

Start   Lvl 1

Lvl 2   Lvl 3

Duration:

(Goal: 30 sec)   Level:

4. Knee to Chest Stretch

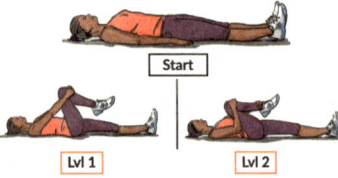

Start

Lvl 1   Lvl 2

Duration:

(Goal: 30 sec each side)   Level:

5. Wig-Wag

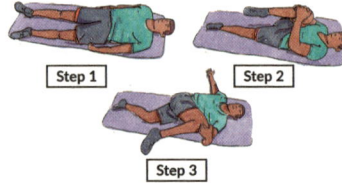

Step 1   Step 2

Step 3

Duration:

(Goal: 30 sec each side)

6. Downward Dog

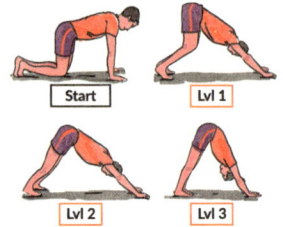

Start   Lvl 1

Lvl 2   Lvl 3

Duration:

(Goal: 30 sec)   Level:

7. Seated Forward Fold Hamstring Stretch

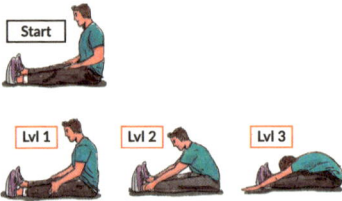

Start

Lvl 1   Lvl 2   Lvl 3

Level:

Duration:

(Goal: 30 sec)

8. Standing Quad Stretch

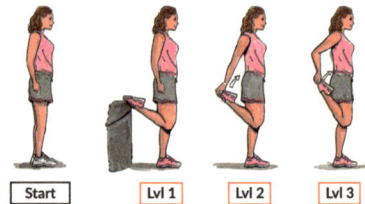

Start   Lvl 1   Lvl 2   Lvl 3

Level:

Duration:

(Goal: 30 sec each side)

9. Hanging Calf Stretch

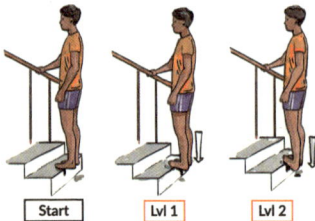

Start   Lvl 1   Lvl 2

Level:

Duration:

(Goal: 30 sec)

10. Standing Wall Calf Stretch w/ Achilles Focus

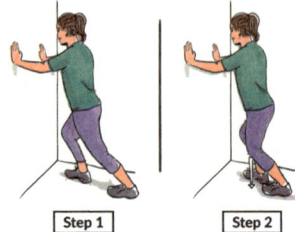

Step 1   Step 2

Duration:

(Goal: 15 sec each side)

Daily Reflection

Benefits I'm Experiencing:

Feel
Lighter

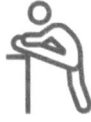

More Freedom
of Movement

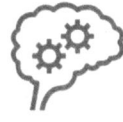

Improved
Mental Clarity

Less
Pain

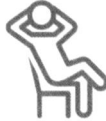

Less
Stressed

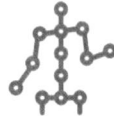

Improved
Posture

Notes On My Body:

Day 20: Dynamic Warm-Up

Full Session Exercise Guide:
habitnest.com/pages/stretching-day-20

1. World's Greatest Stretch

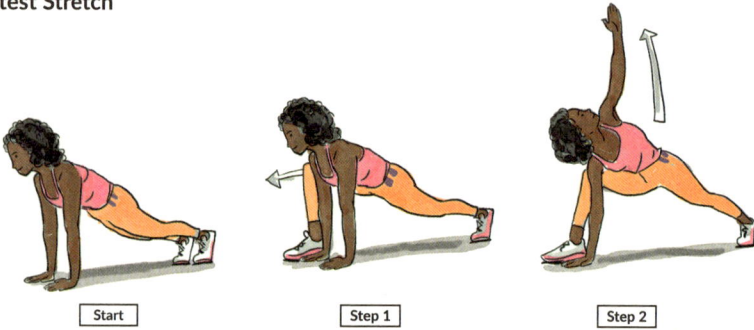

Start | Step 1 | Step 2

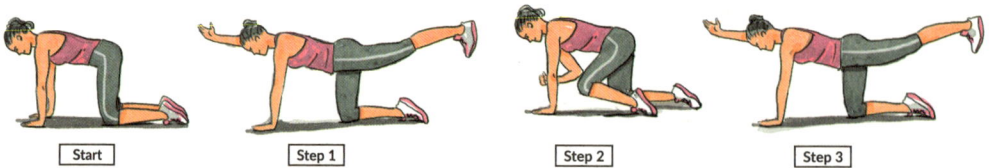

Reps: .... *(Goal: 10-15 each side)*

2. Standing Hamstring Scoop

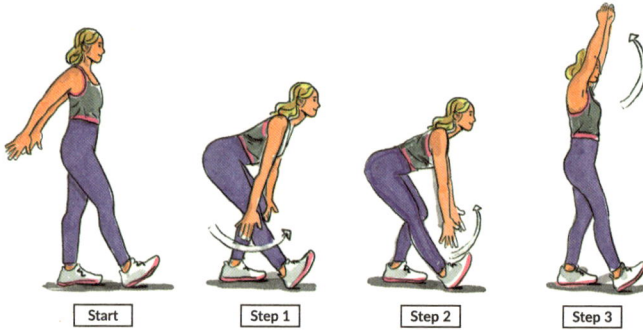

Start | Step 1 | Step 2 | Step 3

Reps: .... *(Goal: 10-15 each side)*

3. Bird-Dog

Start | Step 1 | Step 2 | Step 3

Reps: .... *(Goal: 10-15 each side)*

Day 20: Upper Body

1. Child's Pose

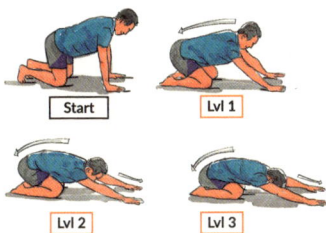

Start Lvl 1 Lvl 2 Lvl 3

Level:

Duration: .... (Goal: 60 sec)

2. Cat-Cow

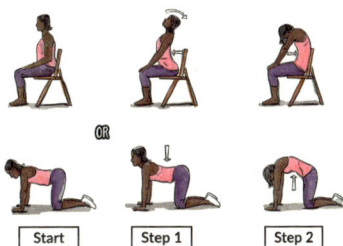

OR

Start Step 1 Step 2

Duration: .... (Goal: 30 sec, alternating)

3. Seated Spinal Twist

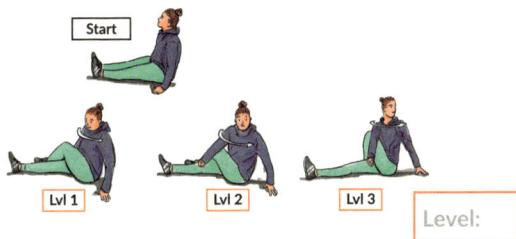

Start Lvl 1 Lvl 2 Lvl 3

Level:

Duration: .... (Goal: 15 sec each side)

4. Cross Arm Shoulder Stretch

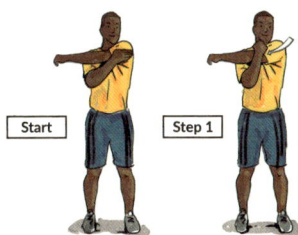

Start Step 1

Duration: .... (Goal: 15 sec each side)

5. Corner Chest Stretch

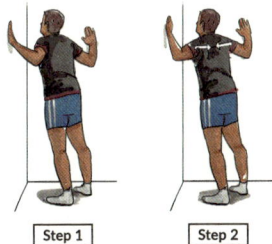

Step 1 Step 2

Duration: .... (Goal: 30 sec)

6. Standing Oblique Stretch

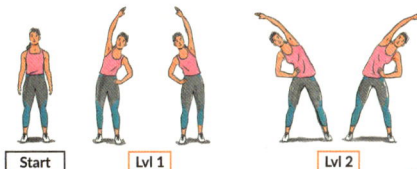

Start Lvl 1 Lvl 2

Level:

Duration: .... (Goal: 15 sec each side)

7. Surface Tricep Stretch

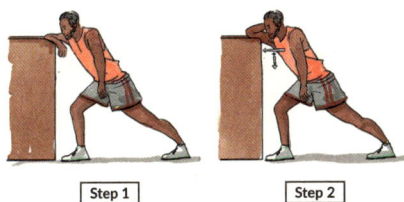

Step 1 Step 2

Duration: .... (Goal: 15 sec each side)

8. Forearm Stretch w/ Hands on Surface

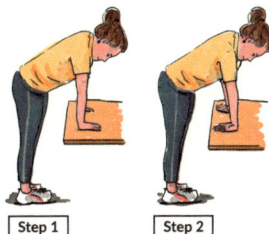

Step 1 Step 2

Level:

Duration: .... (Goal: 15 sec each side)

Day 20: Lower Body

1. Scorpion Pose

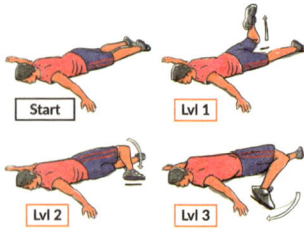

Start   Lvl 1
Lvl 2   Lvl 3

Duration:

(Goal: 30 sec each side)   Level:

2. Butterfly

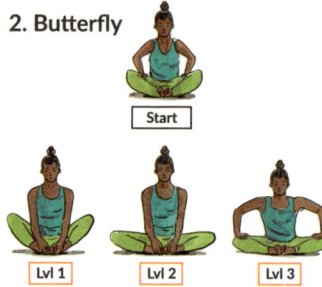

Start
Lvl 1   Lvl 2   Lvl 3

Duration:

(Goal: 30 sec)   Level:

3. Halfway Center Split

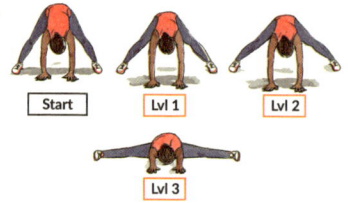

Start   Lvl 1   Lvl 2
Lvl 3

Duration:

(Goal: 30 sec)   Level:

4. Reclining Angle Bound Pose

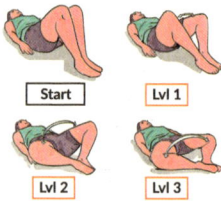

Start   Lvl 1
Lvl 2   Lvl 3

Duration:

(Goal: 30 sec)   Level:

5. Happy Baby Pose

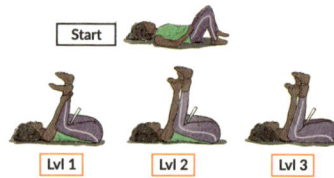

Start
Lvl 1   Lvl 2   Lvl 3

Duration:

(Goal: 30 sec)   Level:

6. Lateral Squat

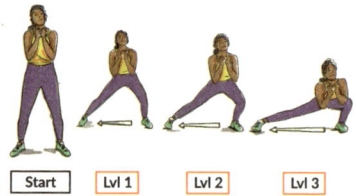

Start   Lvl 1   Lvl 2   Lvl 3

Duration:

(Goal: 30 sec each side)   Level:

7. Lateral Squat w/ Toe Raise

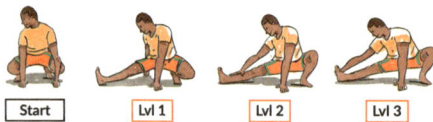

Start   Lvl 1   Lvl 2   Lvl 3

Level:

Duration:

(Goal: 30 sec each side)

8. Lying Quad Stretch

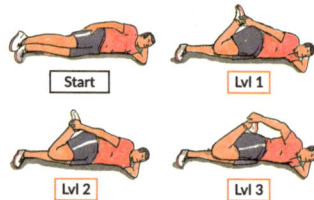

Start   Lvl 1
Lvl 2   Lvl 3

Level:

Duration:

(Goal: 30 sec each side)

9. Pry Squat

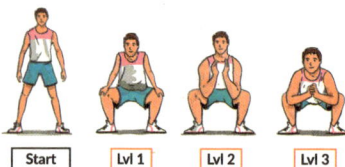

Start   Lvl 1   Lvl 2   Lvl 3

Level:

Duration:

(Goal: 30 sec)

10. Pigeon Stretch

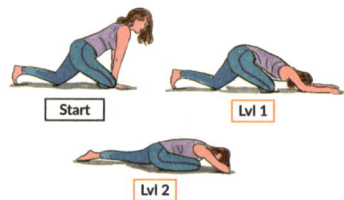

Start   Lvl 1
Lvl 2

Level:

Duration:

(Goal: 30 sec each side)

Daily Reflection

Benefits I'm Experiencing:

Feel
Lighter

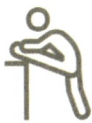

More Freedom
of Movement

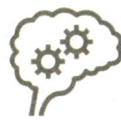

Improved
Mental Clarity

Less
Pain

Less
Stressed

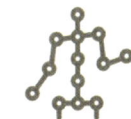

Improved
Posture

Notes On My Body:

Day 21: Dynamic Warm-Up

Full Session Exercise Guide:
habitnest.com/pages/stretching-day-21

1. Inch Worm Walk Out

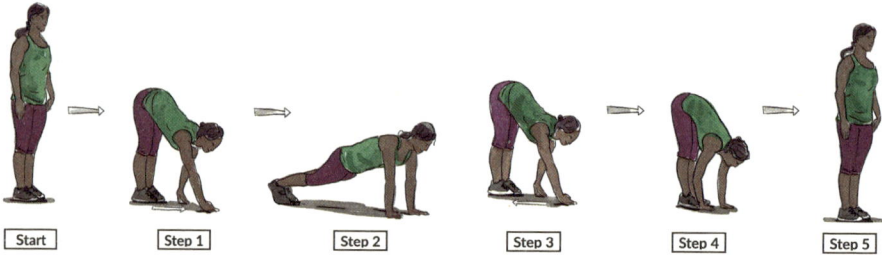

| Start | Step 1 | Step 2 | Step 3 | Step 4 | Step 5 |

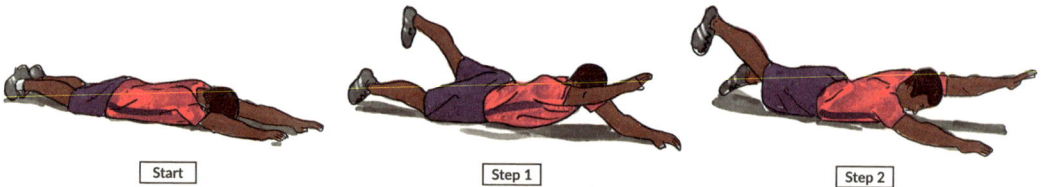

Reps: .... *(Goal: 10-15)*

2. Roundhouse Kick to Squat

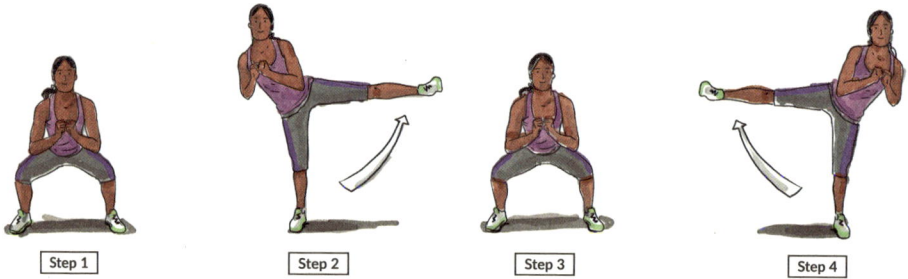

| Step 1 | Step 2 | Step 3 | Step 4 |

Reps: .... *(Goal: 10-15 each side)*

3. Aquaman

| Start | Step 1 | Step 2 |

Reps: .... *(Goal: 10-15)*

Day 21: Upper Body

1. Lateral Side to Side Neck Rotation

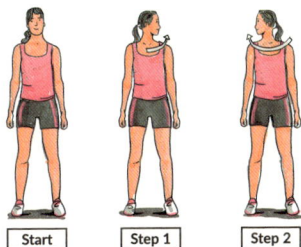

Start   Step 1   Step 2

Duration: *(Goal: 30 sec, alternating)*

2. Up & Down Neck Tilt

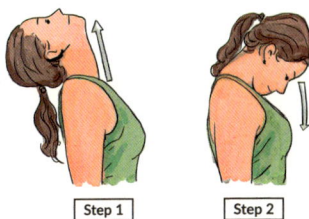

Step 1   Step 2

Duration: *(Goal: 30 sec, alternating)*

3. Side Neck Tilt

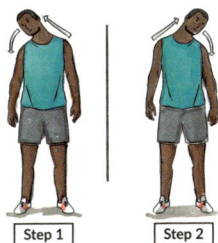

Step 1   Step 2

Duration: *(Goal: 15 sec each side)*

4. Child's Pose

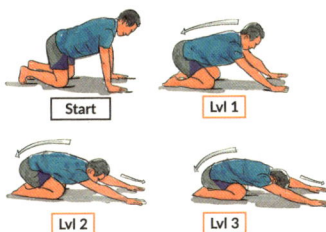

Start   Lvl 1

Lvl 2   Lvl 3

Level:

Duration: *(Goal: 60 sec)*

5. Cat-Cow

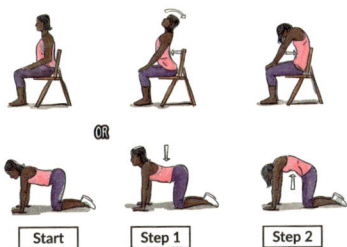

OR

Start   Step 1   Step 2

Duration: *(Goal: 30 sec, alternating)*

6. Floor Angel

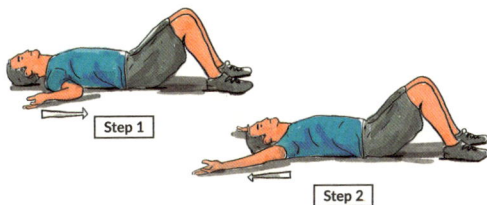

Step 1

Step 2

Duration: *(Goal: 30 sec, alternating)*

7. Locust Pose

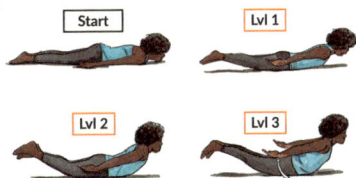

Start   Lvl 1

Lvl 2   Lvl 3

Level:

Duration: *(Goal: 30 sec)*

8. Static Y Hold

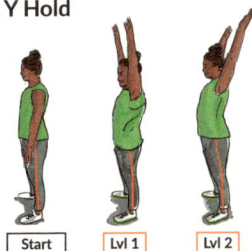

Start   Lvl 1   Lvl 2

Level:

Duration: *(Goal: 30 sec)*

Day 21: Lower Body

1. Standing Quad Stretch

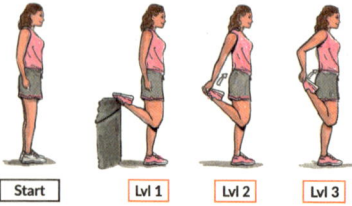

| Start | Lvl 1 | Lvl 2 | Lvl 3 |

Duration:
....

(Goal: 30 sec each side)

Level:

2. Standing Wall Calf Stretch

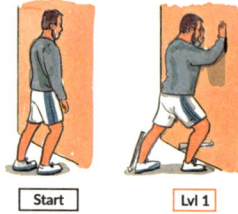

| Start | Lvl 1 |

Duration:
....

(Goal: 15 sec each side)

3. Standing Wall Calf Stretch w/ Achilles Focus

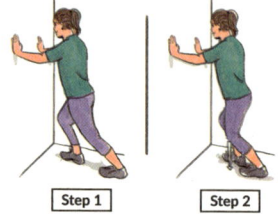

| Step 1 | Step 2 |

Duration:
....

(Goal: 15 sec each side)

4. Seated Single Leg Hamstring Stretch

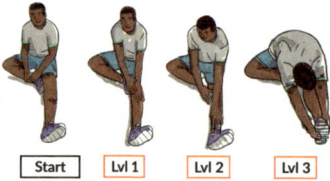

| Start | Lvl 1 | Lvl 2 | Lvl 3 |

Duration:
....

(Goal: 30 sec each side)

Level:

5. Lateral Squat

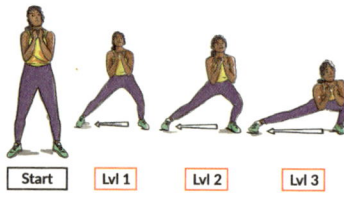

| Start | Lvl 1 | Lvl 2 | Lvl 3 |

Duration:
....

(Goal: 30 sec each side)

Level:

6. Lateral Squat w/ Toe Raise

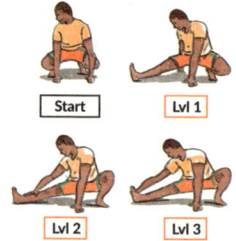

| Start | Lvl 1 |
| Lvl 2 | Lvl 3 |

Duration:
....

(Goal: 30 sec each side)

Level:

7. Figure 4

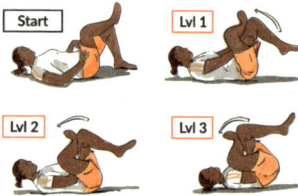

| Start | Lvl 1 |
| Lvl 2 | Lvl 3 |

Level:

Duration:

(Goal: 30 sec each side)

8. Reclining Angle Bound Pose

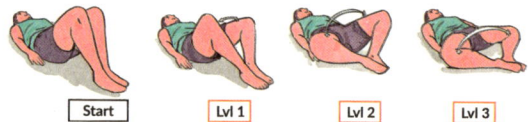

| Start | Lvl 1 | Lvl 2 | Lvl 3 |

Level:

Duration:

(Goal: 30 sec)

9. Runner's Lunge

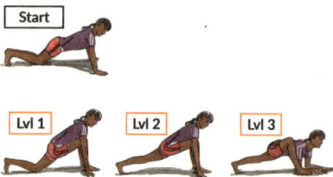

| Start |
| Lvl 1 | Lvl 2 | Lvl 3 |

Level:

Duration:

(Goal: 30 sec each side)

10. Warrior II Pose

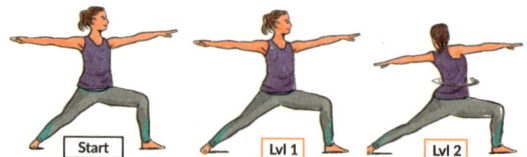

| Start | Lvl 1 | Lvl 2 |

Level:

Duration:

(Goal: 30 sec each side)

Daily Reflection

Benefits I'm Experiencing:

Feel
Lighter

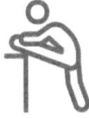

More Freedom
of Movement

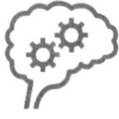

Improved
Mental Clarity

Less
Pain

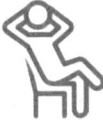

Less
Stressed

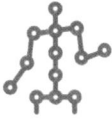

Improved
Posture

Notes On My Body:

....

....

....

....

....

....

....

....

....

You've now completed 21 serious stretching sessions. How are you feeling
about this enormous accomplishment? What's motivating you to keep going?

Recap Questions

1. Which recent stretches do I now know are absolutely essential for me?

2. What stretches felt super uncomfortable at first that I now feel more able to perform?

3. In which body parts do I see the most progress in terms of flexibility and range of motion?

4. Which body parts do I know I need to focus on improving flexibility for?

....

....

....

....

....

....

5. In the last two weeks, what have I learned about my own physical habits and how they play a role in the way my body feels?

....

....

....

....

....

....

Phase 2 Done.

Phase 3:
Days
22 - 66

Rewiring Your Brain

My main stretching goal for this phase:

Phase 3 Overview

You're on fire! 21 days of stretching down and you undoubtedly know the struggle of sticking with a commitment long after the initial motivation wanes. That's one of the most lessons you learn in altering your habits.

Another one of the critical lessons you learn is that anytime you give a certain aspect of your life energy and attention, that part of your life will flourish, or at least be better than it was before.

You've stretched for 21 days, but there are another 45 days left in the journey.

One thing we all do that doesn't make much sense is that we wait for something to go wrong before taking care of it. That's especially true when it comes to our bodies.

Stretching makes your body happier, but when your body does feel good is precisely when this illogical impulse to 'take a break' or let go of the reins kicks in.

When you're feeling good, light, and flexible, you lose sight of why you're doing this in the first place because, well, you already feel pretty good.

In Phase 3, it's really important to battle with yourself to stretch daily, because you don't want to make this something you do only when you feel like you need it.

You want to live a pain free, physically comfortable life, and that means taking care of your body, even when you don't feel the need for it.

In Phase 3, you'll be getting slightly longer routines that border on 20 minutes long, so plan accordingly! You'll still get a dynamic warmup that includes 3 exercises, but now you'll perform 10 upper body stretches and 12 lower body stretches to maximize the impact of each day's routine.

Don't forget that stretching isn't ONLY about how your body feels. It's a time for you to let go of the rest of your life and spend just 10-20 minutes relaxing internally, concentrating on what you're doing, and taking care of yourself so that your day to day life improves mentally and physically.

Day 22: Dynamic Warm-Up

Full Session Exercise Guide:
habitnest.com/pages/stretching-day-22

1. Side Plank w/ Twist

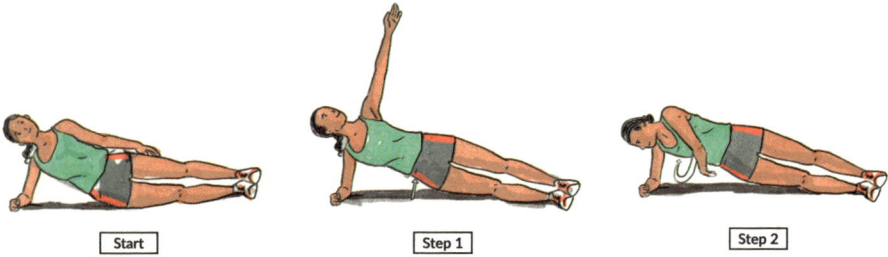

Start

Step 1

Step 2

Reps: .... *(Goal: 10-15 each side)*

2. Good Morning

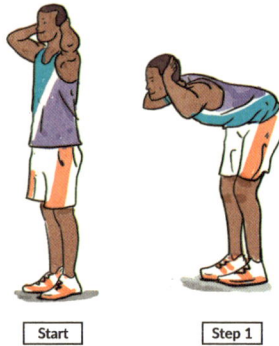

Start

Step 1

Reps: .... *(Goal: 20-30 each side)*

3. Rocking Feet w/ Arm Raise

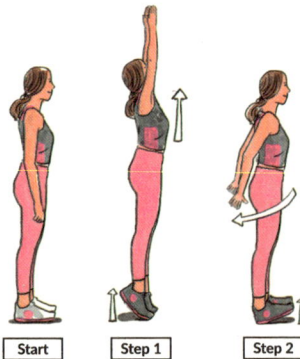

Start

Step 1

Step 2

Reps: .... *(Goal: 10-15 in each direction)*

Day 22: Upper Body

DATE

1. Up & Down Neck Tilt

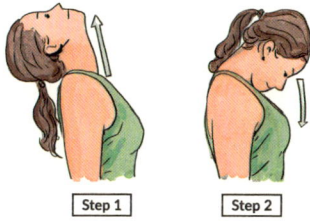

Step 1   Step 2

Duration:

(Goal: 30 sec, alternating)

2. Side Neck Tilt

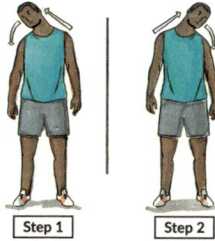

Step 1   Step 2

Duration:

(Goal: 15 sec each side)

3. Forward & Backward Neck Tilt

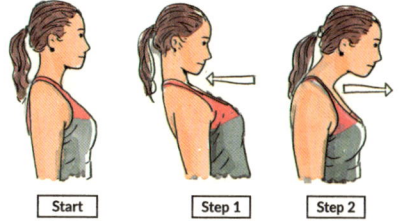

Start   Step 1   Step 2

Duration:

(Goal: 30 sec, alternating)

4. Child's Pose

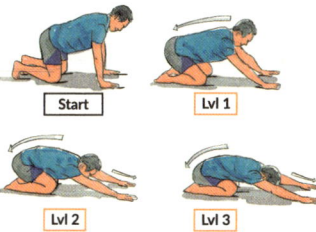

Start   Lvl 1

Lvl 2   Lvl 3

Duration:

(Goal: 60 sec)   Level:

5. Cat-Cow

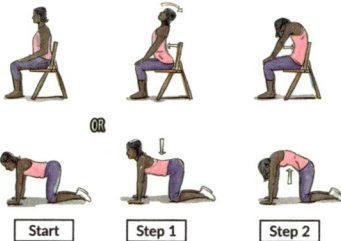

OR

Start   Step 1   Step 2

Duration:

(Goal: 30 sec, alternating)

6. Sphinx/Cobra

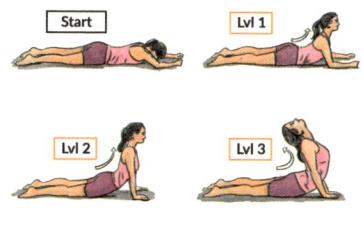

Start   Lvl 1

Lvl 2   Lvl 3

Duration:

(Goal: 30 sec)   Level:

7. Cross Arm Shoulder Stretch

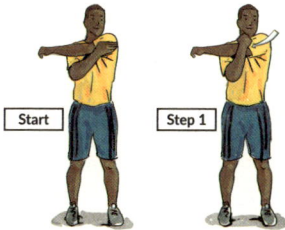

Start   Step 1

Duration: *(Goal: 15 sec each side)*

8. Open Book Chest Stretch

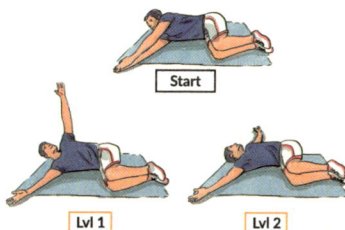

Start

Lvl 1   Lvl 2

Level:

Duration: *(Goal: 30 sec each side)*

9. Standing Oblique Stretch

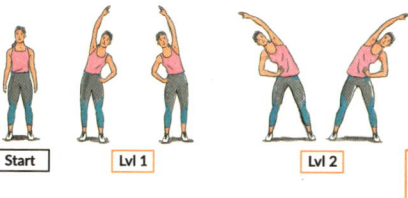

Start   Lvl 1   Lvl 2

Level:

Duration: *(Goal: 15 sec each side)*

10. Surface Tricep Stretch

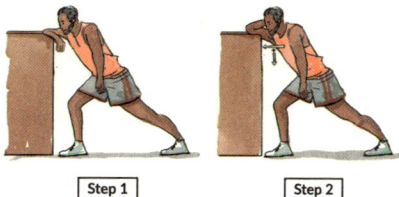

Step 1   Step 2

Duration: *(Goal: 15 sec each side)*

Day 22: Lower Body

1. Frog Pose

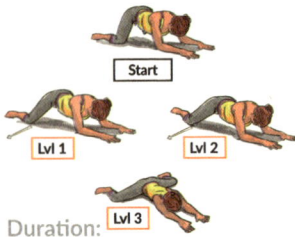

Duration:
....

(Goal: 60 sec)

Level:

2. Runner's Lunge

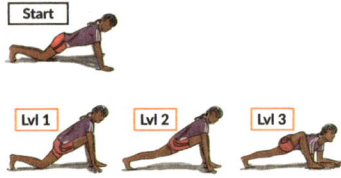

Duration:
....

(Goal: 30 sec each side)

Level:

3. Butterfly

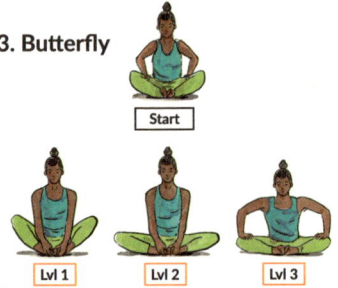

Duration:
....

(Goal: 30 sec)

Level:

4. Scorpion Pose

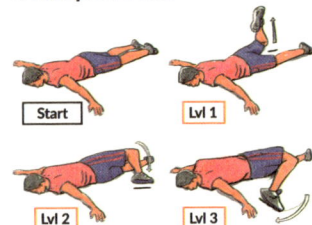

Duration:
....

(Goal: 30 sec each side)

Level:

5. Lying Hip Extension

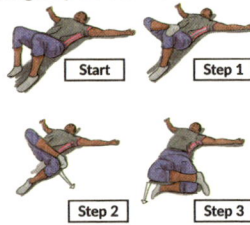

Duration:
....

(Goal: 30 sec each side)

6. Pigeon Stretch

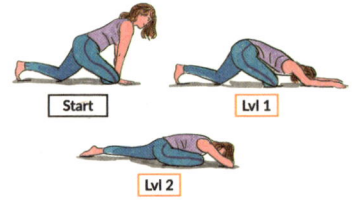

Duration:
....

(Goal: 30 sec each side)

Level:

7. Seated Forward Fold Hamstring Stretch

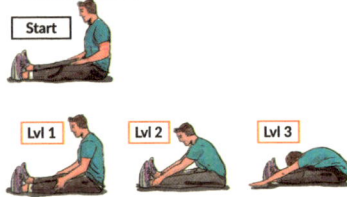

Duration:
....

(Goal: 30 sec)

Level:

8. Lateral Squat

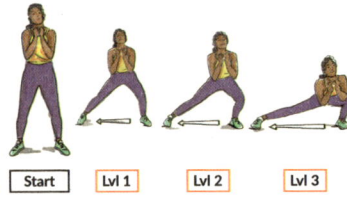

Duration:
....

(Goal: 30 sec each side)

Level:

9. Lateral Squat w/ Toe Raise

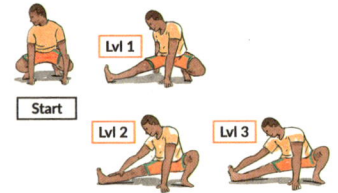

Duration:
....

(Goal: 30 sec each side)

Level:

10. Wig-Wag

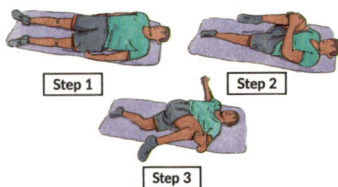

Duration:
....

(Goal: 30 sec each side)

11. Standing Quad Stretch

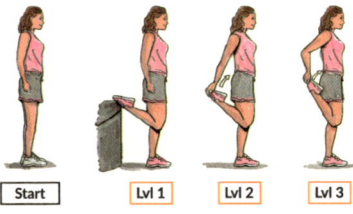

Duration:
....

(Goal: 30 sec each side)

Level:

12. Standing Wall Calf Stretch

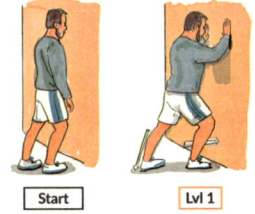

Duration:
....

(Goal: 15 sec each side)

Daily Reflection

Remember - don't take the benefits you're experiencing for granted.

If you step performing your stretching routine and paying closer attention to your body, you WILL revert back to old habits, and the benefits you're feeling will dissipate.

Benefits I'm Experiencing:

Feel
Lighter

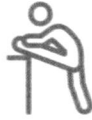

More Freedom
of Movement

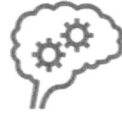

Improved
Mental Clarity

Less
Pain

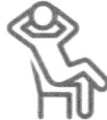

Less
Stressed

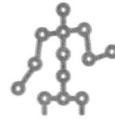

Improved
Posture

Notes On My Body:

....

....

....

....

....

....

....

....

....

Time to set some new goals for Phase 3. Flexibility goals, consistency goals, goals for altering physical habits you've found are problematic... any goals related to your body. List them above.

Day 23: Dynamic Warm-Up

Full Session Exercise Guide:
habitnest.com/pages/stretching-day-23

1. Walking Jacks (or Jumping Jacks)

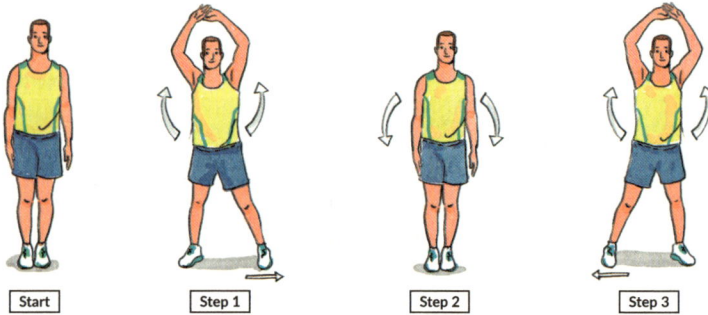

| Start | Step 1 | Step 2 | Step 3 |

Reps: *(Goal: 20-30)*

2. Clam Opener w/ Side Plank

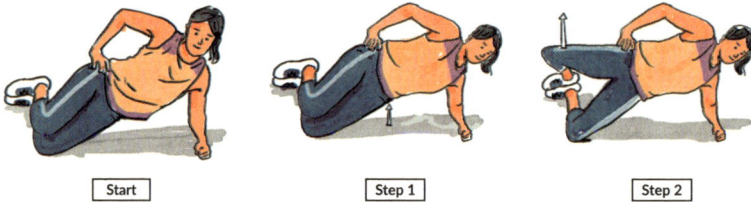

| Start | Step 1 | Step 2 |

Reps: *(Goal: 10-15 each side)*

3. Air Squat to Calf Raise

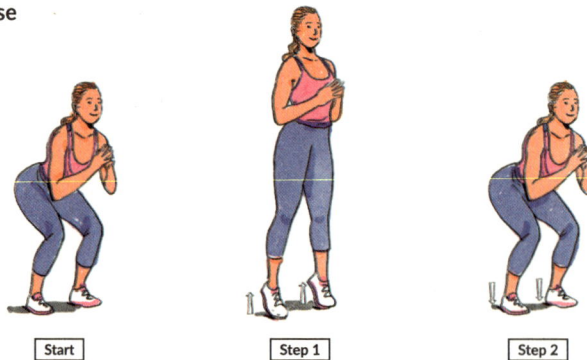

| Start | Step 1 | Step 2 |

Reps: *(Goal: 20-25)*

Day 23: Upper Body

1. Up & Down Neck Tilt

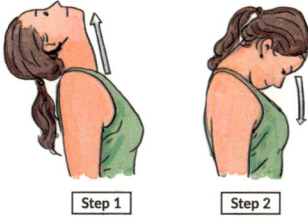

Step 1   Step 2

Duration:
....

(Goal: 30 sec, alternating)

2. Side Neck Tilt

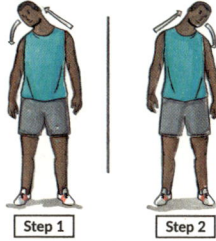

Step 1   Step 2

Duration:
....

(Goal: 15 sec each side)

3. Forward & Backward Neck Tilt

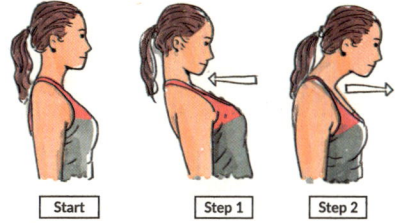

Start   Step 1   Step 2

Duration:
....

(Goal: 30 sec, alternating)

4. Child's Pose

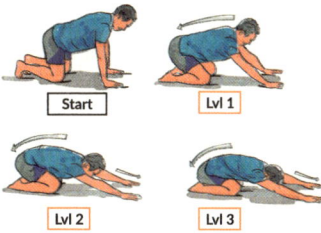

Start   Lvl 1
Lvl 2   Lvl 3

Duration:
....

(Goal: 60 sec)

Level:

5. Cat-Cow

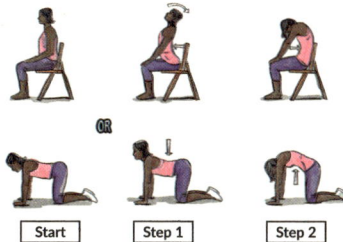

OR

Start   Step 1   Step 2

Duration:
....

(Goal: 30 sec, alternating)

6. Sphinx/Cobra

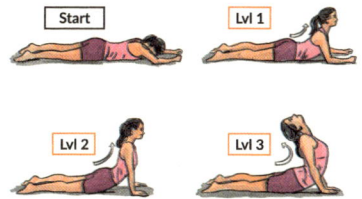

Start   Lvl 1
Lvl 2   Lvl 3

Duration:
....

(Goal: 30 sec)

Level:

7. Cross Arm Shoulder Stretch

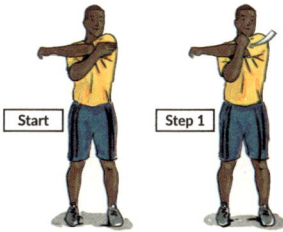

Start   Step 1

Duration:
....

(Goal: 15 sec each side)

8. Open Book Chest Stretch

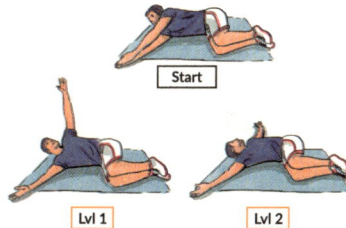

Start

Lvl 1   Lvl 2

Level:

Duration:
....

(Goal: 30 sec each side)

9. Standing Oblique Stretch

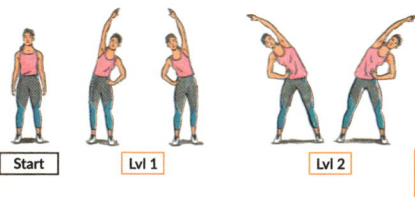

Start   Lvl 1   Lvl 2

Level:

Duration:
....

(Goal: 15 sec each side)

10. Surface Tricep Stretch

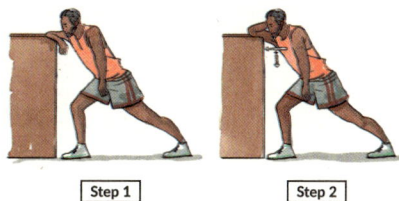

Step 1   Step 2

Duration:
....

(Goal: 15 sec each side)

Day 23: Lower Body

1. Frog Pose

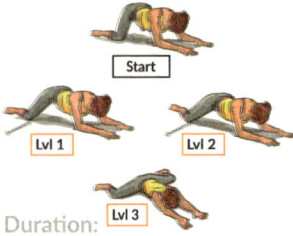

Duration:

(Goal: 60 sec)

Level:

2. Runner's Lunge

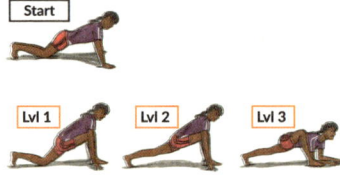

Duration:

(Goal: 30 sec each side)

Level:

3. Butterfly

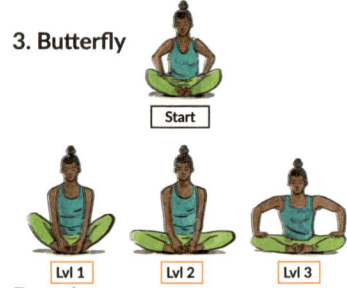

Duration:

(Goal: 30 sec)

Level:

4. Scorpion Pose

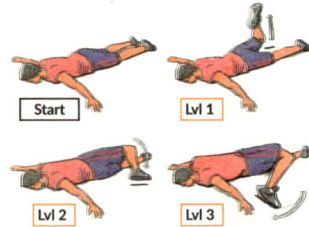

Duration:

(Goal: 30 sec each side)

Level:

5. Lying Hip Extension

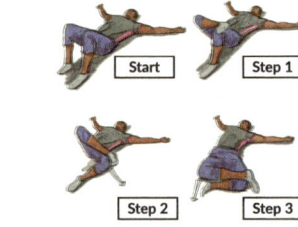

Duration:

(Goal: 30 sec each side)

6. Pigeon Stretch

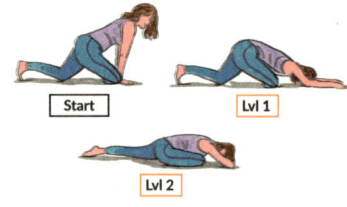

Duration:

(Goal: 30 sec each side)

Level:

7. Seated Forward Fold Hamstring Stretch

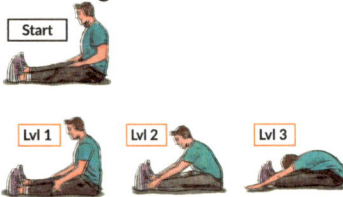

Duration:

(Goal: 30 sec)

Level:

8. Lateral Squat

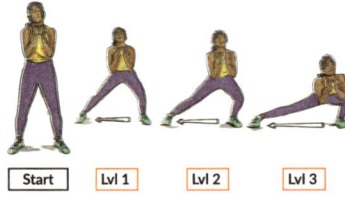

Duration:

(Goal: 30 sec each side)

Level:

9. Lateral Squat w/ Toe Raise

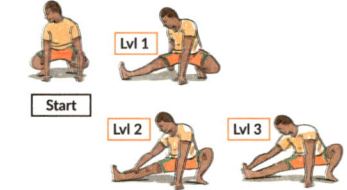

Duration:

(Goal: 30 sec each side)

Level:

10. Wig-Wag

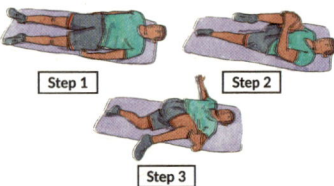

Duration:

(Goal: 30 sec each side)

11. Standing Quad Stretch

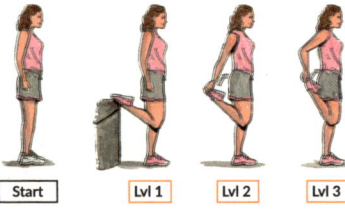

Duration:

(Goal: 30 sec each side)

Level:

12. Standing Wall Calf Stretch

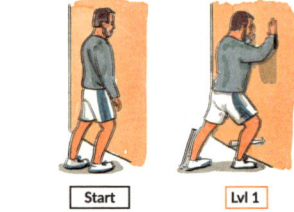

Duration:

(Goal: 15 sec each side)

Daily Reflection

Benefits I'm Experiencing:

Feel
Lighter

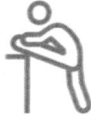

More Freedom
of Movement

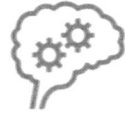

Improved
Mental Clarity

Less
Pain

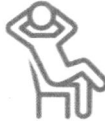

Less
Stressed

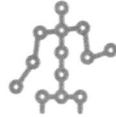

Improved
Posture

Notes On My Body:

Day 24: Dynamic Warm-Up

1. Inch Worm Walk Out

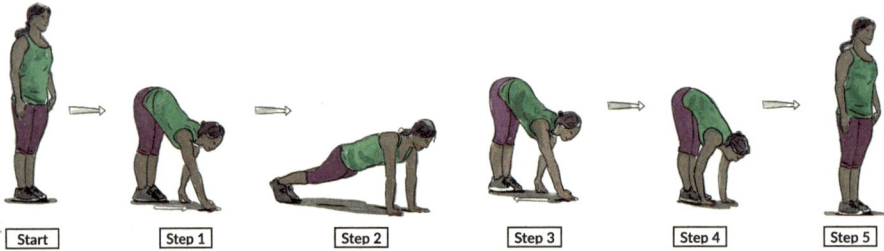

| Start | Step 1 | Step 2 | Step 3 | Step 4 | Step 5 |

Reps: .... *(Goal: 20-30)*

2. Low Lunge w/ Elbow Twist

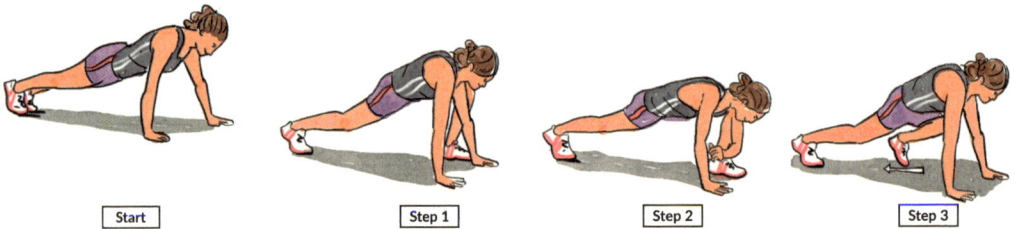

| Start | Step 1 | Step 2 | Step 3 |

Reps: .... *(Goal: 10-15 each side)*

3. Y Raise

| Step 1 | Step 2 |

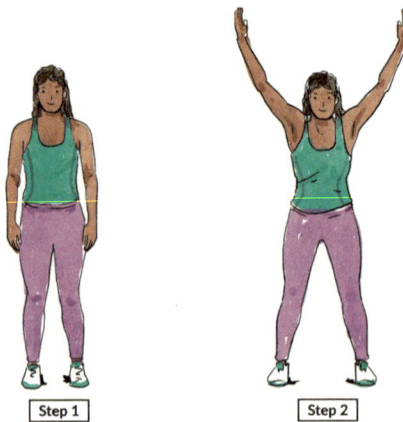

Reps: .... *(Goal: 15-20)*

Day 24: Upper Body

1. Up & Down Neck Tilt

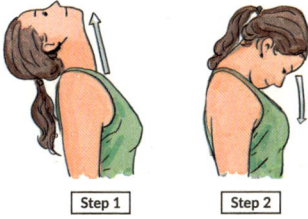

Step 1   Step 2

Duration:

(Goal: 30 sec, alternating)

2. Side Neck Tilt

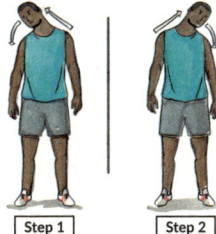

Step 1   Step 2

Duration:

(Goal: 15 sec each side)

3. Forward & Backward Neck Tilt

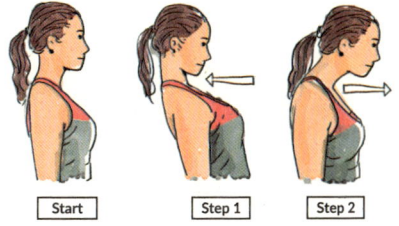

Start   Step 1   Step 2

Duration:

(Goal: 30 sec, alternating)

4. Child's Pose

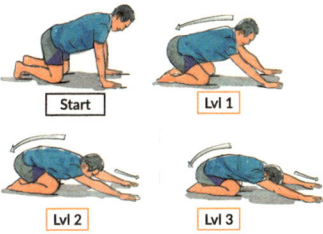

Start   Lvl 1   Lvl 2   Lvl 3

Duration:

(Goal: 60 sec)   Level:

5. Cat-Cow

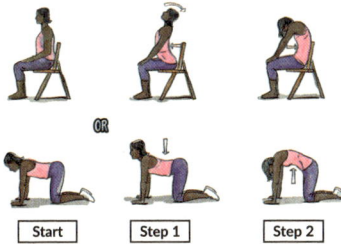

OR

Start   Step 1   Step 2

Duration:

(Goal: 30 sec, alternating)

6. Sphinx/Cobra

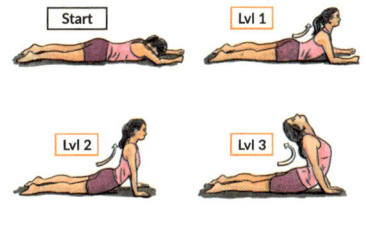

Start   Lvl 1   Lvl 2   Lvl 3

Duration:

(Goal: 30 sec)   Level:

7. Cross Arm Shoulder Stretch

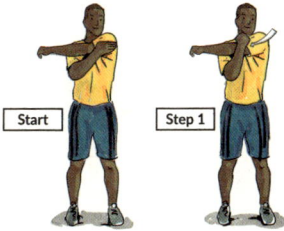

Start   Step 1

Duration: *(Goal: 15 sec each side)*

8. Open Book Chest Stretch

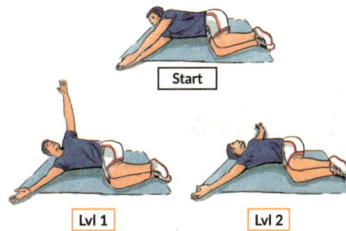

Start   Lvl 1   Lvl 2

Level:

Duration: *(Goal: 30 sec each side)*

9. Standing Oblique Stretch

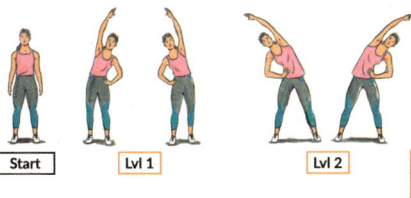

Start   Lvl 1   Lvl 2   Level:

Duration: *(Goal: 15 sec each side)*

10. Surface Tricep Stretch

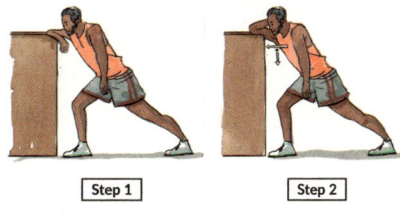

Step 1   Step 2

Duration: *(Goal: 15 sec each side)*

Day 24: Lower Body

1. Frog Pose

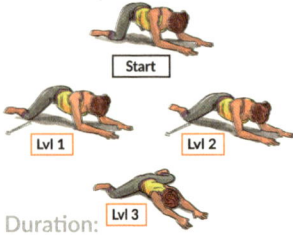

Duration:

(Goal: 60 sec)

Level:

2. Runner's Lunge

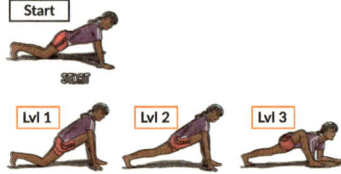

Duration:

(Goal: 30 sec each side)

Level:

3. Butterfly

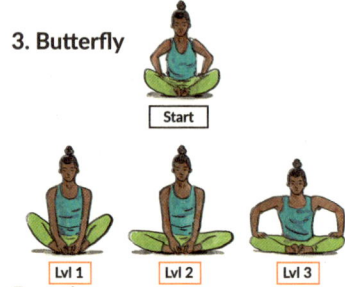

Duration:

(Goal: 30 sec)

Level:

4. Scorpion Pose

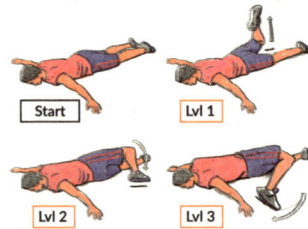

Duration:

(Goal: 30 sec each side)

Level:

5. Lying Hip Extension

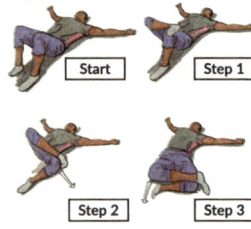

Duration:

(Goal: 30 sec each side)

6. Pigeon Stretch

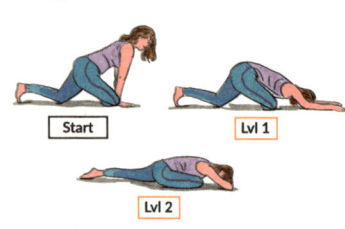

Duration:

(Goal: 30 sec each side)

Level:

7. Seated Forward Fold Hamstring Stretch

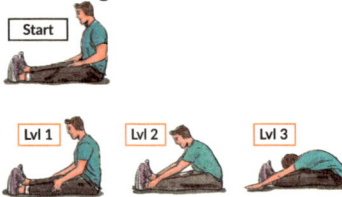

Duration:

(Goal: 30 sec)

Level:

8. Lateral Squat

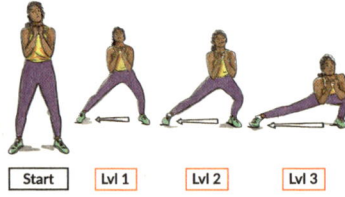

Duration:

(Goal: 30 sec each side)

Level:

9. Lateral Squat w/ Toe Raise

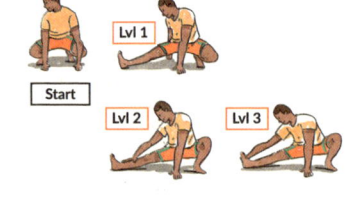

Duration:

(Goal: 30 sec each side)

Level:

10. Wig-Wag

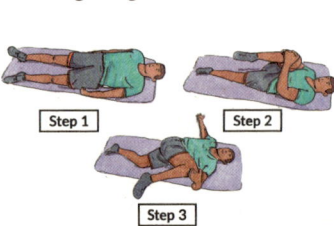

Duration:

(Goal: 30 sec each side)

11. Standing Quad Stretch

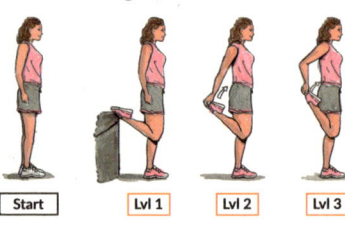

Duration:

(Goal: 30 sec each side)

Level:

12. Standing Wall Calf Stretch

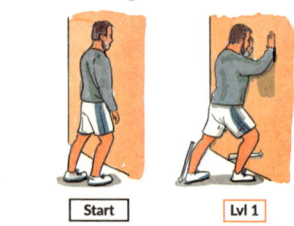

Duration:

(Goal: 15 sec each side)

Daily Reflection

Benefits I'm Experiencing:

Feel
Lighter

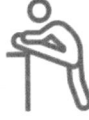

More Freedom
of Movement

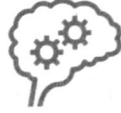

Improved
Mental Clarity

Less
Pain

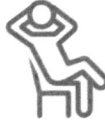

Less
Stressed

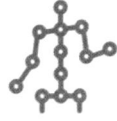

Improved
Posture

Notes On My Body:

Day 25: Dynamic Warm-Up

Full Session Exercise Guide:
habitnest.com/pages/stretching-day-25

1. Glute Bridge

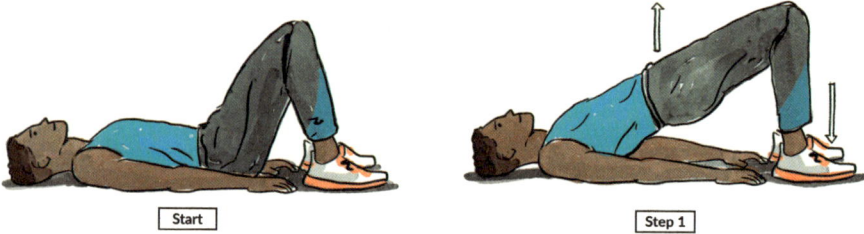

Start

Step 1

Reps: .... (Goal: 20-30)

2. Split Squat

Step 1

Step 2

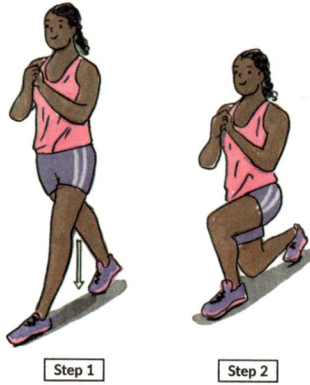

Reps: .... (Goal: 15-20 each side)

3. Mountain Climber

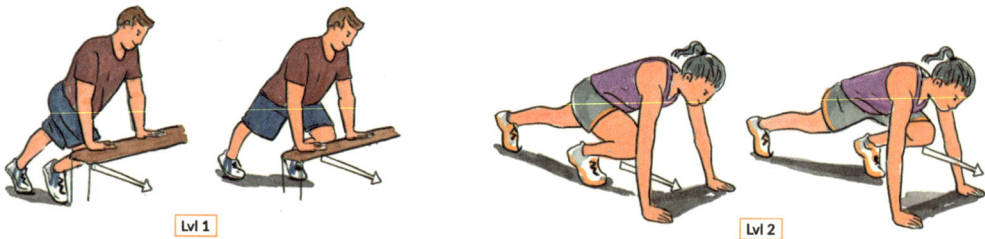

Lvl 1

Lvl 2

Level:

Reps: .... (Goal: 30-40)

146

Day 25: Upper Body

1. Up & Down Neck Tilt

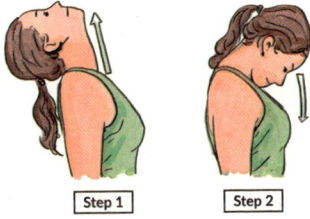

Step 1   Step 2

Duration:
....

(Goal: 30 sec, alternating)

2. Side Neck Tilt

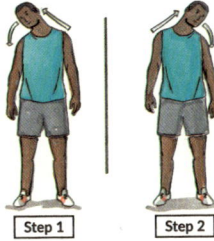

Step 1   Step 2

Duration:
....
(Goal: 15 sec each side)

3. Forward & Backward Neck Tilt

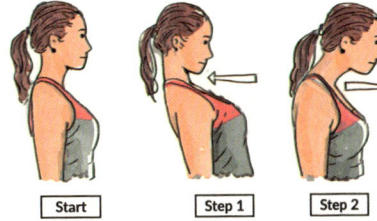

Start   Step 1   Step 2

Duration:
....

(Goal: 30 sec, alternating)

4. Child's Pose

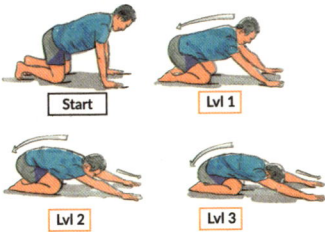

Start   Lvl 1
Lvl 2   Lvl 3

Duration:
....

(Goal: 60 sec)

Level:

5. Cat-Cow

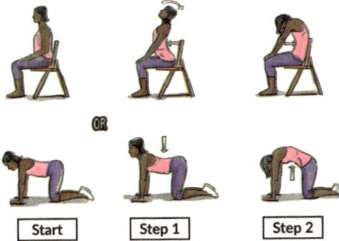

OR

Start   Step 1   Step 2

Duration:
....

(Goal: 30 sec, alternating)

6. Sphinx/Cobra

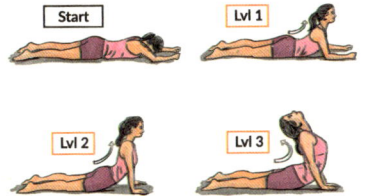

Start   Lvl 1
Lvl 2   Lvl 3

Duration:
....

(Goal: 30 sec)

Level:

7. Cross Arm Shoulder Stretch

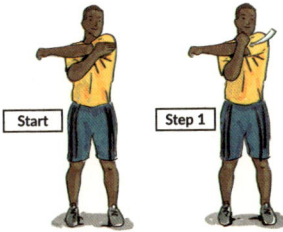

Start   Step 1

Duration:
....
(Goal: 15 sec each side)

8. Open Book Chest Stretch

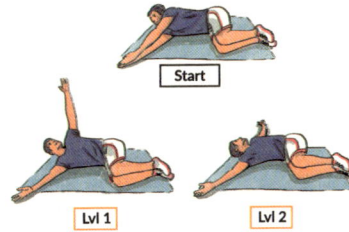

Start

Lvl 1   Lvl 2

Level:

Duration:
....
(Goal: 30 sec each side)

9. Standing Oblique Stretch

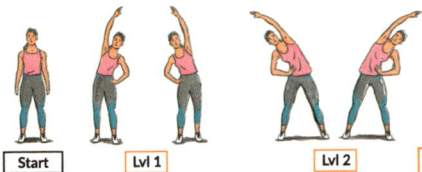

Start   Lvl 1   Lvl 2

Level:

Duration:
....
(Goal: 15 sec each side)

10. Surface Tricep Stretch

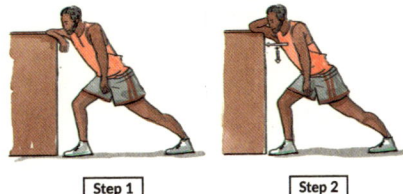

Step 1   Step 2

Duration:
....
(Goal: 15 sec each side)

Day 25: Lower Body

1. Frog Pose

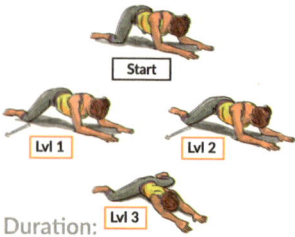

Start
Lvl 1
Lvl 2
Lvl 3

Duration:
....

(Goal: 60 sec)

Level:

2. Runner's Lunge

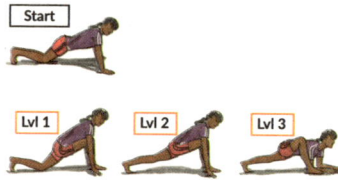

Start
Lvl 1
Lvl 2
Lvl 3

Duration:
....

(Goal: 30 sec each side)

Level:

3. Butterfly

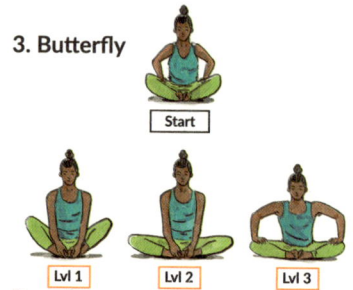

Start
Lvl 1
Lvl 2
Lvl 3

Duration:
....

(Goal: 30 sec)

Level:

4. Scorpion Pose

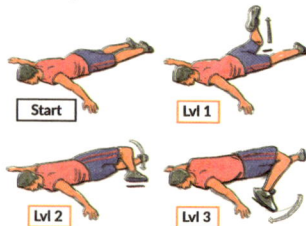

Start
Lvl 1
Lvl 2
Lvl 3

Duration:
....

(Goal: 30 sec each side)

Level:

5. Lying Hip Extension

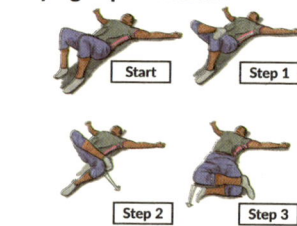

Start
Step 1
Step 2
Step 3

Duration:
....

(Goal: 30 sec each side)

6. Pigeon Stretch

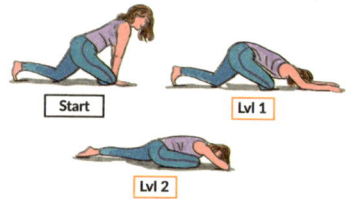

Start
Lvl 1
Lvl 2

Duration:
....

(Goal: 30 sec each side)

Level:

7. Seated Forward Fold Hamstring Stretch

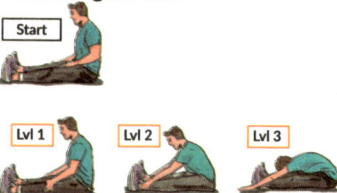

Start
Lvl 1
Lvl 2
Lvl 3

Duration:
....

(Goal: 30 sec)

Level:

8. Lateral Squat

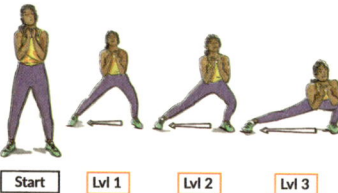

Start
Lvl 1
Lvl 2
Lvl 3

Duration:
....

(Goal: 30 sec each side)

Level:

9. Lateral Squat w/ Toe Raise

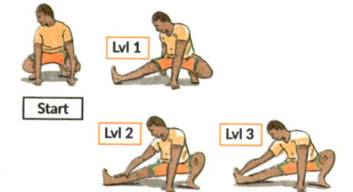

Start
Lvl 1
Lvl 2
Lvl 3

Duration:
....

(Goal: 30 sec each side)

Level:

10. Wig-Wag

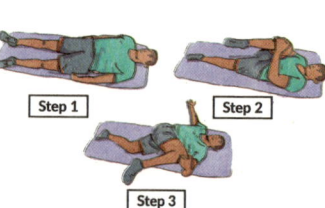

Step 1
Step 2
Step 3

Duration:
....

(Goal: 30 sec each side)

11. Standing Quad Stretch

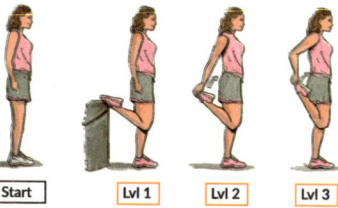

Start
Lvl 1
Lvl 2
Lvl 3

Duration:
....

(Goal: 30 sec each side)

Level:

12. Standing Wall Calf Stretch

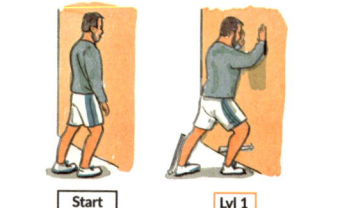

Start
Lvl 1

Duration:
....

(Goal: 15 sec each side)

Daily Reflection

Benefits I'm Experiencing:

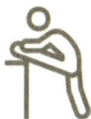

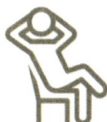

Feel Lighter	More Freedom of Movement	Improved Mental Clarity
Less Pain	Less Stressed	Improved Posture

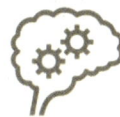

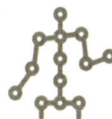

Notes On My Body:

....

....

....

....

....

....

....

....

....

Day 26: Dynamic Warm-Up

Full Session Exercise Guide:
habitnest.com/pages/stretching-day-26

1. World's Greatest Stretch

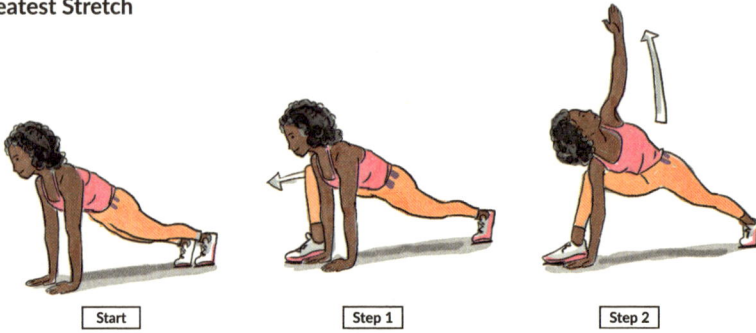

Start   Step 1   Step 2

Reps: *(Goal: 10-15 each side)*

2. High Knees

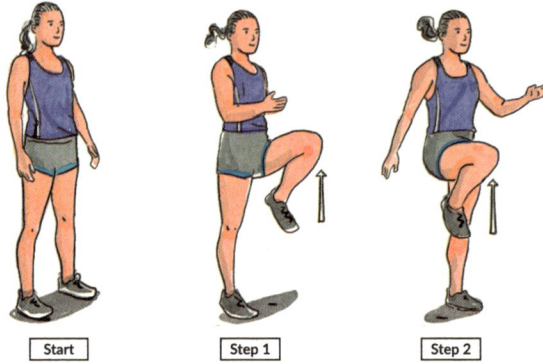

Start   Step 1   Step 2

Reps: *(Goal: 10-15 each side)*

3. Aquaman

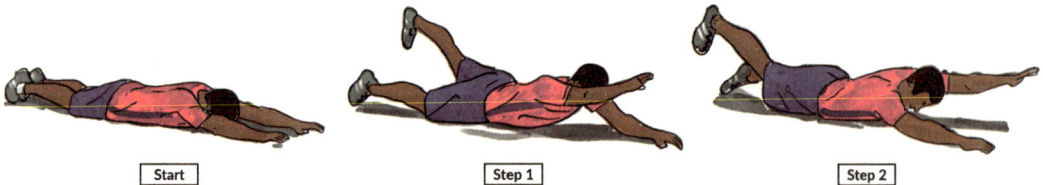

Start   Step 1   Step 2

Reps: *(Goal: 10-15)*

Day 26: Upper Body

1. Up & Down Neck Tilt

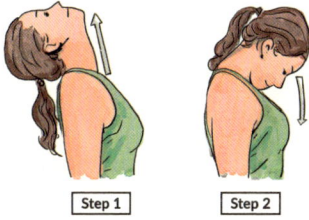

Step 1   Step 2

Duration:
....

(Goal: 30 sec, alternating)

2. Side Neck Tilt

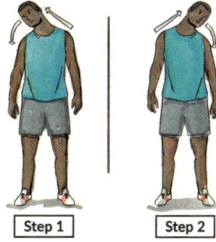

Step 1   Step 2

Duration:
....

(Goal: 15 sec each side)

3. Forward & Backward Neck Tilt

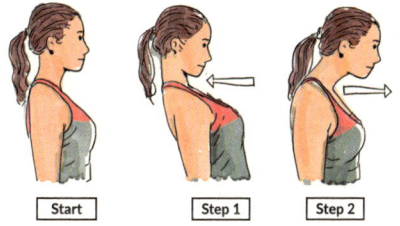

Start   Step 1   Step 2

Duration:
....

(Goal: 30 sec, alternating)

4. Child's Pose

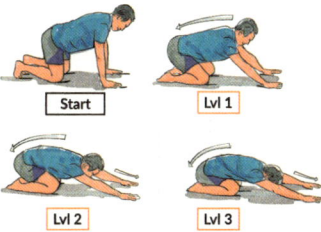

Start   Lvl 1
Lvl 2   Lvl 3

Duration:
....

(Goal: 60 sec)   Level:

5. Cat-Cow

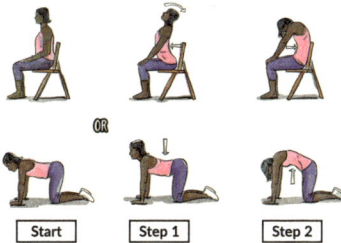

OR

Start   Step 1   Step 2

Duration:
....

(Goal: 30 sec, alternating)

6. Sphinx/Cobra

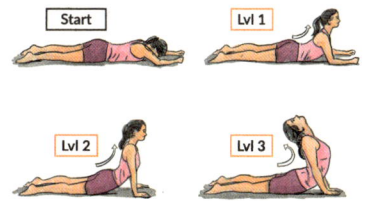

Start   Lvl 1
Lvl 2   Lvl 3

Duration:
....

(Goal: 30 sec)   Level:

7. Cross Arm Shoulder Stretch

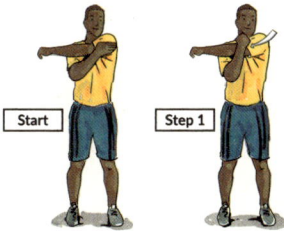

Start   Step 1

Duration:
....
(Goal: 15 sec each side)

8. Open Book Chest Stretch

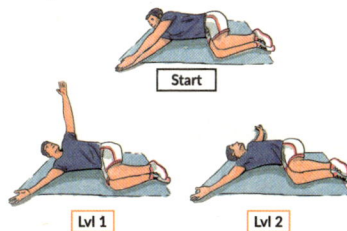

Start

Lvl 1   Lvl 2

Level:

Duration:
....
(Goal: 30 sec each side)

9. Standing Oblique Stretch

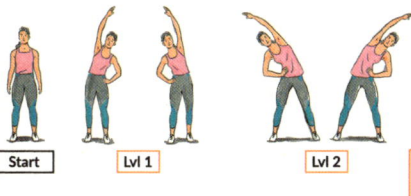

Start   Lvl 1   Lvl 2

Level:

Duration:
....
(Goal: 15 sec each side)

10. Surface Tricep Stretch

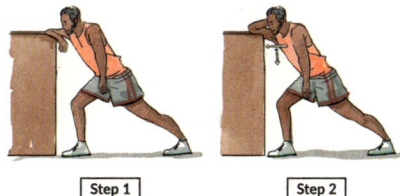

Step 1   Step 2

Duration:
....
(Goal: 15 sec each side)

Day 26: Lower Body

1. Frog Pose

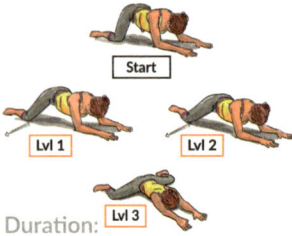

Duration:

(Goal: 60 sec)

Level:

2. Runner's Lunge

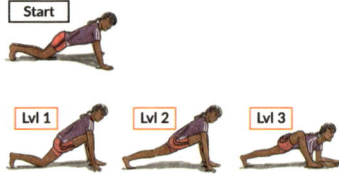

Duration:

(Goal: 30 sec each side)

Level:

3. Butterfly

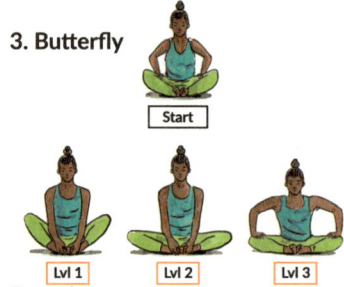

Duration:

(Goal: 30 sec)

Level:

4. Scorpion Pose

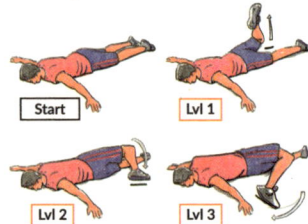

Duration:

(Goal: 30 sec each side)

Level:

5. Lying Hip Extension

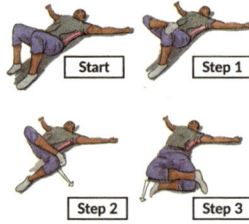

Duration:

(Goal: 30 sec each side)

6. Pigeon Stretch

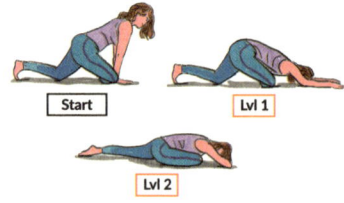

Duration:

(Goal: 30 sec each side)

Level:

7. Seated Forward Fold Hamstring Stretch

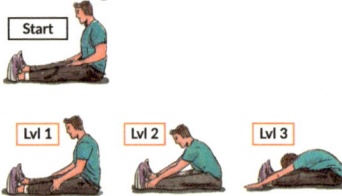

Duration:

(Goal: 30 sec)

Level:

8. Lateral Squat

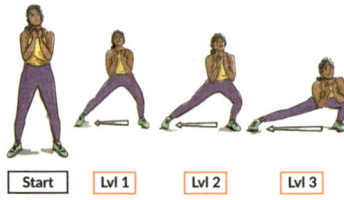

Duration:

(Goal: 30 sec each side)

Level:

9. Lateral Squat w/ Toe Raise

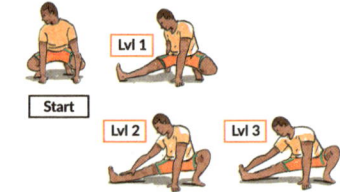

Duration:

(Goal: 30 sec each side)

Level:

10. Wig-Wag

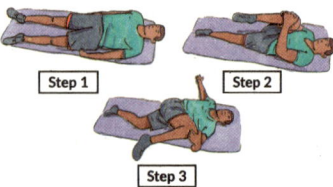

Duration:

(Goal: 30 sec each side)

11. Standing Quad Stretch

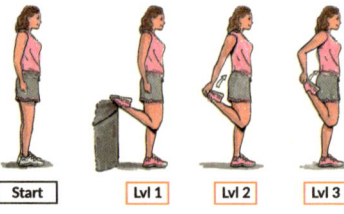

Duration:

(Goal: 30 sec each side)

Level:

12. Standing Wall Calf Stretch

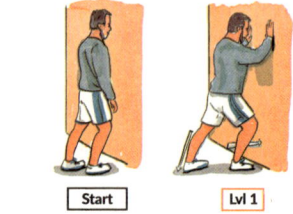

Duration:

(Goal: 15 sec each side)

Daily Reflection

Benefits I'm Experiencing:

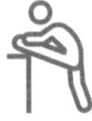

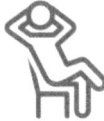

Feel Lighter	More Freedom of Movement	Improved Mental Clarity
Less Pain	Less Stressed	Improved Posture

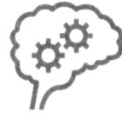

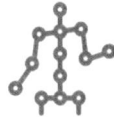

Notes On My Body:

....

....

....

....

....

....

....

....

Day 27: Dynamic Warm-Up

Full Session Exercise Guide:
habitnest.com/pages/stretching-day-27

1. Bird-Dog

| Start | Step 1 | Step 2 | Step 3 |

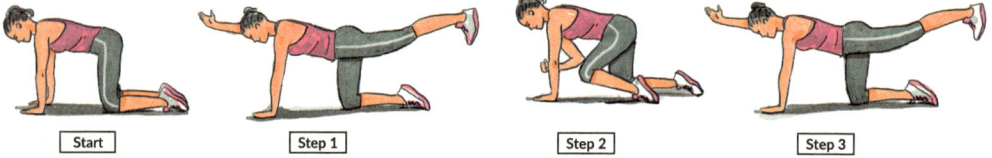

Reps: *(Goal: 10-15 each side)*

2. Good Morning

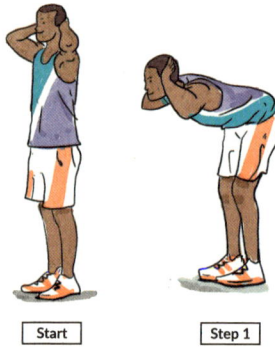

| Start | Step 1 |

Reps: *(Goal: 20-30 each side)*

3. Roundhouse Kick to Squat

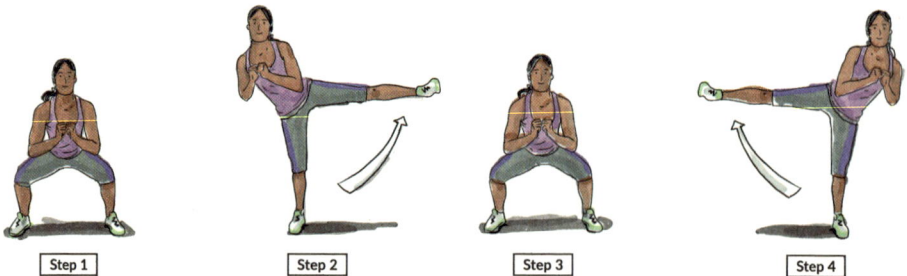

| Step 1 | Step 2 | Step 3 | Step 4 |

Reps: *(Goal: 10-15 each side)*

Day 27: Upper Body

DATE

1. Up & Down Neck Tilt

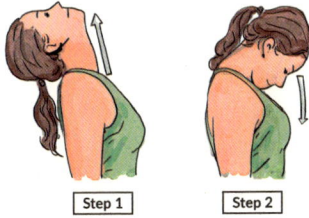

Step 1   Step 2

Duration:
....

(Goal: 30 sec, alternating)

2. Side Neck Tilt

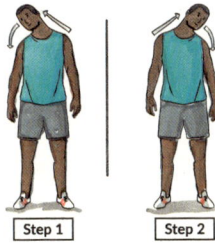

Step 1   Step 2

Duration:
....

(Goal: 15 sec each side)

3. Forward & Backward Neck Tilt

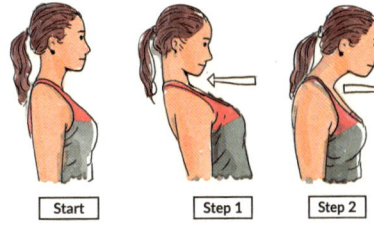

Start   Step 1   Step 2

Duration:
....

(Goal: 30 sec, alternating)

4. Child's Pose

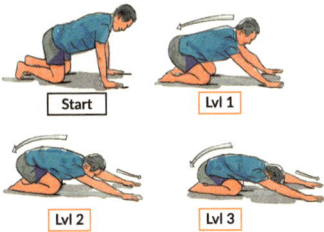

Start   Lvl 1
Lvl 2   Lvl 3

Duration:
....

(Goal: 60 sec)   Level:

5. Cat-Cow

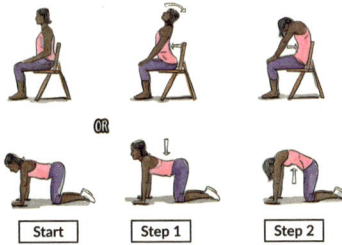

OR

Start   Step 1   Step 2

Duration:
....

(Goal: 30 sec, alternating)

6. Sphinx/Cobra

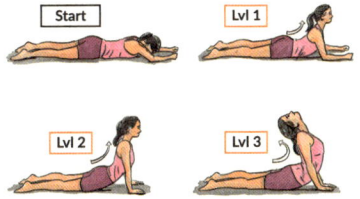

Start   Lvl 1
Lvl 2   Lvl 3

Duration:
....

(Goal: 30 sec)   Level:

7. Cross Arm Shoulder Stretch

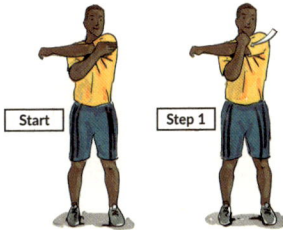

Start   Step 1

Duration:
....

(Goal: 15 sec each side)

8. Open Book Chest Stretch

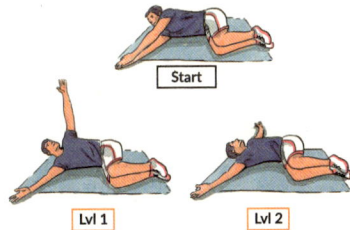

Start

Lvl 1   Lvl 2

Level:

Duration:
....

(Goal: 30 sec each side)

9. Standing Oblique Stretch

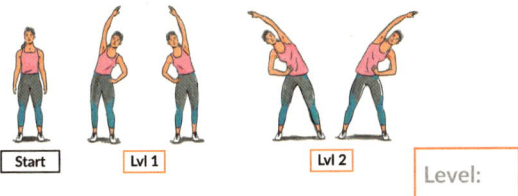

Start   Lvl 1   Lvl 2

Level:

Duration:
....

(Goal: 15 sec each side)

10. Surface Tricep Stretch

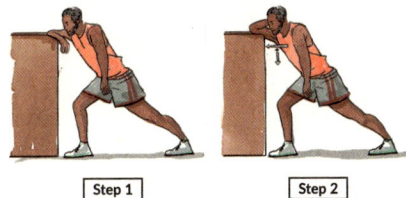

Step 1   Step 2

Duration:
....

(Goal: 15 sec each side)

Day 27: Lower Body

1. Frog Pose

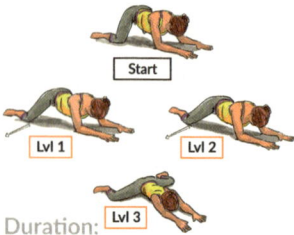

Start

Lvl 1   Lvl 2

Lvl 3

Duration:

(Goal: 60 sec)

Level:

2. Runner's Lunge

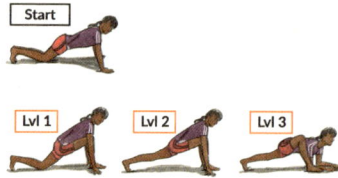

Start

Lvl 1   Lvl 2   Lvl 3

Duration:

(Goal: 30 sec each side)

Level:

3. Butterfly

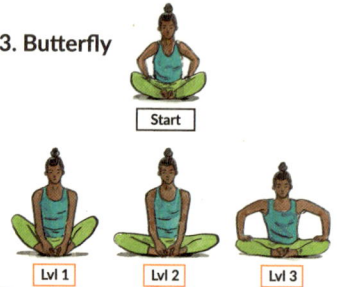

Start

Lvl 1   Lvl 2   Lvl 3

Duration:

(Goal: 30 sec)

Level:

4. Scorpion Pose

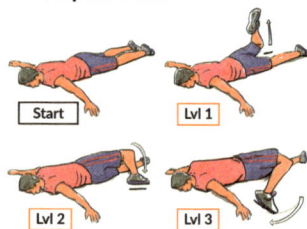

Start   Lvl 1

Lvl 2   Lvl 3

Duration:

(Goal: 30 sec each side)

Level:

5. Lying Hip Extension

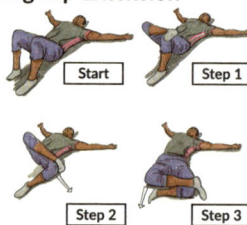

Start   Step 1

Step 2   Step 3

Duration:

(Goal: 30 sec each side)

6. Pigeon Stretch

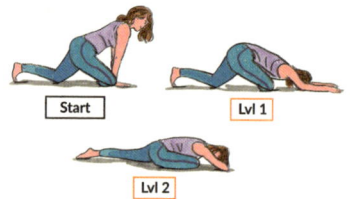

Start   Lvl 1

Lvl 2

Duration:

(Goal: 30 sec each side)

Level:

7. Seated Forward Fold Hamstring Stretch

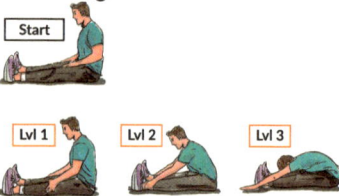

Start

Lvl 1   Lvl 2   Lvl 3

Duration:

(Goal: 30 sec)

Level:

8. Lateral Squat

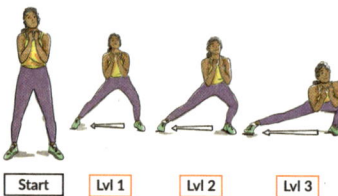

Start   Lvl 1   Lvl 2   Lvl 3

Duration:

(Goal: 30 sec each side)

Level:

9. Lateral Squat w/ Toe Raise

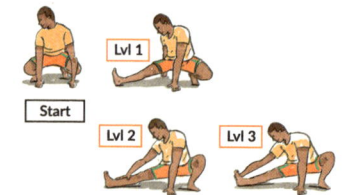

Lvl 1

Start

Lvl 2   Lvl 3

Duration:

(Goal: 30 sec each side)

Level:

10. Wig-Wag

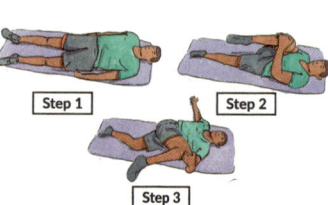

Step 1   Step 2

Step 3

Duration:

(Goal: 30 sec each side)

11. Standing Quad Stretch

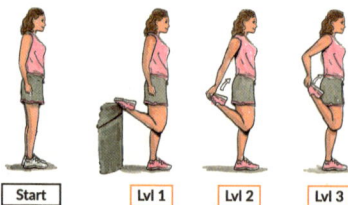

Start   Lvl 1   Lvl 2   Lvl 3

Duration:

(Goal: 30 sec each side)

Level:

12. Standing Wall Calf Stretch

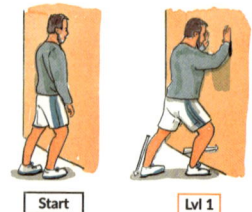

Start   Lvl 1

Duration:

(Goal: 15 sec each side)

Daily Reflection

Benefits I'm Experiencing:

Feel
Lighter

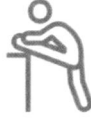

More Freedom
of Movement

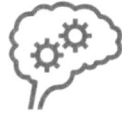

Improved
Mental Clarity

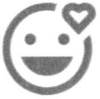

Less
Pain

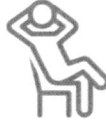

Less
Stressed

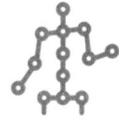

Improved
Posture

Notes On My Body:

Day 28: Dynamic Warm-Up

Full Session Exercise Guide:
habitnest.com/pages/stretching-day-28

1. Side Plank w/ Twist

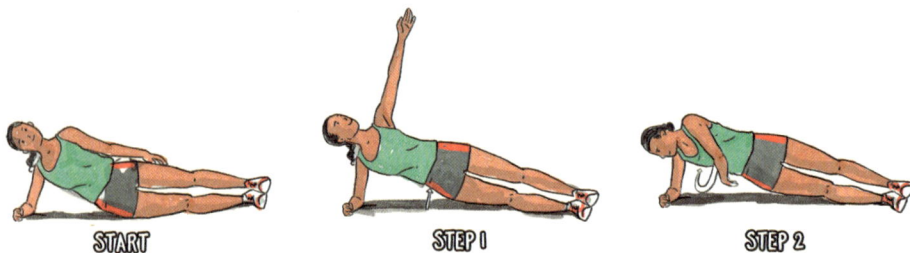

START — STEP 1 — STEP 2

Reps: .... *(Goal: 10-15 each side)*

2. Push-Up

Lvl 1

Lvl 2

Level:

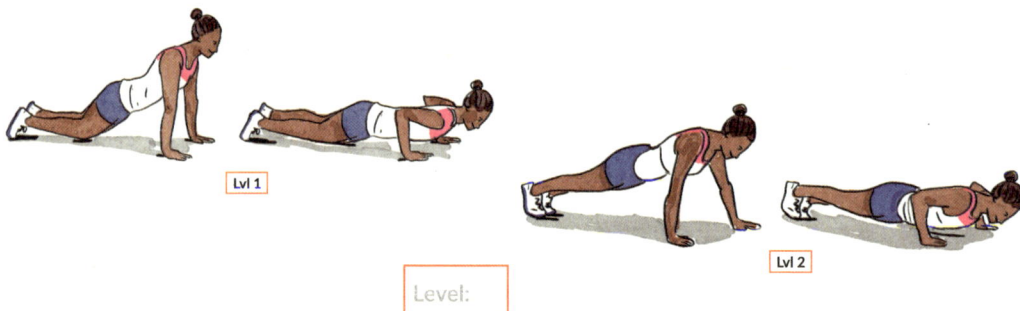

Reps: .... *(Goal: 15-25)*

3. Standing Hamstring Scoop

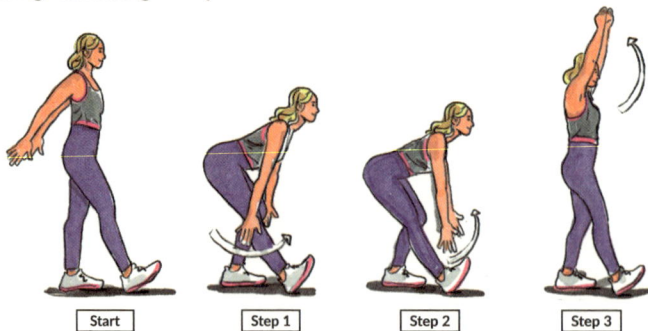

Start — Step 1 — Step 2 — Step 3

Reps: .... *(Goal: 10-15 each side)*

Day 28: Upper Body

1. Up & Down Neck Tilt

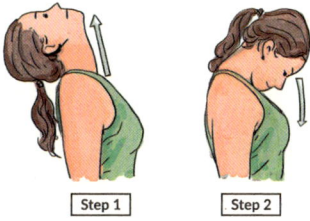

Step 1　　Step 2

Duration:

(Goal: 30 sec, alternating)

2. Side Neck Tilt

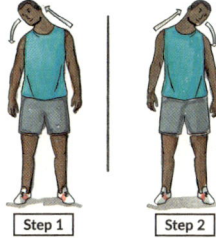

Step 1　　Step 2

Duration:

(Goal: 15 sec each side)

3. Forward & Backward Neck Tilt

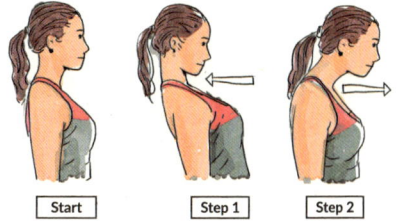

Start　　Step 1　　Step 2

Duration:

(Goal: 30 sec, alternating)

4. Child's Pose

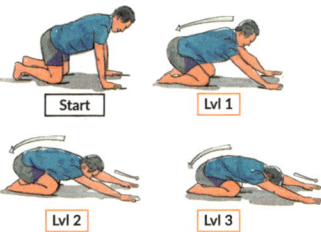

Start　　Lvl 1

Lvl 2　　Lvl 3

Duration:

(Goal: 60 sec)

Level:

5. Cat-Cow

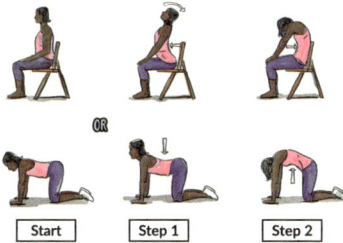

OR

Start　　Step 1　　Step 2

Duration:

(Goal: 30 sec, alternating)

6. Sphinx/Cobra

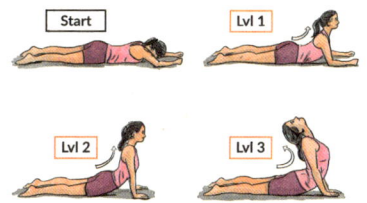

Start　　Lvl 1

Lvl 2　　Lvl 3

Duration:

(Goal: 30 sec)

Level:

7. Cross Arm Shoulder Stretch

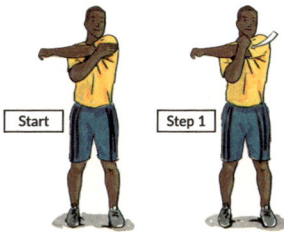

Start　　Step 1

Duration:

(Goal: 15 sec each side)

8. Open Book Chest Stretch

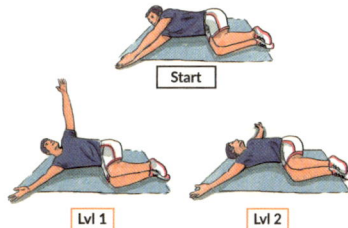

Start

Lvl 1　　Lvl 2

Level:

Duration:

(Goal: 30 sec each side)

9. Standing Oblique Stretch

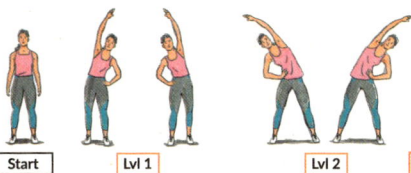

Start　　Lvl 1　　Lvl 2

Level:

Duration:

(Goal: 15 sec each side)

10. Surface Tricep Stretch

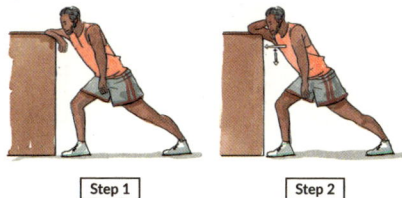

Step 1　　Step 2

Duration:

(Goal: 15 sec each side)

Day 28: Lower Body

1. Frog Pose

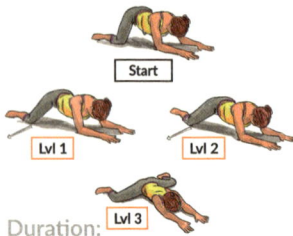

Start

Lvl 1   Lvl 2

Lvl 3

Duration:

(Goal: 60 sec)   Level:

2. Runner's Lunge

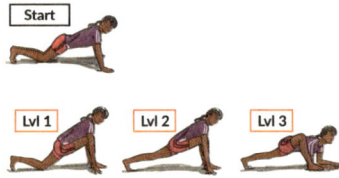

Start

Lvl 1   Lvl 2   Lvl 3

Duration:

(Goal: 30 sec each side)   Level:

3. Butterfly

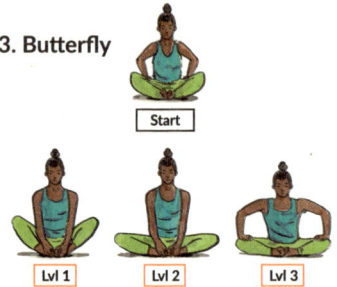

Start

Lvl 1   Lvl 2   Lvl 3

Duration:

(Goal: 30 sec)   Level:

4. Scorpion Pose

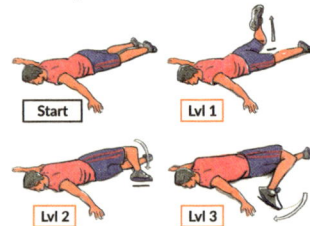

Start   Lvl 1

Lvl 2   Lvl 3

Duration:

(Goal: 30 sec each side)   Level:

5. Lying Hip Extension

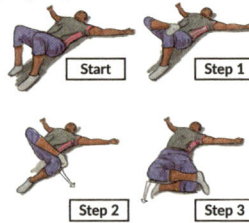

Start   Step 1

Step 2   Step 3

Duration:

(Goal: 30 sec each side)

6. Pigeon Stretch

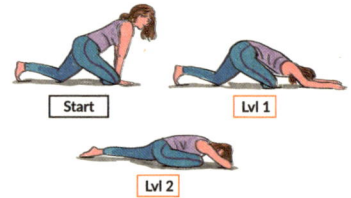

Start   Lvl 1

Lvl 2

Duration:

(Goal: 30 sec each side)   Level:

7. Seated Forward Fold Hamstring Stretch

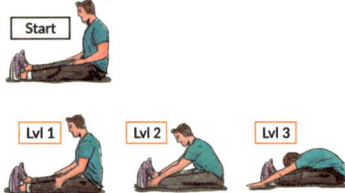

Start

Lvl 1   Lvl 2   Lvl 3

Duration:

(Goal: 30 sec)   Level:

8. Lateral Squat

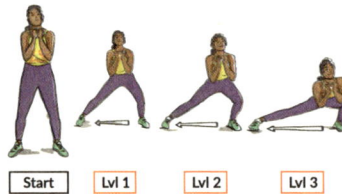

Start   Lvl 1   Lvl 2   Lvl 3

Duration:

(Goal: 30 sec each side)   Level:

9. Lateral Squat w/ Toe Raise

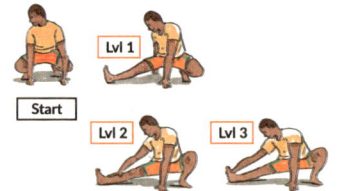

Lvl 1

Start

Lvl 2   Lvl 3

Duration:

(Goal: 30 sec each side)   Level:

10. Wig-Wag

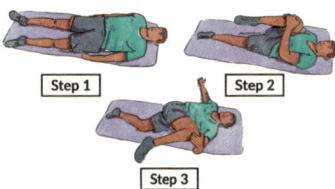

Step 1   Step 2

Step 3

Duration:

(Goal: 30 sec each side)

11. Standing Quad Stretch

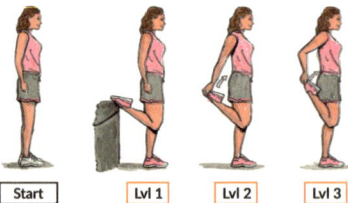

Start   Lvl 1   Lvl 2   Lvl 3

Duration:

(Goal: 30 sec each side)   Level:

12. Standing Wall Calf Stretch

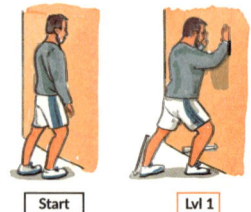

Start   Lvl 1

Duration:

(Goal: 15 sec each side)

Daily Reflection

Benefits I'm Experiencing:

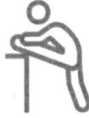

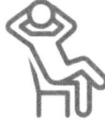

Feel Lighter	More Freedom of Movement	Improved Mental Clarity
Less Pain	Less Stressed	Improved Posture

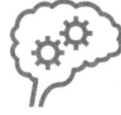

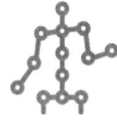

Notes On My Body:

....

....

....

....

....

....

....

....

Day 29: Dynamic Warm-Up

Full Session Exercise Guide:
habitnest.com/pages/stretching-day-29

1. Pike Push-Up

Lvl 1

Lvl 2

Level:

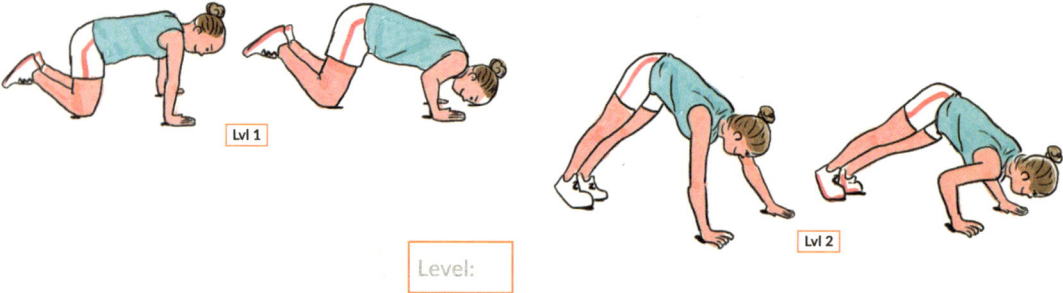

Reps: *(Goal: 15-25)*

2. World's Greatest Stretch

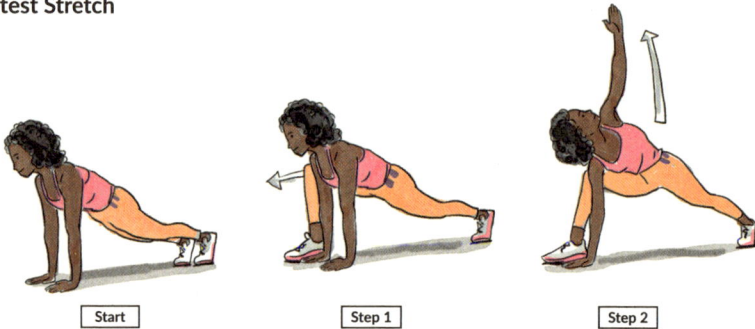

Start

Step 1

Step 2

Reps: *(Goal: 10-15 each side)*

3. Standing Hip Circles

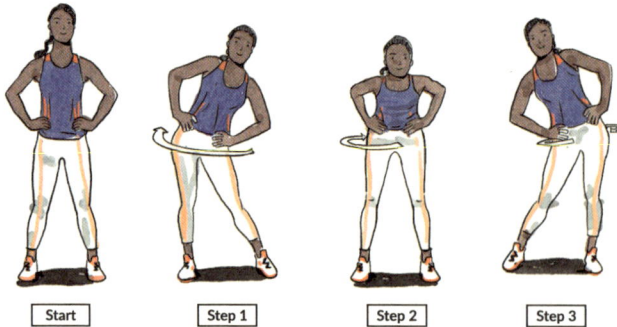

Start

Step 1

Step 2

Step 3

Reps: *(Goal: 10-15 in each direction)*

162

Day 29: Upper Body

1. Lateral Side to Side Neck Rotation

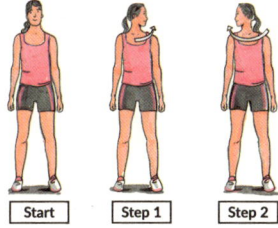

Start Step 1 Step 2

Duration:

(Goal: 30 sec, alternating)

2. Side Neck Stretch w/ Upside Down Palm on Wall

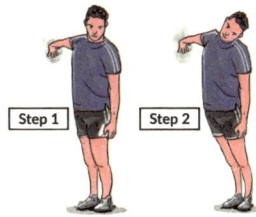

Step 1 Step 2

Duration:

(Goal: 15 sec each side)

3. Levator Scap Neck Stretch

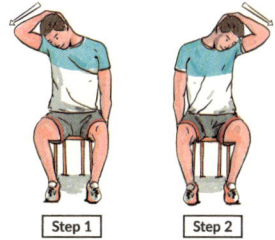

Step 1 Step 2

Duration:

(Goal: 15 sec each side)

4. Seated Forward Curl

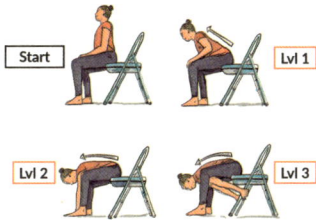

Start Lvl 1 Lvl 2 Lvl 3

Duration:

(Goal: 30 sec)

Level:

5. Seated Spinal Twist

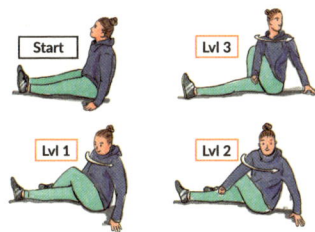

Start Lvl 3 Lvl 1 Lvl 2

Duration:

(Goal: 15 sec each side)

Level:

6. Wall Lat Stretch

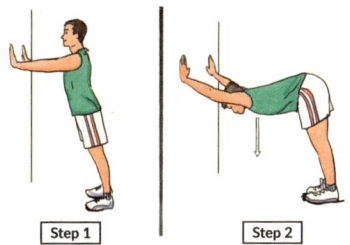

Step 1 Step 2

Duration:

(Goal: 15 sec each side)

7. Corner Chest Stretch

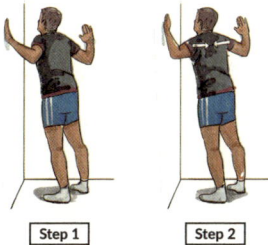

Step 1 Step 2

Duration:

(Goal: 30 sec)

8. Thread the Needle Shoulder Stretch

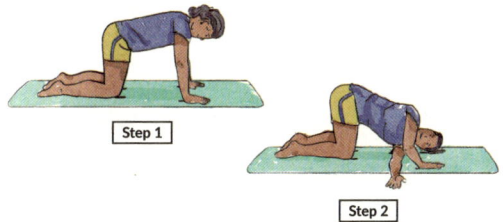

Step 1 Step 2

Duration:

(Goal: 15 sec each side)

9. Behind the Back Tricep Extension

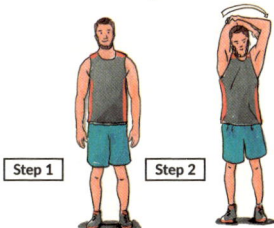

Step 1 Step 2

Duration:

(Goal: 15 sec each side)

10. Lying Full Body Extension

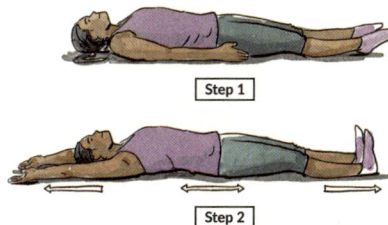

Step 1 Step 2

Duration:

(Goal: 30 sec)

Day 29: Lower Body

1. Warrior II Pose

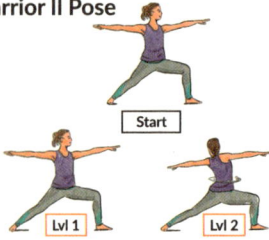

Duration:

(Goal: 30 sec each side) Level:

2. Reverse Tabletop

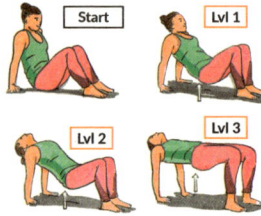

Duration:

(Goal: 30 sec) Level:

3. Reclining Angle Bound Pose

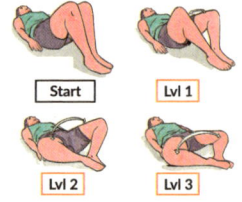

Duration:

(Goal: 30 sec) Level:

4. Pry Squat

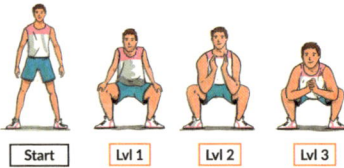

Duration:

(Goal: 30 sec) Level:

5. Frog Pose

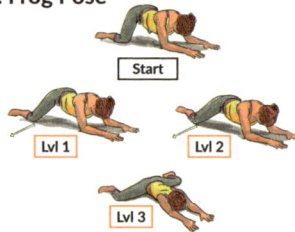

Duration:

(Goal: 60 sec) Level:

6. Figure 4

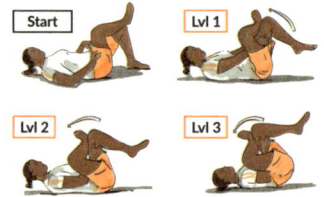

Duration:

(Goal: 30 sec each side) Level:

7. Downward Dog

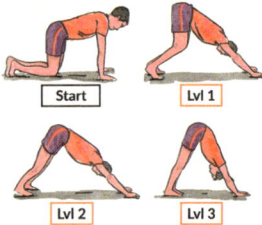

Duration:

(Goal: 30 sec) Level:

8. Seated Single Leg Hamstring Stretch

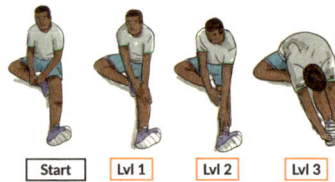

Duration:

(Goal: 30 sec each side) Level:

9. Knee to Chest Stretch

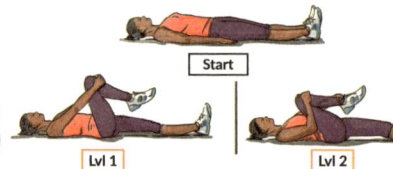

Duration:

(Goal: 30 sec each side) Level:

10. Extended Triangle Pose

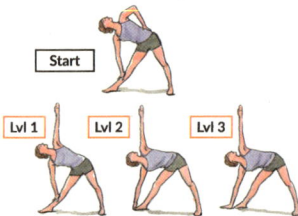

Duration:

(Goal: 30 sec each side) Level:

11. Kneeling Quad Stretch

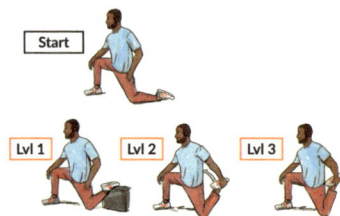

Duration:

(Goal: 30 sec each side) Level:

12. Hanging Calf Stretch

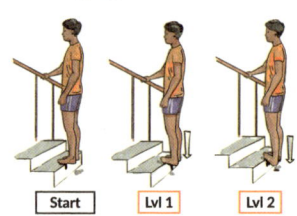

Duration:

(Goal: 30 sec) Level:

Daily Reflection

Benefits I'm Experiencing:

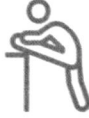

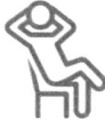

Feel Lighter	More Freedom of Movement	Improved Mental Clarity
Less Pain	Less Stressed	Improved Posture

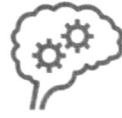

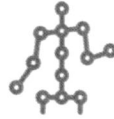

Notes On My Body:

_____

_____

_____

_____

_____

_____

_____

_____

_____

Day 30: Dynamic Warm-Up

Full Session Exercise Guide:
habitnest.com/pages/stretching-day-30

1. Inch Worm Walk Out

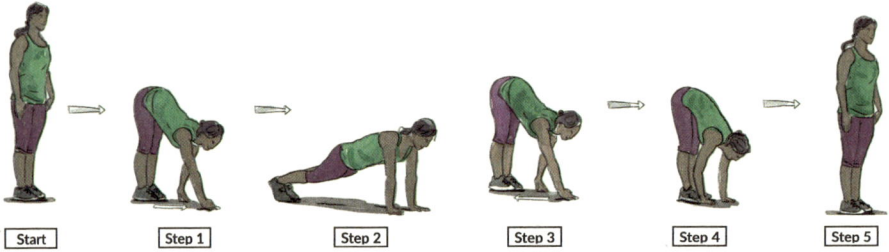

| Start | Step 1 | Step 2 | Step 3 | Step 4 | Step 5 |

Reps: .... *(Goal: 10-20)*

2. Bird-Dog

| Start | Step 1 | Step 2 | Step 3 |

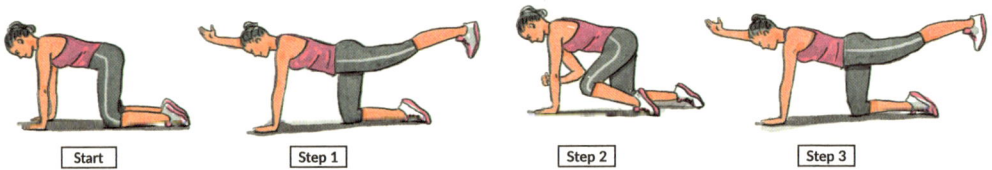

Reps: .... *(Goal: 10-15 each side)*

3. Glute Bridge

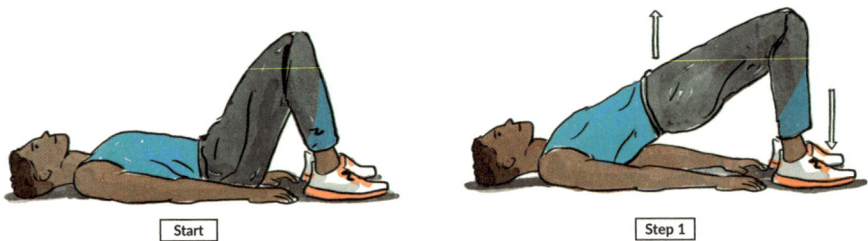

| Start | Step 1 |

Reps: .... *(Goal: 25-35)*

Day 30: Upper Body

DATE

1. Lateral Side to Side Neck Rotation

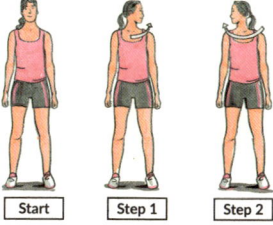

Start | Step 1 | Step 2

Duration:

(Goal: 30 sec, alternating)

2. Side Neck Stretch w/ Upside Down Palm on Wall

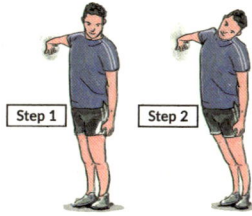

Step 1 | Step 2

Duration:

(Goal: 15 sec each side)

3. Levator Scap Neck Stretch

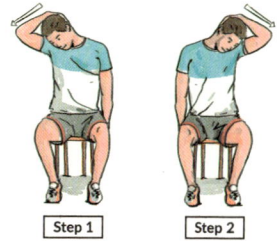

Step 1 | Step 2

Duration:

(Goal: 15 sec each side)

4. Seated Forward Curl

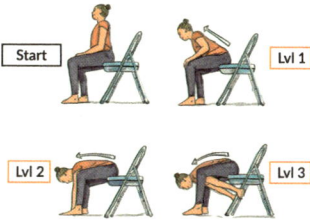

Start | Lvl 1 | Lvl 2 | Lvl 3

Duration:

(Goal: 30 sec)

Level:

5. Seated Spinal Twist

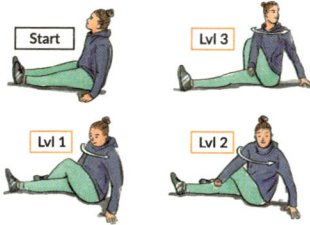

Start | Lvl 3 | Lvl 1 | Lvl 2

Duration:

(Goal: 15 sec each side)

Level:

6. Wall Lat Stretch

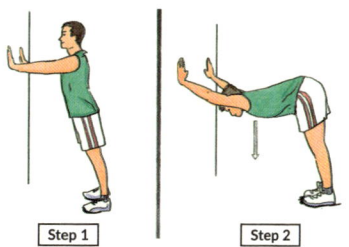

Step 1 | Step 2

Duration:

(Goal: 15 sec each side)

7. Corner Chest Stretch

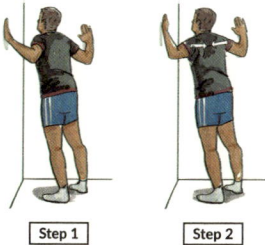

Step 1 | Step 2

Duration:

(Goal: 30 sec)

8. Thread the Needle Shoulder Stretch

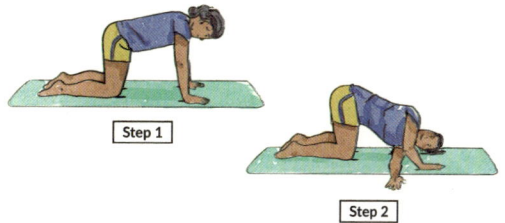

Step 1 | Step 2

Duration:

(Goal: 15 sec each side)

9. Behind the Back Tricep Extension

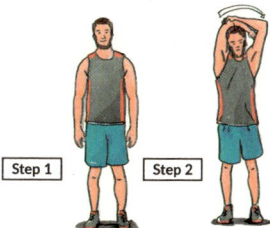

Step 1 | Step 2

Duration:

(Goal: 15 sec each side)

10. Lying Full Body Extension

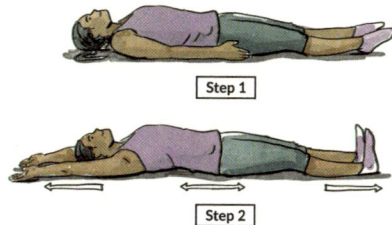

Step 1 | Step 2

Duration:

(Goal: 30 sec)

Day 30: Lower Body

1. Warrior II Pose

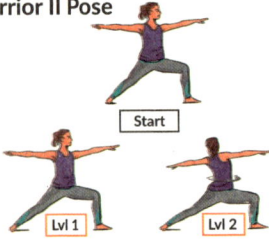

Duration: ....

(Goal: 30 sec each side) Level:

2. Reverse Tabletop

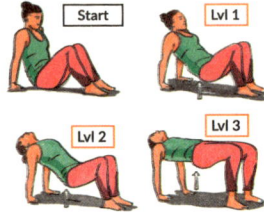

Duration: ....

(Goal: 30 sec) Level:

3. Reclining Angle Bound Pose

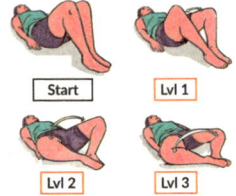

Duration: ....

(Goal: 30 sec) Level:

4. Pry Squat

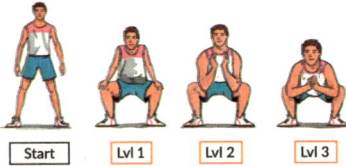

Duration: ....

(Goal: 30 sec) Level:

5. Frog Pose

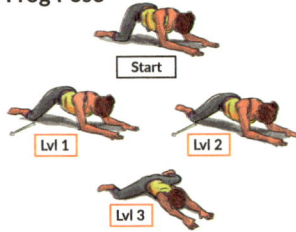

Duration: ....

(Goal: 60 sec) Level:

6. Figure 4

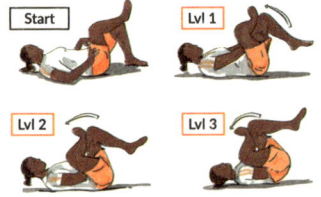

Duration: ....

(Goal: 30 sec each side) Level:

7. Downward Dog

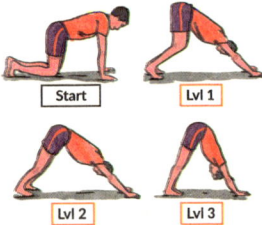

Duration: ....

(Goal: 30 sec) Level:

8. Seated Single Leg Hamstring Stretch

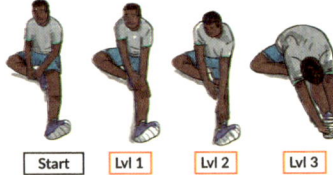

Duration: ....

(Goal: 30 sec each side) Level:

9. Knee to Chest Stretch

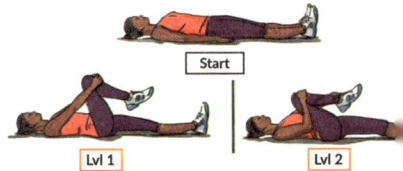

Duration: ....

(Goal: 30 sec each side) Level:

10. Extended Triangle Pose

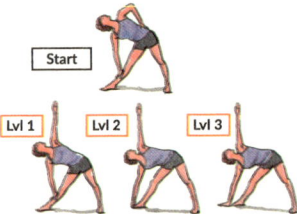

Duration: ....

(Goal: 30 sec each side) Level:

11. Kneeling Quad Stretch

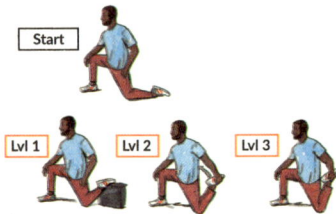

Duration: ....

(Goal: 30 sec each side) Level:

12. Hanging Calf Stretch

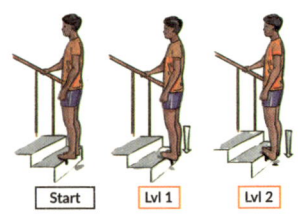

Duration: ....

(Goal: 30 sec) Level:

Daily Reflection

Benefits I'm Experiencing:

Feel
Lighter

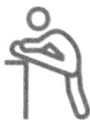

More Freedom
of Movement

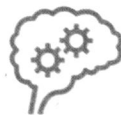

Improved
Mental Clarity

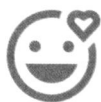

Less
Pain

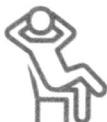

Less
Stressed

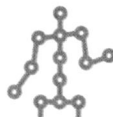

Improved
Posture

Notes On My Body:

Day 31: Dynamic Warm-Up

Full Session Exercise Guide:
habitnest.com/pages/stretching-day-31

1. Y Raise

Step 1

Step 2

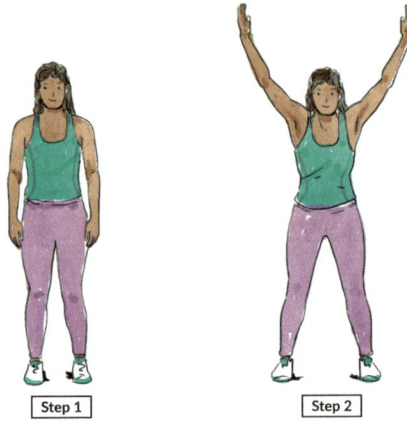

Reps: *(Goal: 15-25)*

2. Bird-Dog

Start   Step 1   Step 2   Step 3

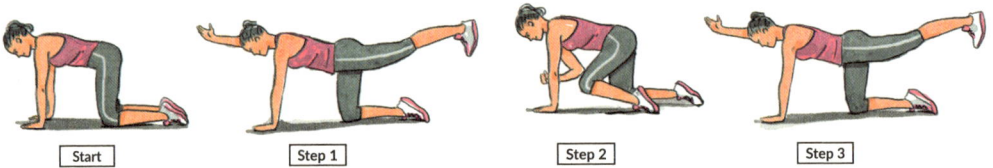

Reps: *(Goal: 10-15 each side)*

3. Air Squat to Calf Raise

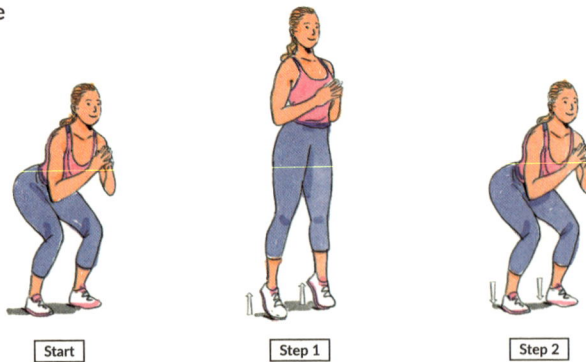

Start   Step 1   Step 2

Reps: *(Goal: 15-25)*

Day 31: Upper Body

1. Lateral Side to Side Neck Rotation

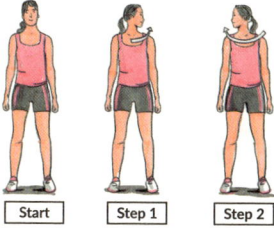

Start   Step 1   Step 2

Duration:

(Goal: 30 sec, alternating)

2. Side Neck Stretch w/ Upside Down Palm on Wall

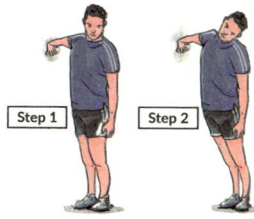

Step 1   Step 2

Duration:

(Goal: 15 sec each side)

3. Levator Scap Neck Stretch

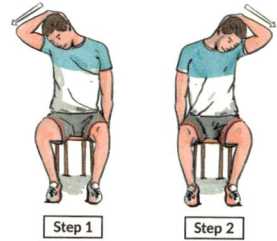

Step 1   Step 2

Duration:

(Goal: 15 sec each side)

4. Seated Forward Curl

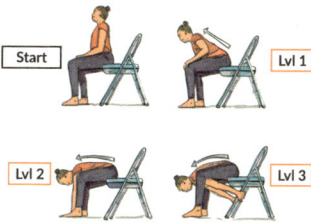

Start   Lvl 1

Lvl 2   Lvl 3

Duration:

(Goal: 30 sec)   Level:

5. Seated Spinal Twist

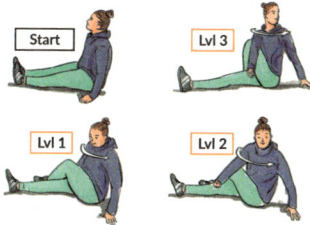

Start   Lvl 3

Lvl 1   Lvl 2

Duration:

(Goal: 15 sec each side)   Level:

6. Wall Lat Stretch

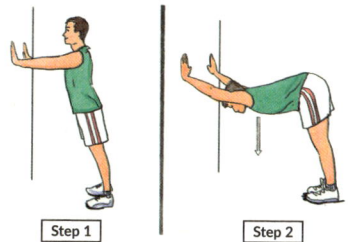

Step 1   Step 2

Duration:

(Goal: 15 sec each side)

7. Corner Chest Stretch

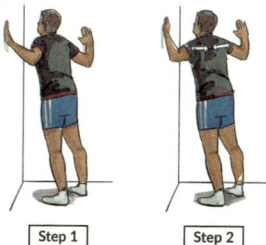

Step 1   Step 2

Duration:

(Goal: 30 sec)

8. Thread the Needle Shoulder Stretch

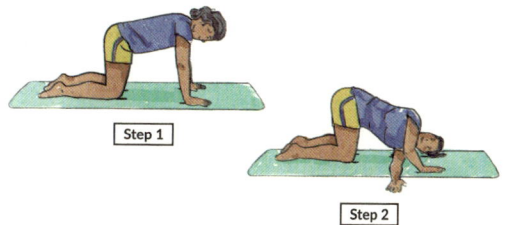

Step 1

Step 2

Duration:

(Goal: 15 sec each side)

9. Behind the Back Tricep Extension

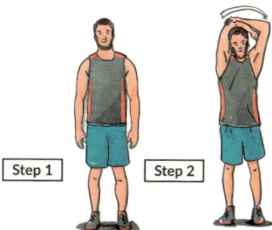

Step 1   Step 2

Duration:

(Goal: 15 sec each side)

10. Lying Full Body Extension

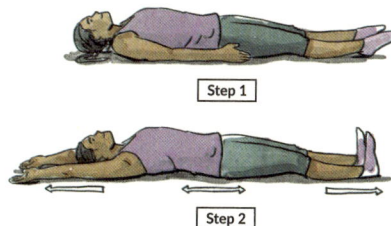

Step 1

Step 2

Duration:

(Goal: 30 sec)

Day 31: Lower Body

1. Warrior II Pose

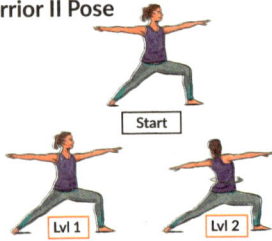

Duration:

(Goal: 30 sec each side)

Level:

2. Reverse Tabletop

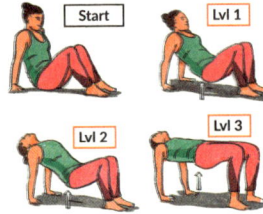

Duration:

(Goal: 30 sec)

Level:

3. Reclining Angle Bound Pose

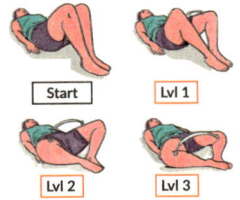

Duration:

(Goal: 30 sec)

Level:

4. Pry Squat

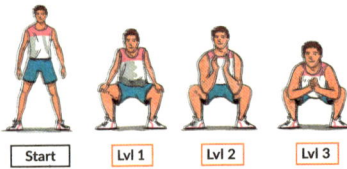

Duration:

(Goal: 30 sec)

Level:

5. Frog Pose

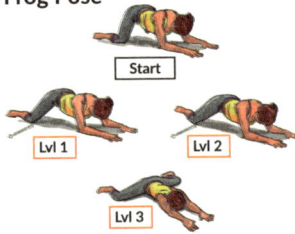

Duration:

(Goal: 60 sec)

Level:

6. Figure 4

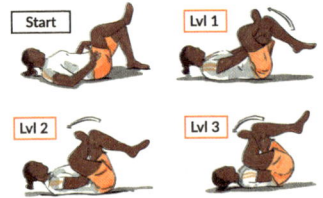

Duration:

(Goal: 30 sec each side)

Level:

7. Downward Dog

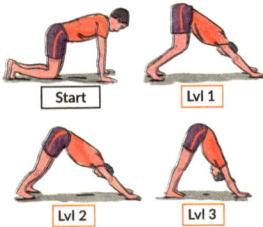

Duration:

(Goal: 30 sec)

Level:

8. Seated Single Leg Hamstring Stretch

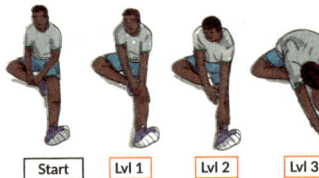

Duration:

(Goal: 30 sec each side)

Level:

9. Knee to Chest Stretch

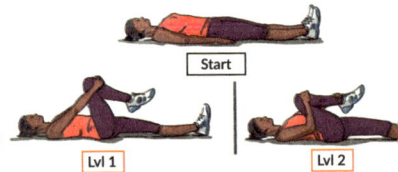

Duration:

(Goal: 30 sec each side)

Level:

10. Extended Triangle Pose

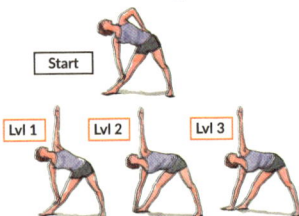

Duration:

(Goal: 30 sec each side)

Level:

11. Kneeling Quad Stretch

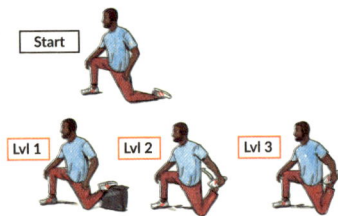

Duration:

(Goal: 30 sec each side)

Level:

12. Hanging Calf Stretch

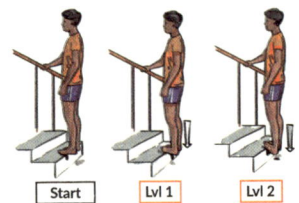

Duration:

(Goal: 30 sec)

Level:

Daily Reflection

Benefits I'm Experiencing:

Feel
Lighter

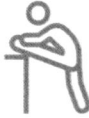

More Freedom
of Movement

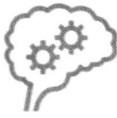

Improved
Mental Clarity

Less
Pain

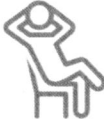

Less
Stressed

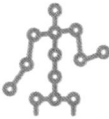

Improved
Posture

Notes On My Body:

Day 32: Dynamic Warm-Up

Full Session Exercise Guide:
habitnest.com/pages/stretching-day-32

1. Inch Worm Walk Out

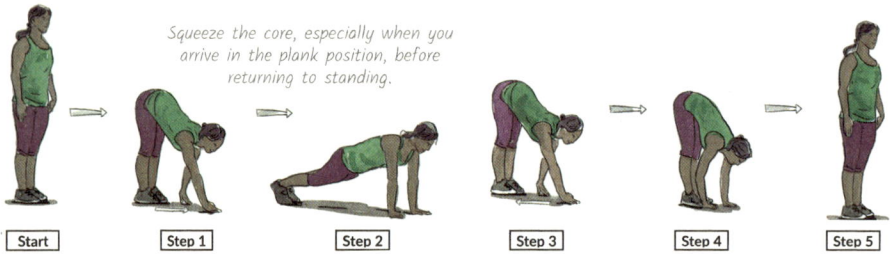

Squeeze the core, especially when you arrive in the plank position, before returning to standing.

Start → Step 1 → Step 2 Step 3 → Step 4 → Step 5

Reps: _____ *(Goal: 10-20)*

2. Clam Opener w/ Side Plank

Nothing wrong with taking a rest as you're completing your repetitions for each side!

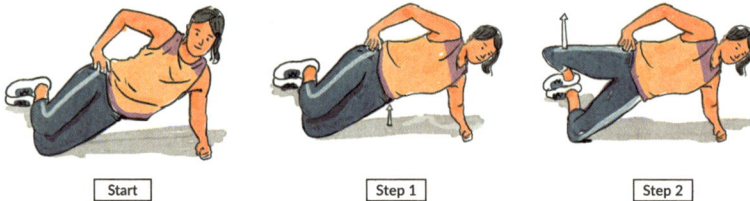

Start Step 1 Step 2

Reps: _____ *(Goal: 10-15 each side)*

3. Low Lunge w/ Elbow Twist

Here, you'll feel the stretch in the hip/groin area on your straight leg, and in your back on the same side. It feels good, so you can pause for a moment when you're reaching your elbow down!

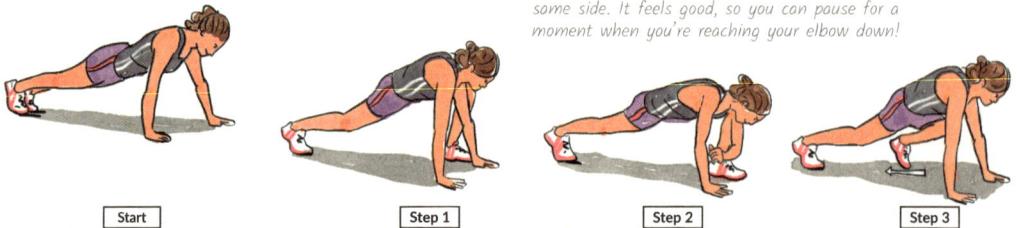

Start Step 1 Step 2 Step 3

Reps: _____ *(Goal: 10-15 each side)*

Day 32: Upper Body

1. Lateral Side to Side Neck Rotation

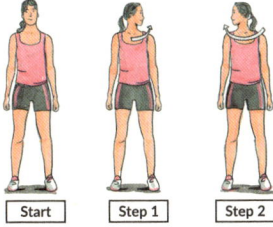

Start   Step 1   Step 2

Duration:

(Goal: 30 sec, alternating)

2. Side Neck Stretch w/ Upside Down Palm on Wall

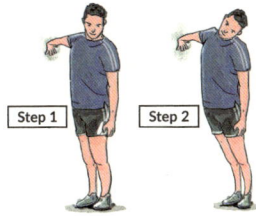

Step 1   Step 2

Duration:

(Goal: 15 sec each side)

3. Levator Scap Neck Stretch

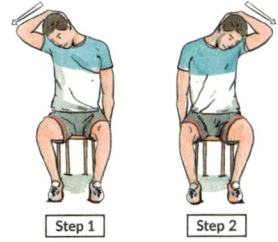

Step 1   Step 2

Duration:

(Goal: 15 sec each side)

4. Seated Forward Curl

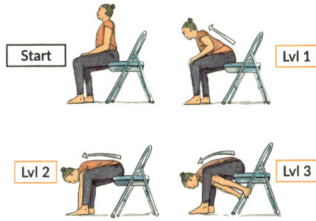

Start   Lvl 1
Lvl 2   Lvl 3

Duration:

(Goal: 30 sec)   Level:

5. Seated Spinal Twist

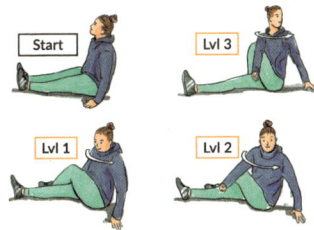

Start   Lvl 3
Lvl 1   Lvl 2

Duration:

(Goal: 15 sec each side)   Level:

6. Wall Lat Stretch

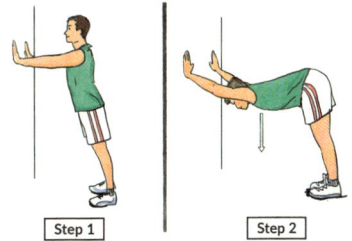

Step 1   Step 2

Duration:

(Goal: 15 sec each side)

7. Corner Chest Stretch

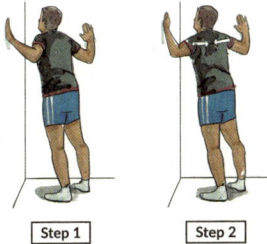

Step 1   Step 2

Duration:

(Goal: 30 sec)

8. Thread the Needle Shoulder Stretch

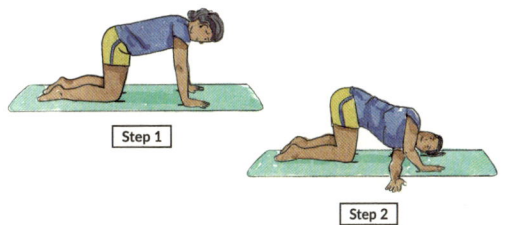

Step 1   Step 2

Duration:

(Goal: 15 sec each side)

9. Behind the Back Tricep Extension

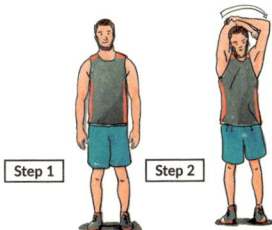

Step 1   Step 2

Duration:

(Goal: 15 sec each side)

10. Lying Full Body Extension

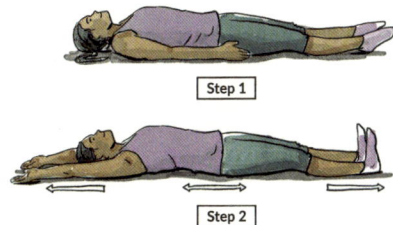

Step 1   Step 2

Duration:

(Goal: 30 sec)

Day 32: Lower Body

1. Warrior II Pose

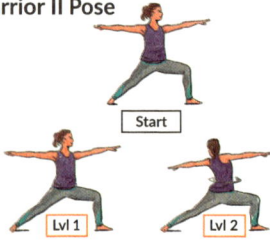

Duration:
....

(Goal: 30 sec each side) | Level:

2. Reverse Tabletop

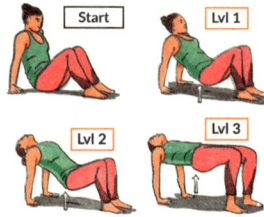

Duration:
....

(Goal: 30 sec) | Level:

3. Reclining Angle Bound Pose

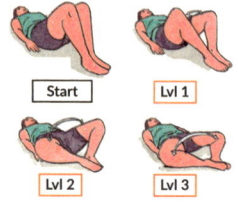

Duration:
....

(Goal: 30 sec) | Level:

4. Pry Squat

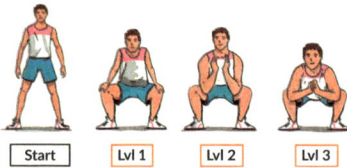

Duration:
....

(Goal: 30 sec) | Level:

5. Frog Pose

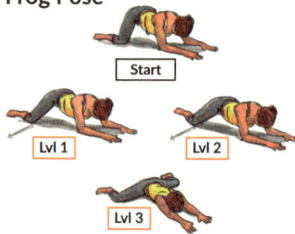

Duration:
....

(Goal: 60 sec) | Level:

6. Figure 4

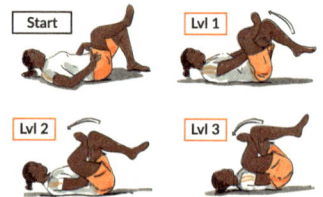

Duration:
....

(Goal: 30 sec each side) | Level:

7. Downward Dog

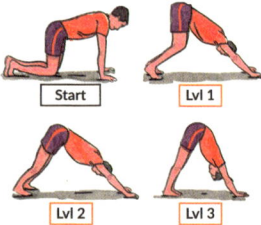

Duration:
....

(Goal: 30 sec) | Level:

8. Seated Single Leg Hamstring Stretch

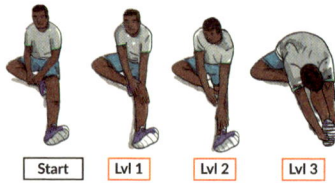

Duration:
....

(Goal: 30 sec each side) | Level:

9. Knee to Chest Stretch

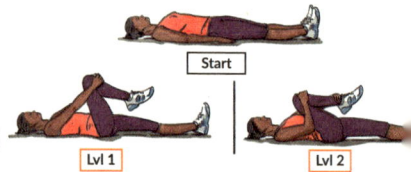

Duration:
....

(Goal: 30 sec each side) | Level:

10. Extended Triangle Pose

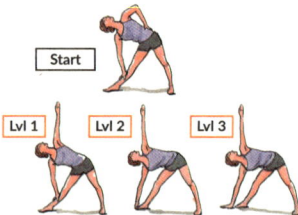

Duration:
....

(Goal: 30 sec each side) | Level:

11. Kneeling Quad Stretch

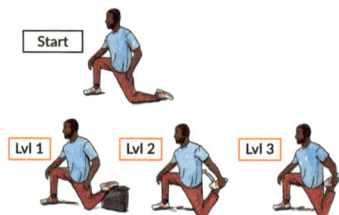

Duration:
....

(Goal: 30 sec each side) | Level:

12. Hanging Calf Stretch

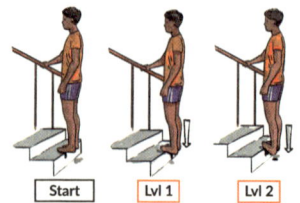

Duration:
....

(Goal: 30 sec) | Level:

Daily Reflection

Benefits I'm Experiencing:

Feel
Lighter

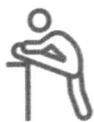

More Freedom
of Movement

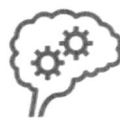

Improved
Mental Clarity

Less
Pain

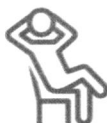

Less
Stressed

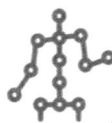

Improved
Posture

Notes On My Body:

....

....

....

....

....

....

....

....

When you really commit to and stick with a goal you've set for yourself, it comes with the awesome benefit of an altered attitude about your own ability to accomplish goals you set for yourself. Have you noticed a shift in attitude as a result of sticking with your stretching routines?

Day 33: Dynamic Warm-Up

Full Session Exercise Guide:
habitnest.com/pages/stretching-day-33

1. World's Greatest Stretch

You will learn to LOVE this movement.
Take it slowly the first few times you do it.

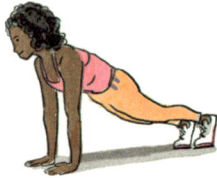 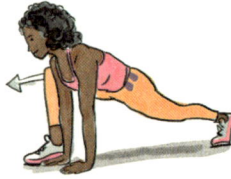 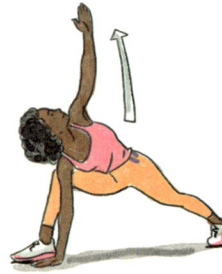

Start   Step 1   Step 2

Reps: ....   *(Goal: 10-20)*

2. Good Morning

One of the best full body warmup exercises!
You're bending at the hip, and the knees.
Everything else maintains posture.

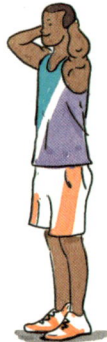 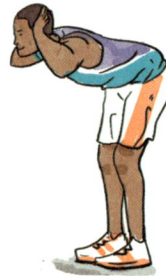

Start   Step 1

Reps: ....   *(Goal: 10-20)*

3. Standing Hip Circles

Open up as widely
as possible in back
and in front!

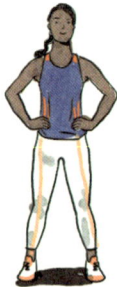 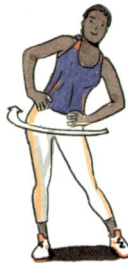 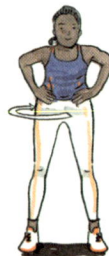 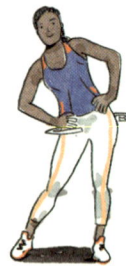

Start   Step 1   Step 2   Step 3

Reps: ....   *(Goal: 10-15 in each direction)*

Day 33: Upper Body

1. Lateral Side to Side Neck Rotation

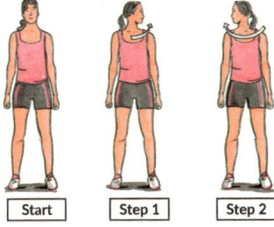

Start Step 1 Step 2

Duration:

(Goal: 30 sec, alternating)

2. Side Neck Stretch w/ Upside Down Palm on Wall

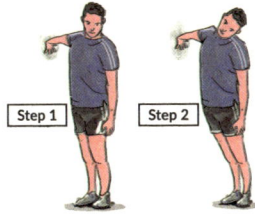

Step 1 Step 2

Duration:

(Goal: 15 sec each side)

3. Levator Scap Neck Stretch

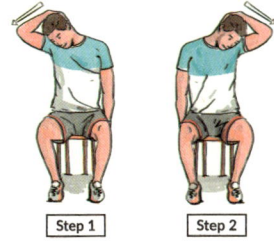

Step 1 Step 2

Duration:

(Goal: 15 sec each side)

4. Seated Forward Curl

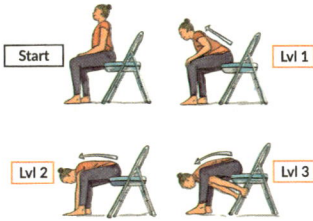

Start Lvl 1 Lvl 2 Lvl 3

Duration:

(Goal: 30 sec) Level:

5. Seated Spinal Twist

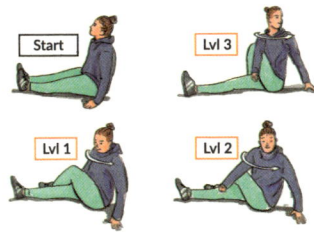

Start Lvl 3 Lvl 1 Lvl 2

Duration:

(Goal: 15 sec each side) Level:

6. Wall Lat Stretch

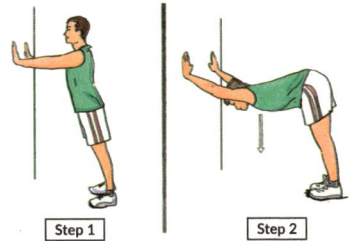

Step 1 Step 2

Duration:

(Goal: 15 sec each side)

7. Corner Chest Stretch

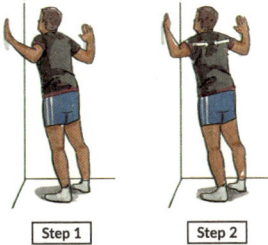

Step 1 Step 2

Duration:

(Goal: 30 sec)

8. Thread the Needle Shoulder Stretch

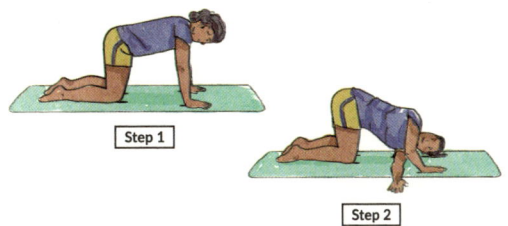

Step 1 Step 2

Duration:

(Goal: 15 sec each side)

9. Behind the Back Tricep Extension

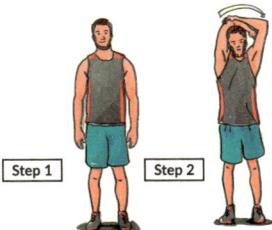

Step 1 Step 2

Duration:

(Goal: 15 sec each side)

10. Lying Full Body Extension

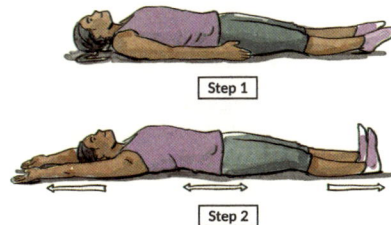

Step 1 Step 2

Duration:

(Goal: 30 sec)

179

Day 33: Lower Body

1. Warrior II Pose

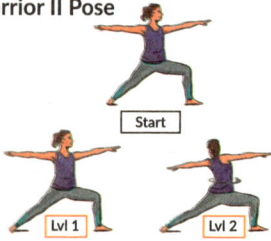

Start
Lvl 1
Lvl 2

Duration:
....

(Goal: 30 sec each side)

Level:

2. Reverse Tabletop

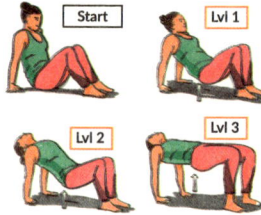

Start
Lvl 1
Lvl 2
Lvl 3

Duration:
....

(Goal: 30 sec)

Level:

3. Reclining Angle Bound Pose

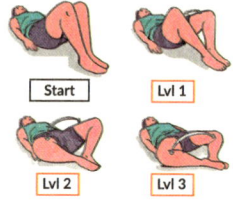

Start
Lvl 1
Lvl 2
Lvl 3

Duration:
....

(Goal: 30 sec)

Level:

4. Pry Squat

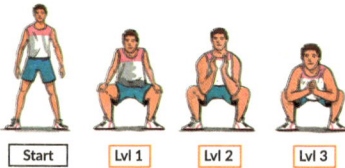

Start
Lvl 1
Lvl 2
Lvl 3

Duration:
....

(Goal: 30 sec)

Level:

5. Frog Pose

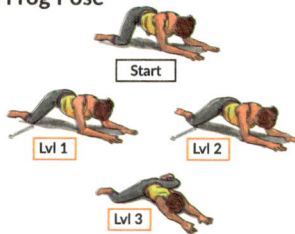

Start
Lvl 1
Lvl 2
Lvl 3

Duration:
....

(Goal: 60 sec)

Level:

6. Figure 4

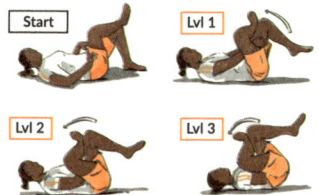

Start
Lvl 1
Lvl 2
Lvl 3

Duration:
....

(Goal: 30 sec each side)

Level:

7. Downward Dog

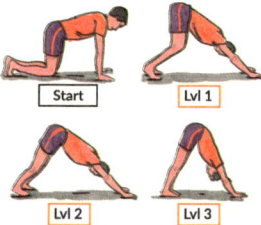

Start
Lvl 1
Lvl 2
Lvl 3

Duration:
....

(Goal: 30 sec)

Level:

8. Seated Single Leg Hamstring Stretch

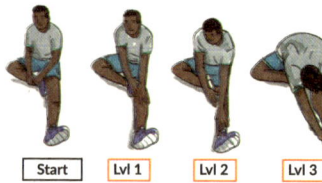

Start
Lvl 1
Lvl 2
Lvl 3

Duration:
....

(Goal: 30 sec each side)

Level:

9. Knee to Chest Stretch

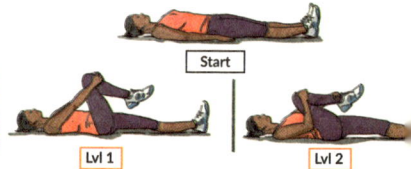

Start
Lvl 1
Lvl 2

Duration:
....

(Goal: 30 sec each side)

Level:

10. Extended Triangle Pose

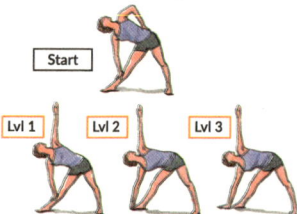

Start
Lvl 1
Lvl 2
Lvl 3

Duration:
....

(Goal: 30 sec each side)

Level:

11. Kneeling Quad Stretch

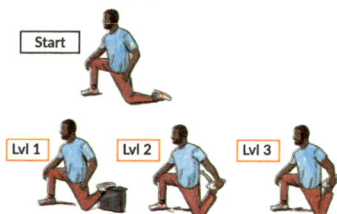

Start
Lvl 1
Lvl 2
Lvl 3

Duration:
....

(Goal: 30 sec each side)

Level:

12. Hanging Calf Stretch

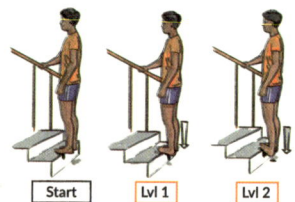

Start
Lvl 1
Lvl 2

Duration:
....

(Goal: 30 sec)

Level:

Daily Reflection

Benefits I'm Experiencing:

Feel
Lighter

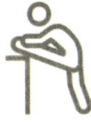

More Freedom
of Movement

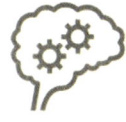

Improved
Mental Clarity

Less
Pain

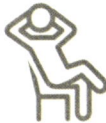

Less
Stressed

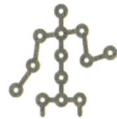

Improved
Posture

Notes On My Body:

Day 34: Dynamic Warm-Up

1. Standing Hamstring Scoop

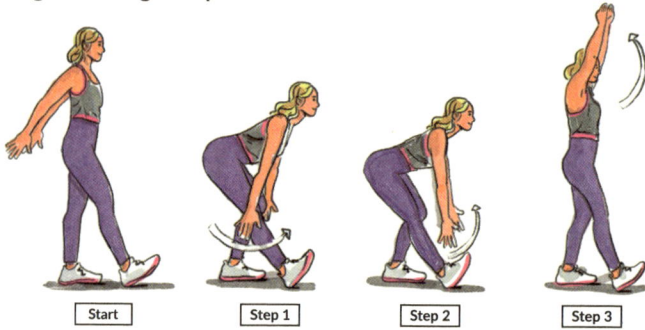

| Start | Step 1 | Step 2 | Step 3 |

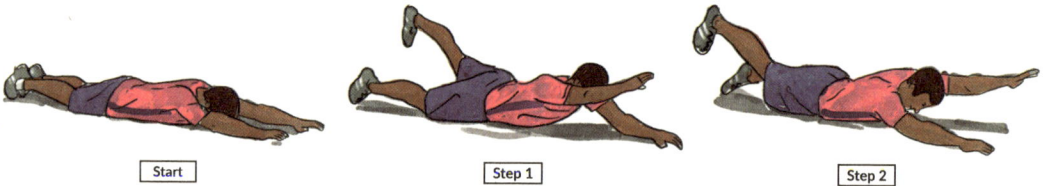

Reps: .... *(Goal: 10-20 each side)* ....

2. Aquaman

| Start | Step 1 | Step 2 |

Reps: .... *(Goal: 10-20)* ....

3. Towel Snatch

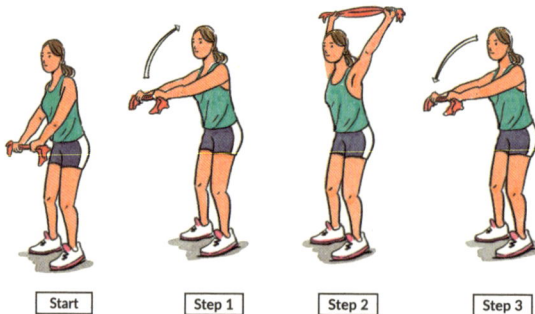

| Start | Step 1 | Step 2 | Step 3 |

Reps: .... *(Goal: 10-20)* ....

Day 34: Upper Body

DATE

1. Lateral Side to Side Neck Rotation

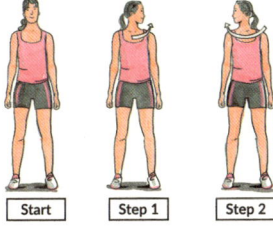

Start | Step 1 | Step 2

Duration:

(Goal: 30 sec, alternating)

2. Side Neck Stretch w/ Upside Down Palm on Wall

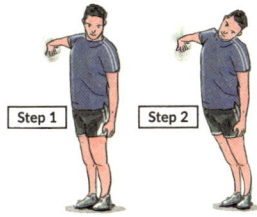

Step 1 | Step 2

Duration:

(Goal: 15 sec each side)

3. Levator Scap Neck Stretch

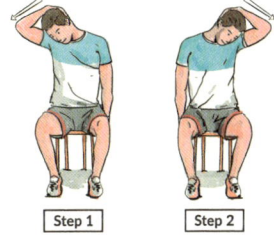

Step 1 | Step 2

Duration:

(Goal: 15 sec each side)

4. Seated Forward Curl

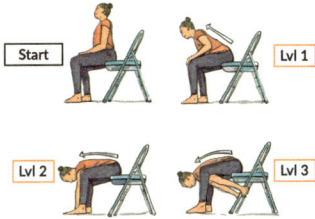

Start | Lvl 1 | Lvl 2 | Lvl 3

Duration:

(Goal: 30 sec)

Level:

5. Seated Spinal Twist

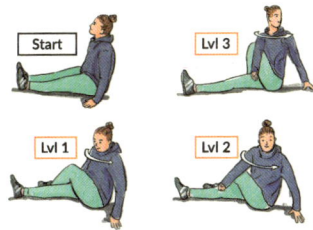

Start | Lvl 3 | Lvl 1 | Lvl 2

Duration:

(Goal: 15 sec each side)

Level:

6. Wall Lat Stretch

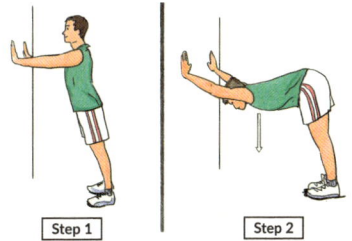

Step 1 | Step 2

Duration:

(Goal: 15 sec each side)

7. Corner Chest Stretch

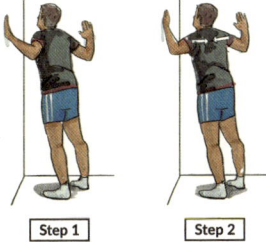

Step 1 | Step 2

Duration:

(Goal: 30 sec)

8. Thread the Needle Shoulder Stretch

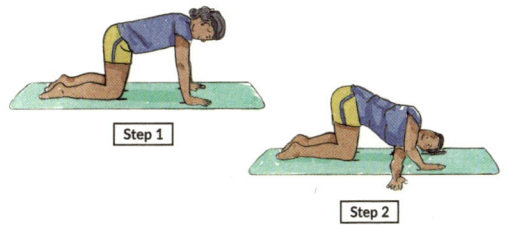

Step 1 | Step 2

Duration:

(Goal: 15 sec each side)

9. Behind the Back Tricep Extension

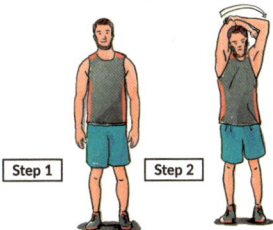

Step 1 | Step 2

Duration:

(Goal: 15 sec each side)

10. Lying Full Body Extension

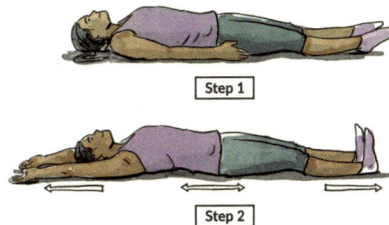

Step 1 | Step 2

Duration:

(Goal: 30 sec)

183

Day 34: Lower Body

1. Warrior II Pose

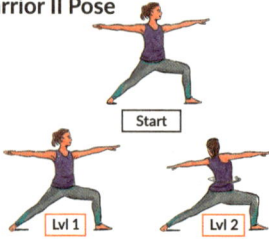

Start
Lvl 1
Lvl 2

Duration:
....

(Goal: 30 sec each side)

Level:

2. Reverse Tabletop

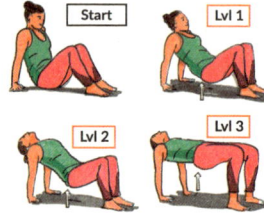

Start
Lvl 1
Lvl 2
Lvl 3

Duration:
....

(Goal: 30 sec)

Level:

3. Reclining Angle Bound Pose

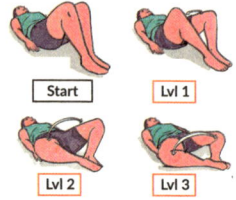

Start
Lvl 1
Lvl 2
Lvl 3

Duration:
....

(Goal: 30 sec)

Level:

4. Pry Squat

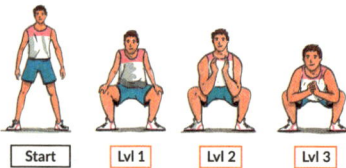

Start
Lvl 1
Lvl 2
Lvl 3

Duration:
....

(Goal: 30 sec)

Level:

5. Frog Pose

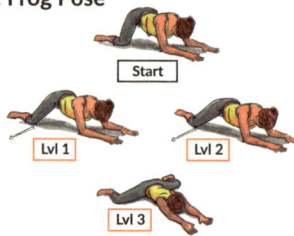

Start
Lvl 1
Lvl 2
Lvl 3

Duration:
....

(Goal: 60 sec)

Level:

6. Figure 4

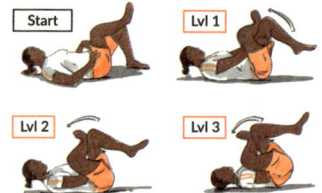

Start
Lvl 1
Lvl 2
Lvl 3

Duration:
....

(Goal: 30 sec each side)

Level:

7. Downward Dog

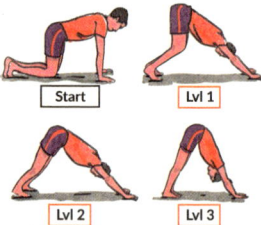

Start
Lvl 1
Lvl 2
Lvl 3

Duration:
....

(Goal: 30 sec)

Level:

8. Seated Single Leg Hamstring Stretch

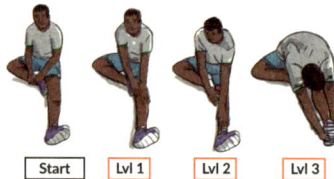

Start
Lvl 1
Lvl 2
Lvl 3

Duration:
....

(Goal: 30 sec each side)

Level:

9. Knee to Chest Stretch

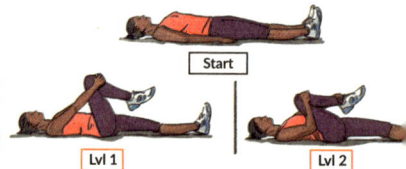

Start
Lvl 1
Lvl 2

Duration:
....

(Goal: 30 sec each side)

Level:

10. Extended Triangle Pose

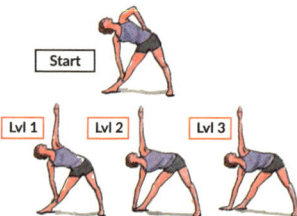

Start
Lvl 1
Lvl 2
Lvl 3

Duration:
....

(Goal: 30 sec each side)

Level:

11. Kneeling Quad Stretch

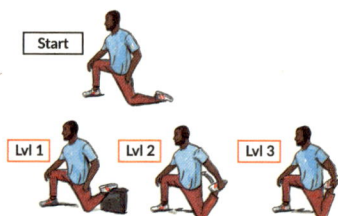

Start
Lvl 1
Lvl 2
Lvl 3

Duration:
....

(Goal: 30 sec each side)

Level:

12. Hanging Calf Stretch

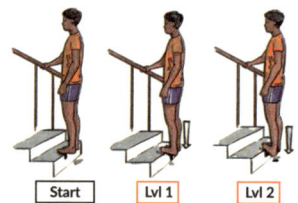

Start
Lvl 1
Lvl 2

Duration:
....

(Goal: 30 sec)

Level:

Daily Reflection

Benefits I'm Experiencing:

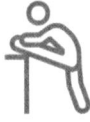

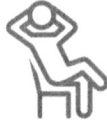

Feel Lighter	More Freedom of Movement	Improved Mental Clarity
Less Pain	Less Stressed	Improved Posture

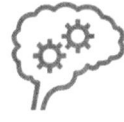

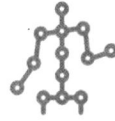

Notes On My Body:

_____

_____

_____

_____

_____

_____

_____

_____

Day 35: Dynamic Warm-Up

Full Session Exercise Guide:
habitnest.com/pages/stretching-day-35

1. World's Greatest Stretch

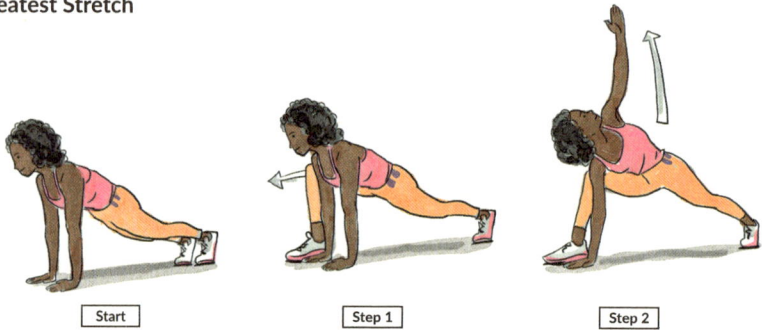

| Start | Step 1 | Step 2 |

Reps: .... (Goal: 10-20)

2. Mountain Climber

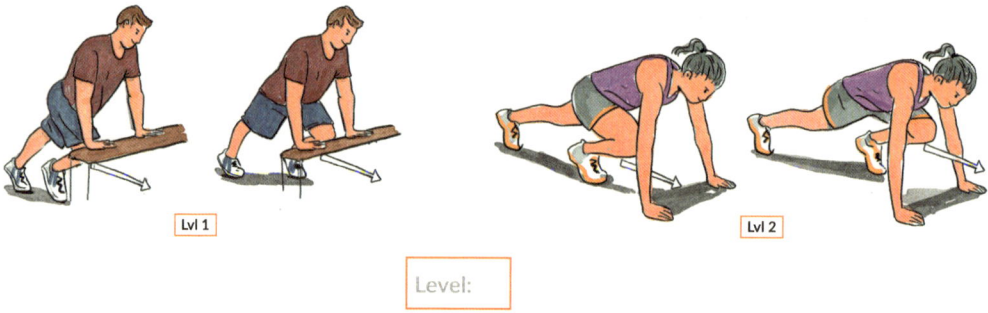

| Lvl 1 | | Lvl 2 |

Level:

Reps: .... (Goal: 20-30 each side)

3. Clam Opener w/ Side Plank

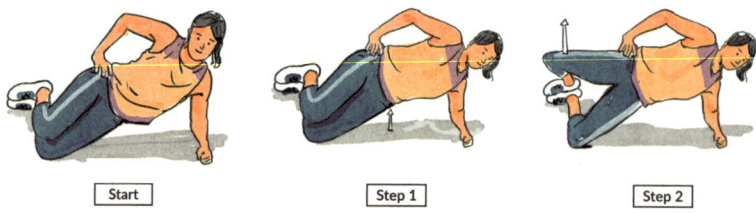

| Start | Step 1 | Step 2 |

Reps: .... (Goal: 10-15 each side)

Day 35: Upper Body

1. Lateral Side to Side Neck Rotation

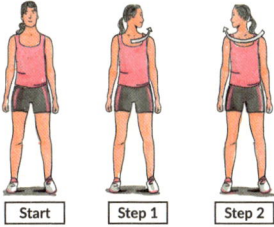

Start | Step 1 | Step 2

Duration:

(Goal: 30 sec, alternating)

2. Side Neck Stretch w/ Upside Down Palm on Wall

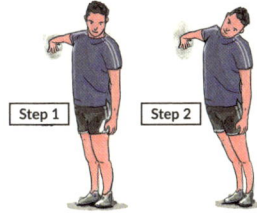

Step 1 | Step 2

Duration:

(Goal: 15 sec each side)

3. Levator Scap Neck Stretch

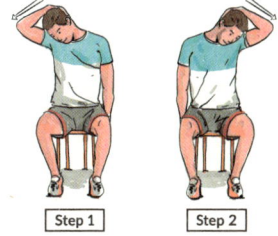

Step 1 | Step 2

Duration:

(Goal: 15 sec each side)

4. Seated Forward Curl

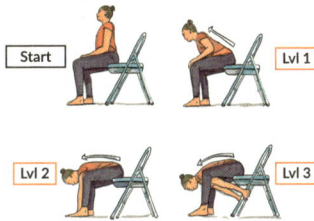

Start | Lvl 1 | Lvl 2 | Lvl 3

Duration:

(Goal: 30 sec)

Level:

5. Seated Spinal Twist

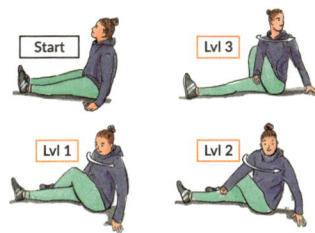

Start | Lvl 3 | Lvl 1 | Lvl 2

Duration:

(Goal: 15 sec each side)

Level:

6. Wall Lat Stretch

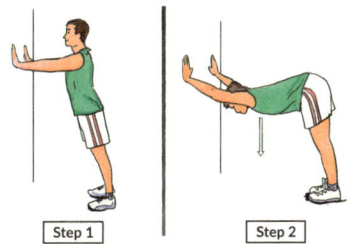

Step 1 | Step 2

Duration:

(Goal: 15 sec each side)

7. Corner Chest Stretch

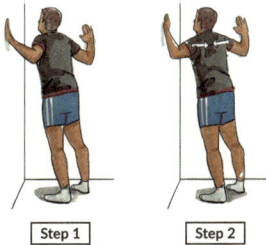

Step 1 | Step 2

Duration:

(Goal: 30 sec)

8. Thread the Needle Shoulder Stretch

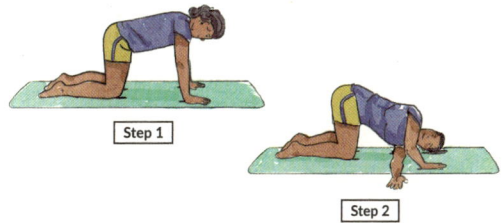

Step 1 | Step 2

Duration:

(Goal: 15 sec each side)

9. Behind the Back Tricep Extension

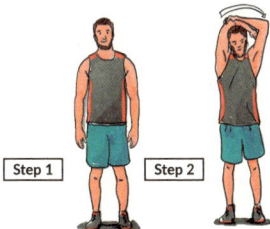

Step 1 | Step 2

Duration:

(Goal: 15 sec each side)

10. Lying Full Body Extension

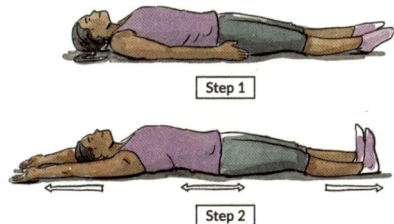

Step 1 | Step 2

Duration:

(Goal: 30 sec)

Day 35: Lower Body

1. Warrior II Pose

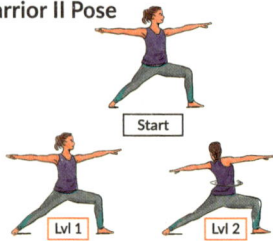
Start
Lvl 1
Lvl 2

Duration:

(Goal: 30 sec each side)

Level:

2. Reverse Tabletop

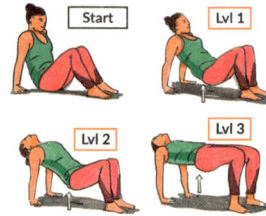
Start
Lvl 1
Lvl 2
Lvl 3

Duration:

(Goal: 30 sec)

Level:

3. Reclining Angle Bound Pose

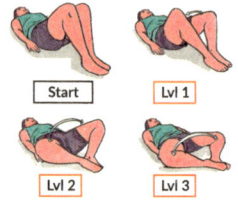
Start
Lvl 1
Lvl 2
Lvl 3

Duration:

(Goal: 30 sec)

Level:

4. Pry Squat

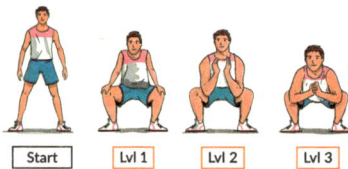
Start
Lvl 1
Lvl 2
Lvl 3

Duration:

(Goal: 30 sec)

Level:

5. Frog Pose

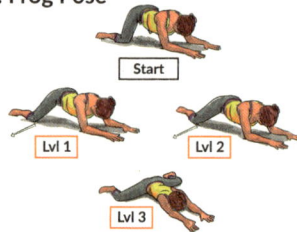
Start
Lvl 1
Lvl 2
Lvl 3

Duration:

(Goal: 60 sec)

Level:

6. Figure 4

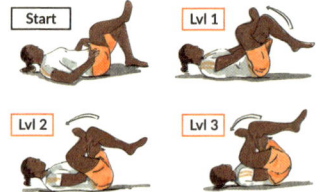
Start
Lvl 1
Lvl 2
Lvl 3

Duration:

(Goal: 30 sec each side)

Level:

7. Downward Dog

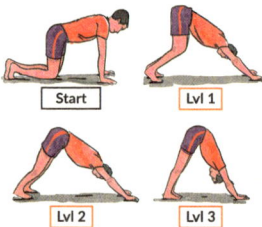
Start
Lvl 1
Lvl 2
Lvl 3

Duration:

(Goal: 30 sec)

Level:

8. Seated Single Leg Hamstring Stretch

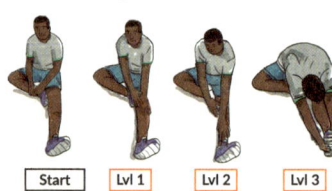
Start
Lvl 1
Lvl 2
Lvl 3

Duration:

(Goal: 30 sec each side)

Level:

9. Knee to Chest Stretch

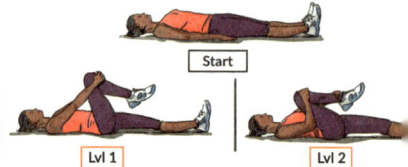
Start
Lvl 1
Lvl 2

Duration:

(Goal: 30 sec each side)

Level:

10. Extended Triangle Pose

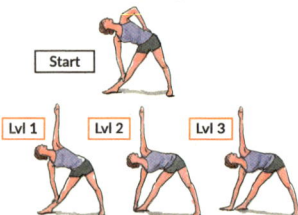
Start
Lvl 1
Lvl 2
Lvl 3

Duration:

(Goal: 30 sec each side)

Level:

11. Kneeling Quad Stretch

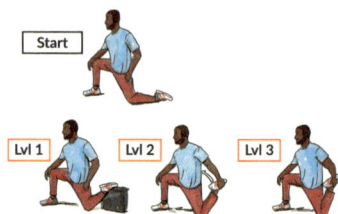
Start
Lvl 1
Lvl 2
Lvl 3

Duration:

(Goal: 30 sec each side)

Level:

12. Hanging Calf Stretch

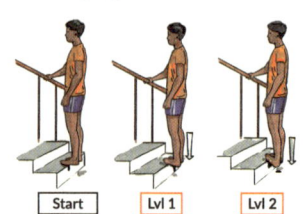
Start
Lvl 1
Lvl 2

Duration:

(Goal: 30 sec)

Level:

Daily Reflection

Benefits I'm Experiencing:

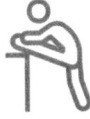

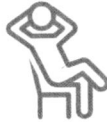

Feel Lighter	More Freedom of Movement	Improved Mental Clarity
Less Pain	Less Stressed	Improved Posture

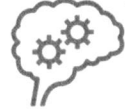

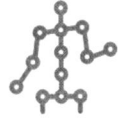

Notes On My Body:

Day 36: Dynamic Warm-Up

Full Session Exercise Guide:

habitnest.com/pages/stretching-day-36

1. Rocking Feet w/ Arm Raise

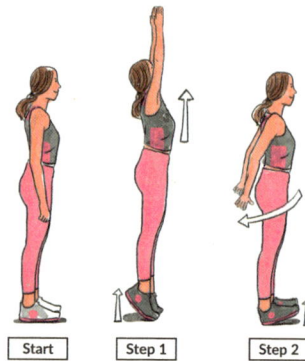

Start   Step 1   Step 2

Reps: *(Goal: 10-20 in each direction)*

2. Plank w/ Shoulder Tap

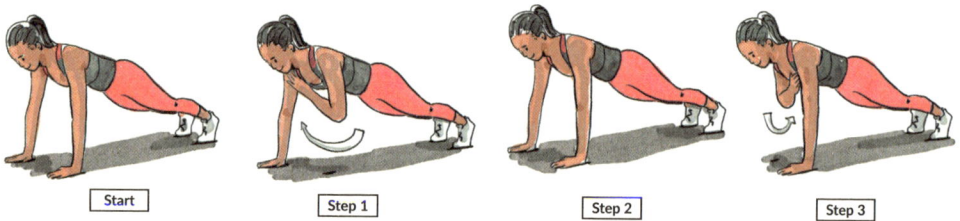

Start   Step 1   Step 2   Step 3

Reps: *(Goal: 10-20 each side)*

3. Split Squat

Step 1   Step 2

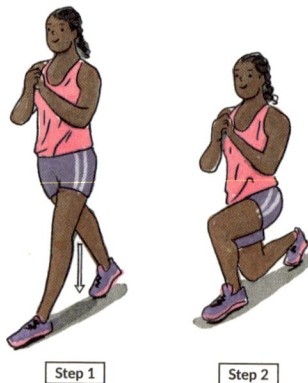

Reps: *(Goal: 15-20 each side)*

Day 36: Upper Body

1. Up & Down Neck Tilt

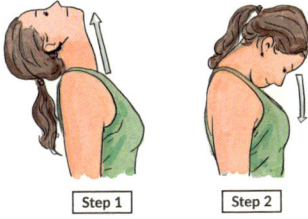

Step 1   Step 2

Duration:

(Goal: 30 sec, alternating)

2. Side Neck Tilt

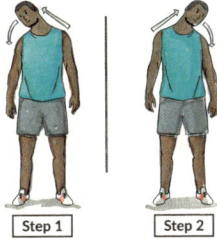

Step 1   Step 2

Duration:

(Goal: 15 sec each side)

3. Forward & Backward Neck Tilt

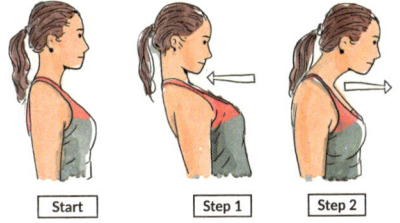

Start   Step 1   Step 2

Duration:

(Goal: 30 sec, alternating)

4. Child's Pose

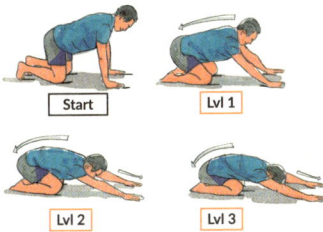

Start   Lvl 1
Lvl 2   Lvl 3

Duration:

(Goal: 60 sec)   Level:

5. Cat-Cow

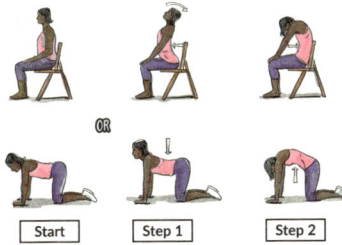

OR

Start   Step 1   Step 2

Duration:

(Goal: 30 sec, alternating)

6. Seated Spinal Twist

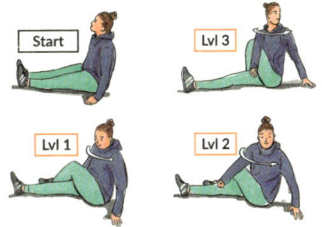

Start   Lvl 3
Lvl 1   Lvl 2

Duration:

(Goal: 15 sec each side)   Level:

7. Leaning Long Arm Shoulder Stretch

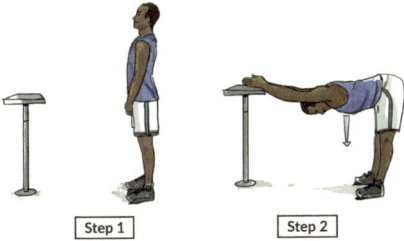

Step 1   Step 2

Duration: *(Goal: 30 sec)*

8. Floor Angel

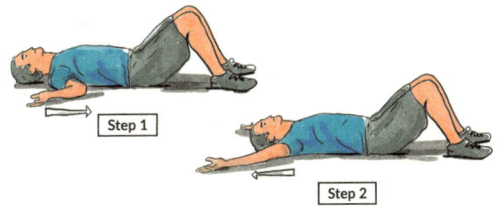

Step 1
Step 2

Duration: *(Goal: 30 sec, alternating)*

9. Behind the Back Elbow to Elbow Grip

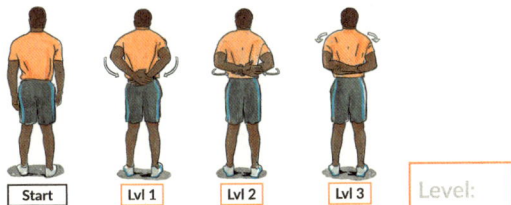

Start   Lvl 1   Lvl 2   Lvl 3

Level:

Duration: *(Goal: 30 sec)*

10. Locust Pose

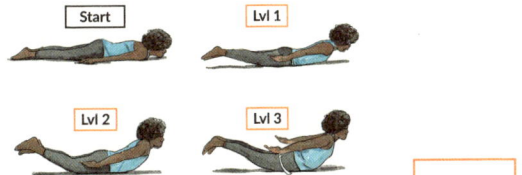

Start   Lvl 1
Lvl 2   Lvl 3

Level:

Duration: *(Goal: 30 sec)*

Day 36: Lower Body

1. Runner's Lunge

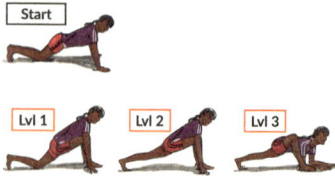

Duration:

(Goal: 30 sec each side)   Level:

2. Lying Hip Extension

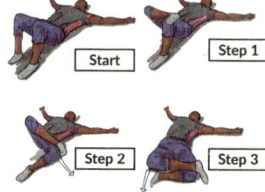

Duration:

(Goal: 30 sec each side)

3. Butterfly

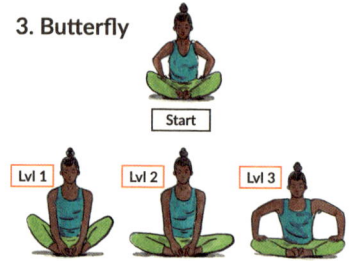

Duration:

(Goal: 30 sec)   Level:

4. Scorpion Pose

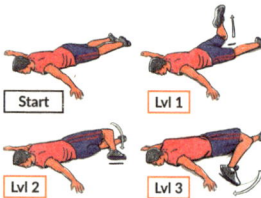

Duration:

(Goal: 30 sec each side)   Level:

5. Happy Baby Pose

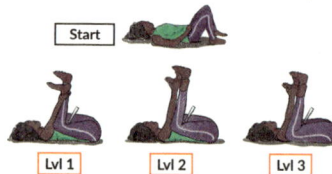

Duration:

(Goal: 30 sec)   Level:

6. Pigeon Stretch

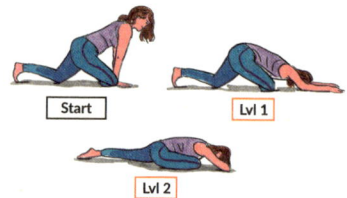

Duration:

(Goal: 30 sec each side)   Level:

7. Figure 4

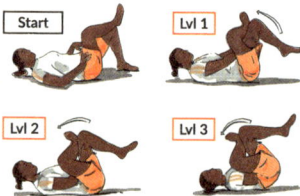

Duration:

(Goal: 30 sec each side)   Level:

8. Halfway Center Split

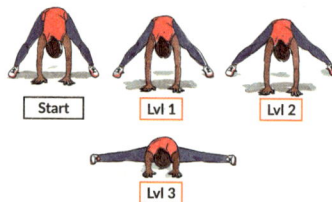

Duration:

(Goal: 30 sec)   Level:

9. Lying Hamstring Extension

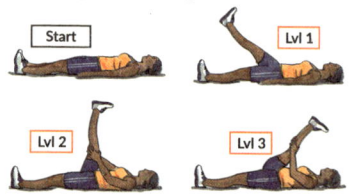

Duration:

(Goal: 30 sec each side)   Level:

10. Seated Forward Fold Hamstring Stretch

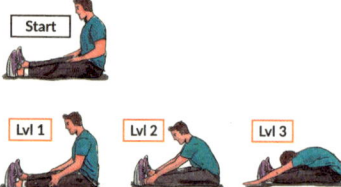

Duration:

(Goal: 30 sec)   Level:

11. Lying Quad Stretch

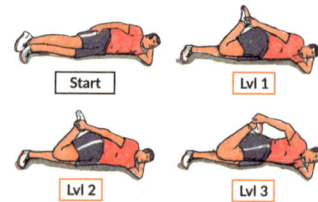

Duration:

(Goal: 30 sec each side)   Level:

12. Standing Wall Calf Stretch w/ Achilles Focus

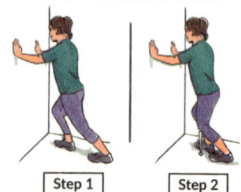

Duration:

(Goal: 15 sec each side)

Daily Reflection

Benefits I'm Experiencing:

Feel
Lighter

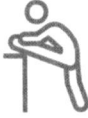

More Freedom
of Movement

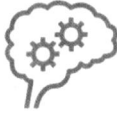

Improved
Mental Clarity

Less
Pain

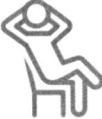

Less
Stressed

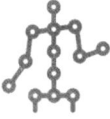

Improved
Posture

Notes On My Body:

Day 37: Dynamic Warm-Up

Full Session Exercise Guide:
habitnest.com/pages/stretching-day-37

1. Inch Worm Walk Out

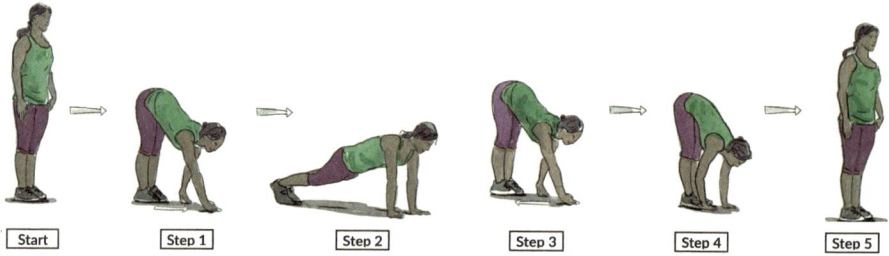

| Start | Step 1 | Step 2 | Step 3 | Step 4 | Step 5 |

Reps: *(Goal: 10-20)*

2. Good Morning

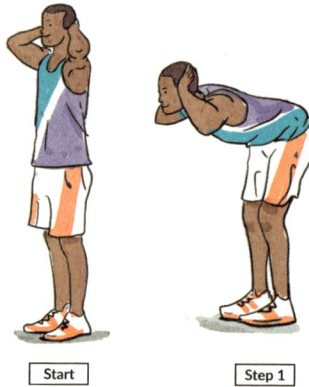

| Start | Step 1 |

Reps: *(Goal: 15-20)*

3. Knee Hug

| Start | Step 1 | Step 2 |

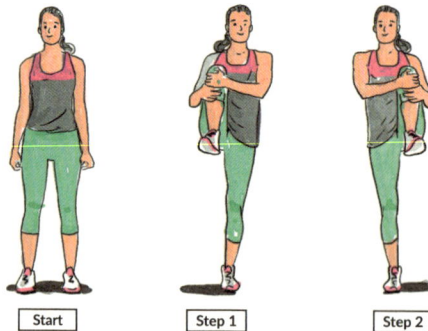

Reps: *(Goal: 10-15 each side)*

194

Day 37: Upper Body

1. Up & Down Neck Tilt

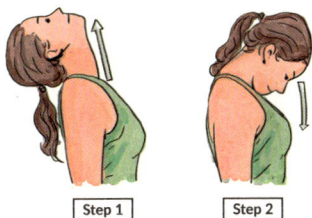

Step 1   Step 2

Duration:

(Goal: 30 sec, alternating)

2. Side Neck Tilt

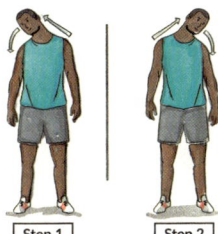

Step 1   Step 2

Duration:

(Goal: 15 sec each side)

3. Forward & Backward Neck Tilt

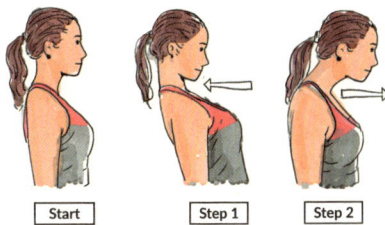

Start   Step 1   Step 2

Duration:

(Goal: 30 sec, alternating)

4. Child's Pose

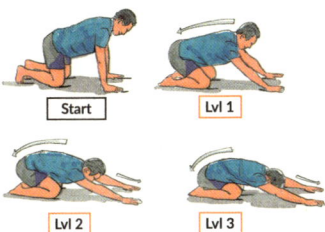

Start   Lvl 1
Lvl 2   Lvl 3

Duration:

(Goal: 60 sec)   Level:

5. Cat-Cow

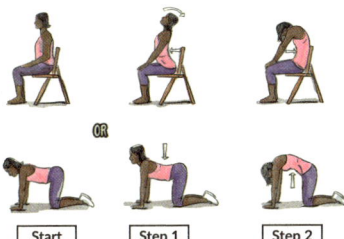

OR

Start   Step 1   Step 2

Duration:

(Goal: 30 sec, alternating)

6. Seated Spinal Twist

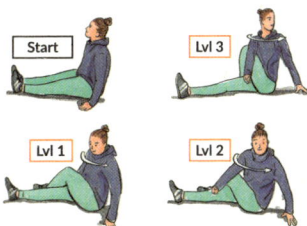

Start   Lvl 3
Lvl 1   Lvl 2

Duration:

(Goal: 15 sec each side)   Level:

7. Leaning Long Arm Shoulder Stretch

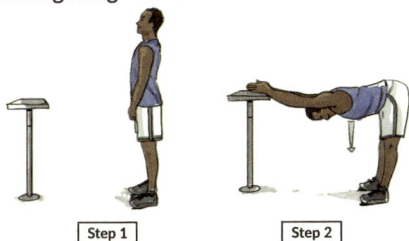

Step 1   Step 2

Duration:

(Goal: 30 sec)

8. Floor Angel

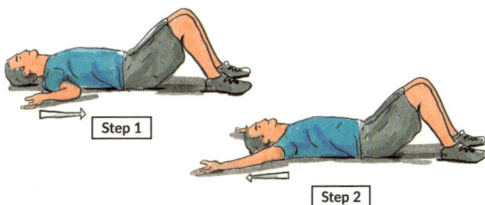

Step 1   Step 2

Duration:

(Goal: 30 sec, alternating)

9. Behind the Back Elbow to Elbow Grip

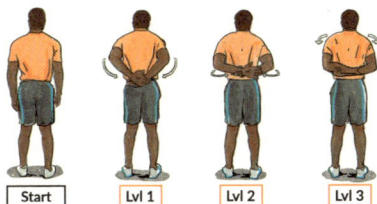

Start   Lvl 1   Lvl 2   Lvl 3

Level:

Duration:

(Goal: 30 sec)

10. Locust Pose

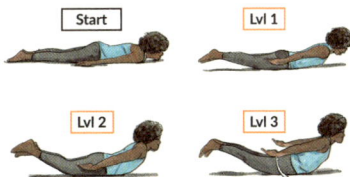

Start   Lvl 1
Lvl 2   Lvl 3

Level:

Duration:

(Goal: 30 sec)

Day 37: Lower Body

1. Runner's Lunge

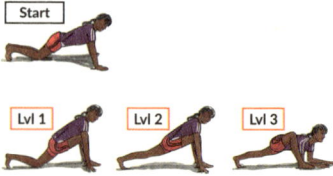

Duration:
....

(Goal: 30 sec each side)

Level:

2. Lying Hip Extension

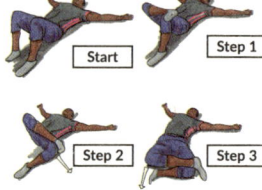

Duration:
....

(Goal: 30 sec each side)

3. Butterfly

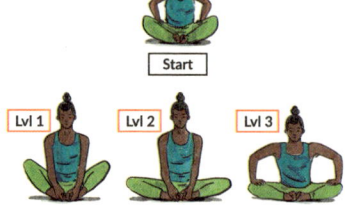

Duration:
....

(Goal: 30 sec)

Level:

4. Scorpion Pose

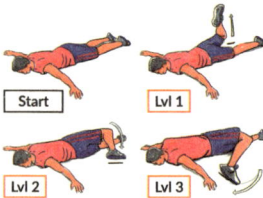

Duration:
....

(Goal: 30 sec each side)

Level:

5. Happy Baby Pose

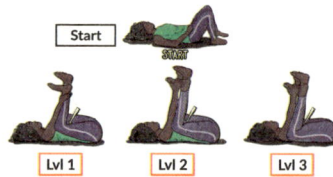

Duration:
....

(Goal: 30 sec)

Level:

6. Pigeon Stretch

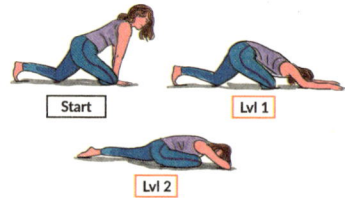

Duration:
....

(Goal: 30 sec each side)

Level:

7. Figure 4

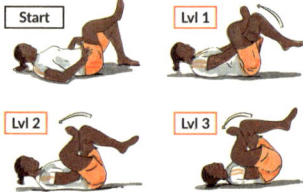

Duration:
....

(Goal: 30 sec each side)

Level:

8. Halfway Center Split

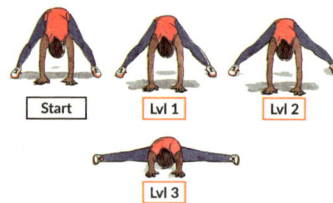

Duration:
....

(Goal: 30 sec)

Level:

9. Lying Hamstring Extension

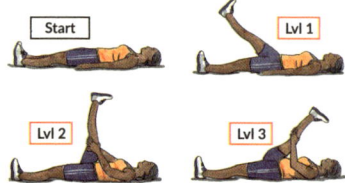

Duration:
....

(Goal: 30 sec each side)

Level:

10. Seated Forward Fold Hamstring Stretch

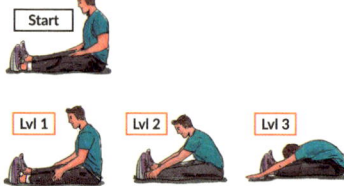

Duration:
....

(Goal: 30 sec)

Level:

11. Lying Quad Stretch

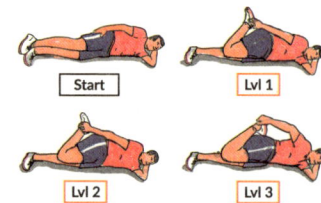

Duration:
....

(Goal: 30 sec each side)

Level:

12. Standing Wall Calf Stretch w/ Achilles Focus

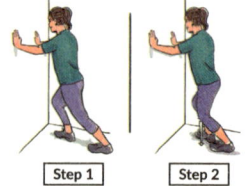

Duration:
....

(Goal: 15 sec each side)

Daily Reflection

Benefits I'm Experiencing:

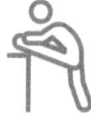

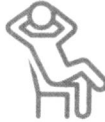

Feel Lighter	More Freedom of Movement	Improved Mental Clarity
Less Pain	Less Stressed	Improved Posture

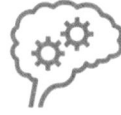

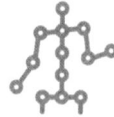

Notes On My Body:

_____

_____

_____

_____

_____

_____

_____

_____

Today, remind yourself WHY you began this journey.

Day 38: Dynamic Warm-Up

1. Side Plank w/ Twist

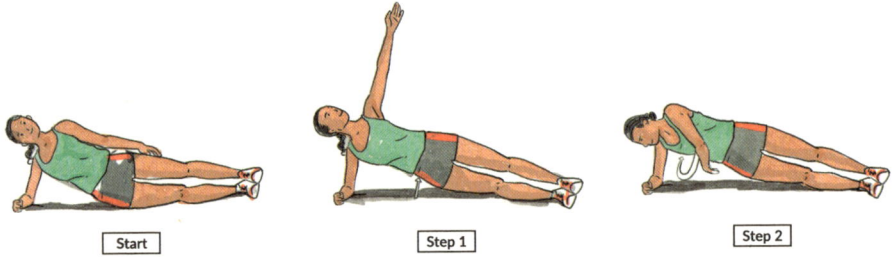

Start | Step 1 | Step 2

Reps: *(Goal: 10-15 each side)*

2. Roundhouse Kick to Squat

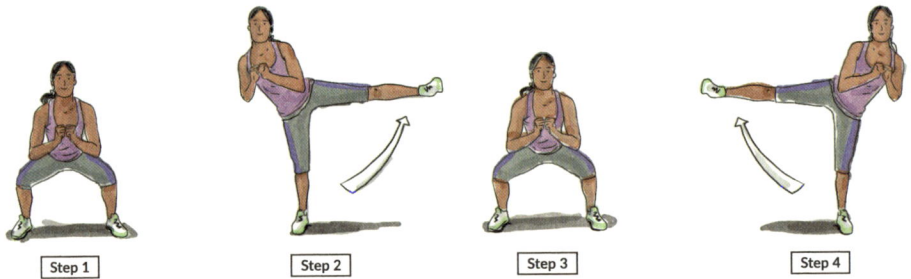

Step 1 | Step 2 | Step 3 | Step 4

Reps: *(Goal: 10-15 each side)*

3. Glute Bridge

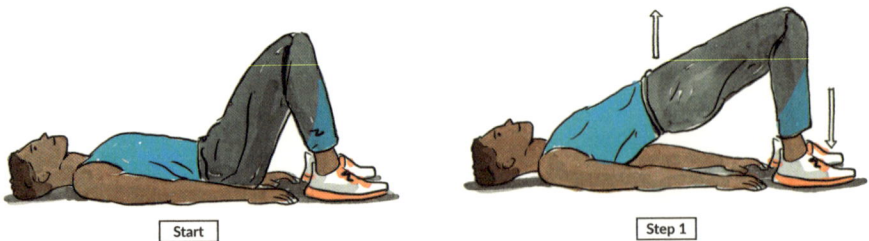

Start | Step 1

Reps: *(Goal: 25-35)*

Day 38: Upper Body

1. Up & Down Neck Tilt

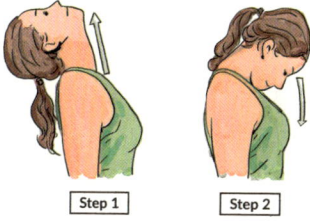

Step 1   Step 2

Duration:
....

(Goal: 30 sec, alternating)

2. Side Neck Tilt

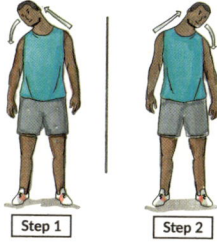

Step 1   Step 2

Duration:
....

(Goal: 15 sec each side)

3. Forward & Backward Neck Tilt

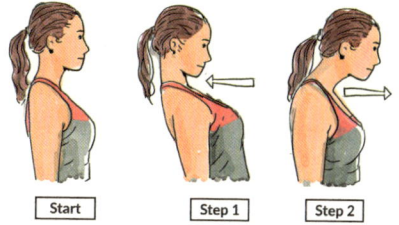

Start   Step 1   Step 2

Duration:
....

(Goal: 30 sec, alternating)

4. Child's Pose

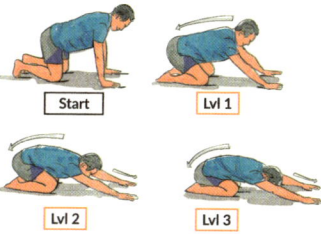

Start   Lvl 1

Lvl 2   Lvl 3

Duration:
....

(Goal: 60 sec)   Level:

5. Cat-Cow

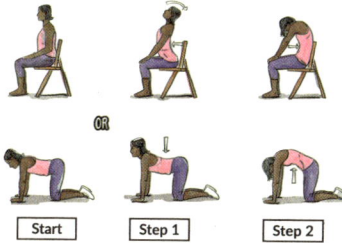

OR

Start   Step 1   Step 2

Duration:
....

(Goal: 30 sec, alternating)

6. Seated Spinal Twist

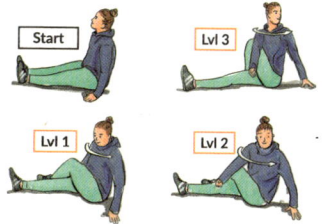

Start   Lvl 3

Lvl 1   Lvl 2

Duration:
....

(Goal: 15 sec each side)   Level:

7. Leaning Long Arm Shoulder Stretch

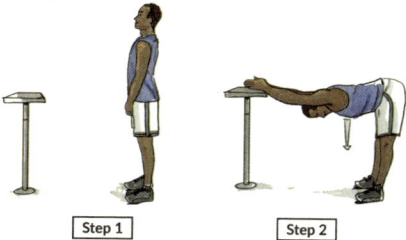

Step 1   Step 2

Duration:
....   *(Goal: 30 sec)*

8. Floor Angel

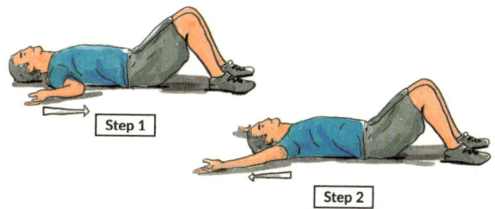

Step 1

Step 2

Duration:
....   *(Goal: 30 sec, alternating)*

9. Behind the Back Elbow to Elbow Grip

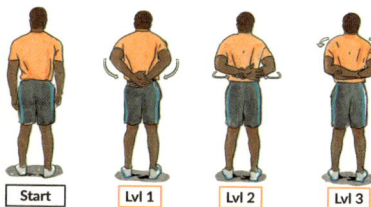

Start   Lvl 1   Lvl 2   Lvl 3   Level:

Duration:
....   *(Goal: 30 sec)*

10. Locust Pose

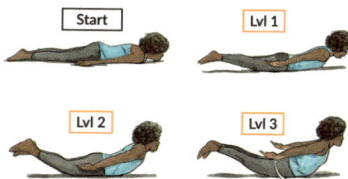

Start   Lvl 1

Lvl 2   Lvl 3

Level:

Duration:
....   *(Goal: 30 sec)*

Day 38: Lower Body

1. Runner's Lunge

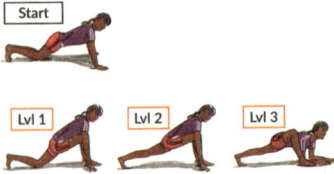

Duration:
....

(Goal: 30 sec each side)   Level:

2. Lying Hip Extension

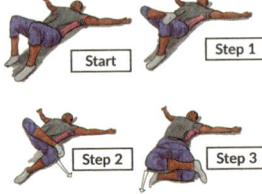

Duration:
....

(Goal: 30 sec each side)

3. Butterfly

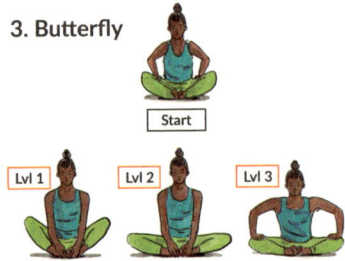

Duration:
....

(Goal: 30 sec)   Level:

4. Scorpion Pose

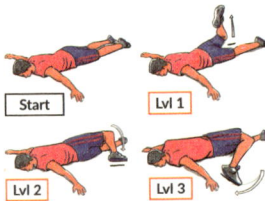

Duration:
....

(Goal: 30 sec each side)   Level:

5. Happy Baby Pose

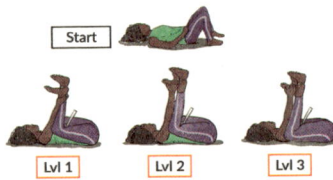

Duration:
....

(Goal: 30 sec)   Level:

6. Pigeon Stretch

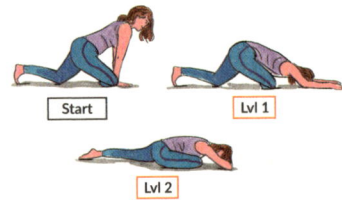

Duration:
....

(Goal: 30 sec each side)   Level:

7. Figure 4

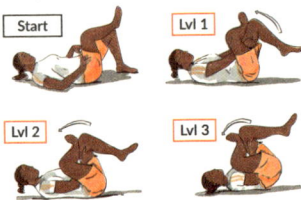

Duration:
....

(Goal: 30 sec each side)   Level:

8. Halfway Center Split

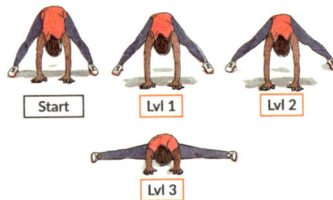

Duration:
....

(Goal: 30 sec)   Level:

9. Lying Hamstring Extension

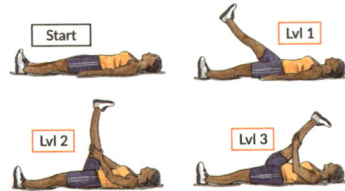

Duration:
....

(Goal: 30 sec each side)   Level:

10. Seated Forward Fold Hamstring Stretch

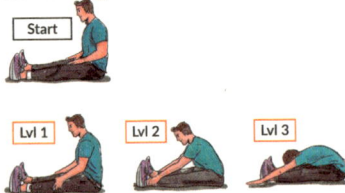

Duration:
....

(Goal: 30 sec)   Level:

11. Lying Quad Stretch

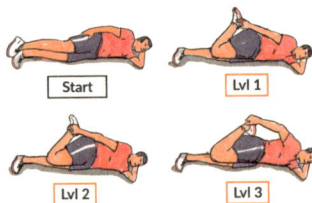

Duration:
....

(Goal: 30 sec each side)   Level:

12. Standing Wall Calf Stretch w/ Achilles Focus

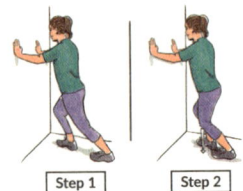

Duration:
....

(Goal: 15 sec each side)

Daily Reflection

Benefits I'm Experiencing:

Feel
Lighter

More Freedom
of Movement

Improved
Mental Clarity

Less
Pain

Less
Stressed

Improved
Posture

Notes On My Body:

Examples, examples, examples. How are the benefits you're tapping actually manifesting in your life and impacting your quality of life in a real, tangible way?

Day 39: Dynamic Warm-Up

Full Session Exercise Guide:
habitnest.com/pages/stretching-day-39

1. Walking Jacks (or Jumping Jacks)

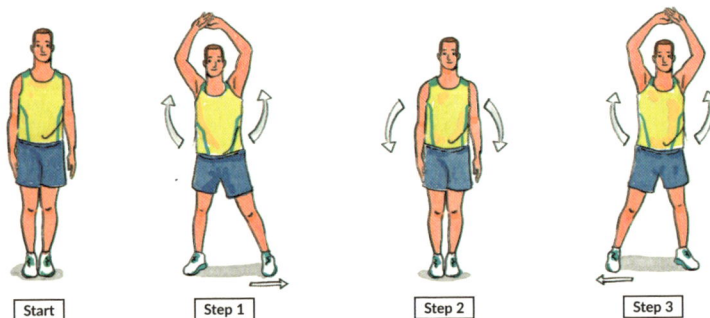

| Start | Step 1 | Step 2 | Step 3 |

Reps: .... *(Goal: 20-30)*

2. Bird-Dog

| Start | Step 1 | Step 2 | Step 3 |

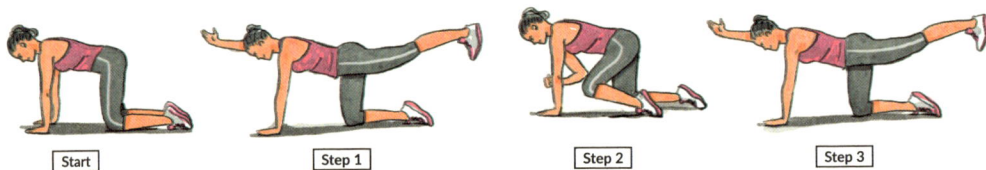

Reps: .... *(Goal: 10-15 each side)*

3. Speed Skater Arms

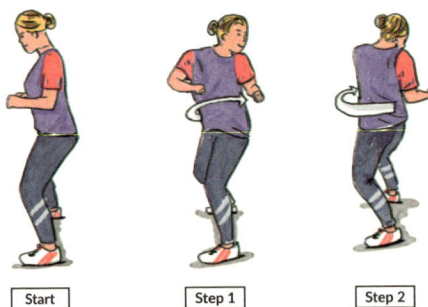

| Start | Step 1 | Step 2 |

Reps: .... *(Goal: 25-30)*

Day 39: Upper Body

DATE

1. Up & Down Neck Tilt

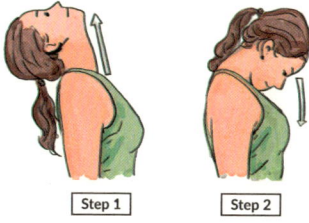

Step 1 Step 2

Duration:

(Goal: 30 sec, alternating)

2. Side Neck Tilt

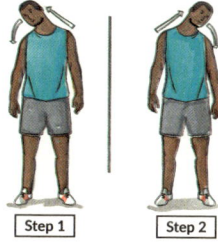

Step 1 Step 2

Duration:

(Goal: 15 sec each side)

3. Forward & Backward Neck Tilt

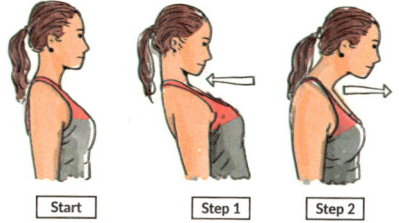

Start Step 1 Step 2

Duration:

(Goal: 30 sec, alternating)

4. Child's Pose

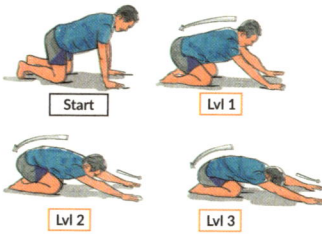

Start Lvl 1 Lvl 2 Lvl 3

Duration:

(Goal: 60 sec) Level:

5. Cat-Cow

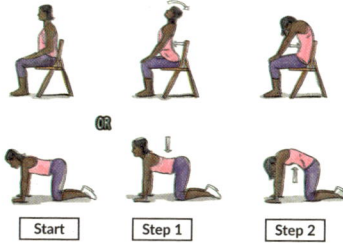

OR

Start Step 1 Step 2

Duration:

(Goal: 30 sec, alternating)

6. Seated Spinal Twist

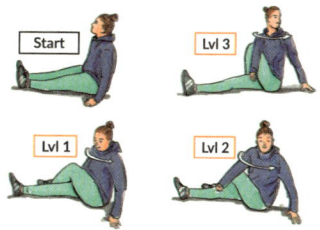

Start Lvl 3 Lvl 1 Lvl 2

Duration:

(Goal: 15 sec each side) Level:

7. Leaning Long Arm Shoulder Stretch

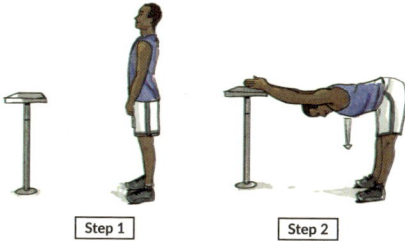

Step 1 Step 2

Duration: *(Goal: 30 sec)*

8. Floor Angel

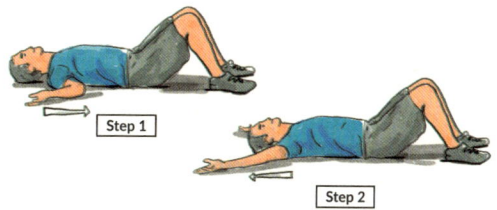

Step 1 Step 2

Duration: *(Goal: 30 sec, alternating)*

9. Behind the Back Elbow to Elbow Grip

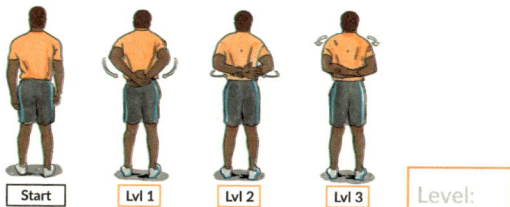

Start Lvl 1 Lvl 2 Lvl 3 Level:

Duration: *(Goal: 30 sec)*

10. Locust Pose

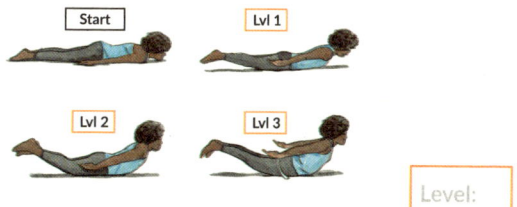

Start Lvl 1 Lvl 2 Lvl 3 Level:

Duration: *(Goal: 30 sec)*

Day 39: Lower Body

1. Runner's Lunge

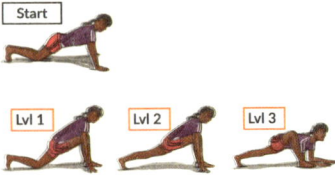

Duration:

(Goal: 30 sec each side) Level:

2. Lying Hip Extension

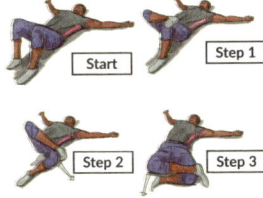

Duration:

(Goal: 30 sec each side)

3. Butterfly

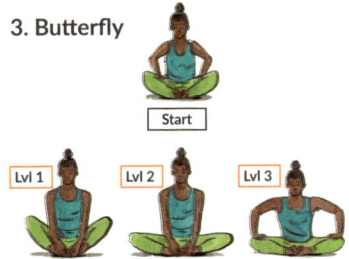

Duration:

(Goal: 30 sec) Level:

4. Scorpion Pose

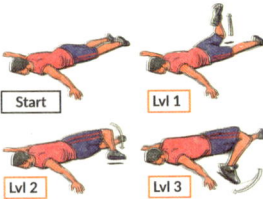

Duration:

(Goal: 30 sec each side) Level:

5. Happy Baby Pose

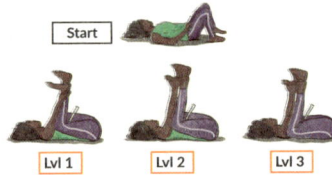

Duration:

(Goal: 30 sec) Level:

6. Pigeon Stretch

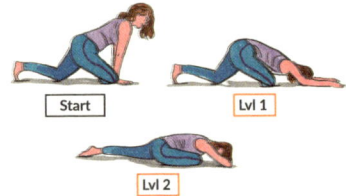

Duration:

(Goal: 30 sec each side) Level:

7. Figure 4

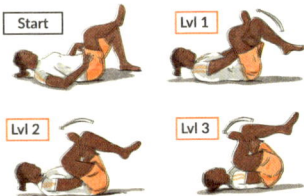

Duration:

(Goal: 30 sec each side) Level:

8. Halfway Center Split

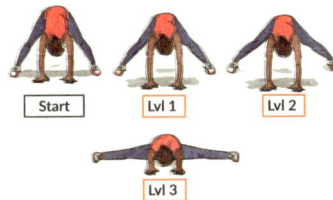

Duration:

(Goal: 30 sec) Level:

9. Lying Hamstring Extension

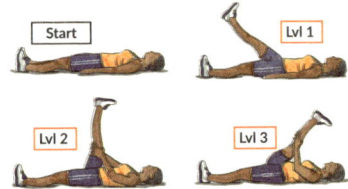

Duration:

(Goal: 30 sec each side) Level:

10. Seated Forward Fold Hamstring Stretch

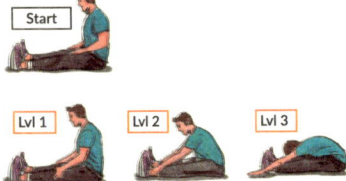

Duration:

(Goal: 30 sec) Level:

11. Lying Quad Stretch

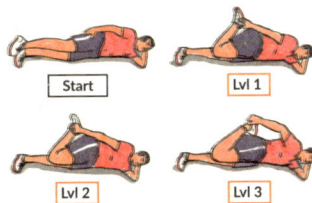

Duration:

(Goal: 30 sec each side) Level:

12. Standing Wall Calf Stretch w/ Achilles Focus

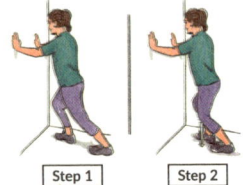

Duration:

(Goal: 15 sec each side)

Daily Reflection

Benefits I'm Experiencing:

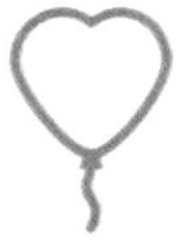

Feel
Lighter

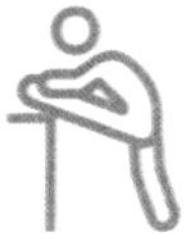

More Freedom
of Movement

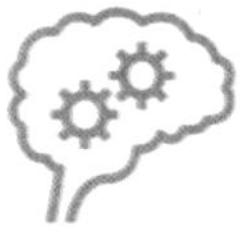

Improved
Mental Clarity

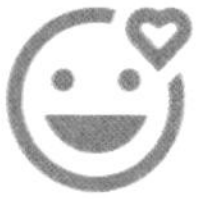

Less
Pain

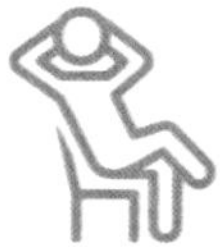

Less
Stressed

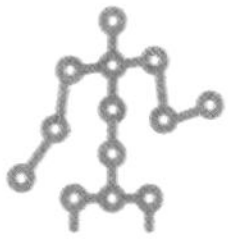

Improved
Posture

Notes On My Body:

Day 40: Dynamic Warm-Up

Full Session Exercise Guide:
habitnest.com/pages/stretching-day-40

1. Plank w/ Shoulder Tap

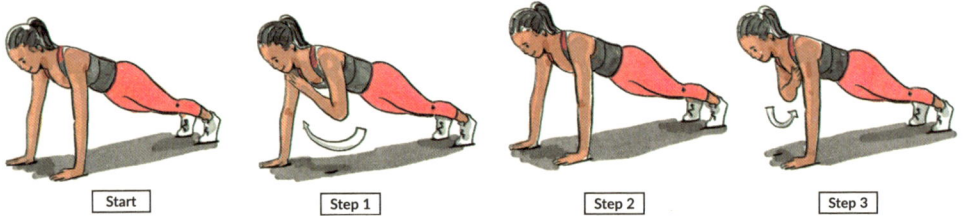

| Start | Step 1 | Step 2 | Step 3 |

Reps: .... *(Goal: 10-20 each side)*

2. Mountain Climber

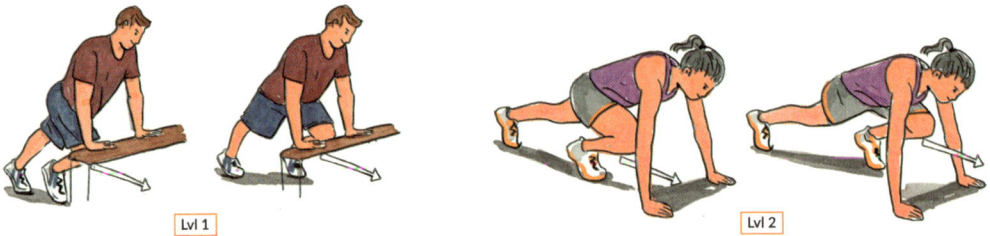

Lvl 1   Lvl 2

Level:

Reps: .... *(Goal: 20-30 each side)*

3. Good Morning

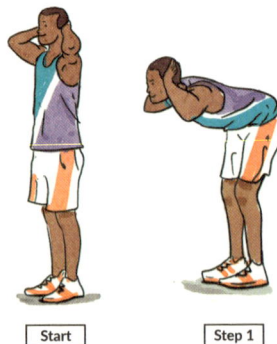

Start   Step 1

Reps: .... *(Goal: 15-20)*

Day 40: Upper Body

1. Up & Down Neck Tilt

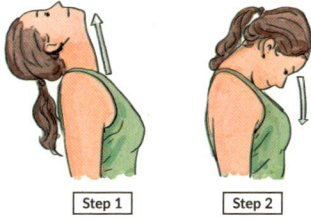

Step 1   Step 2

Duration:

(Goal: 30 sec, alternating)

2. Side Neck Tilt

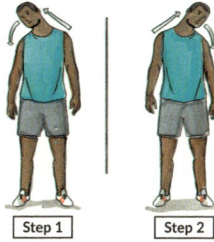

Step 1   Step 2

Duration:

(Goal: 15 sec each side)

3. Forward & Backward Neck Tilt

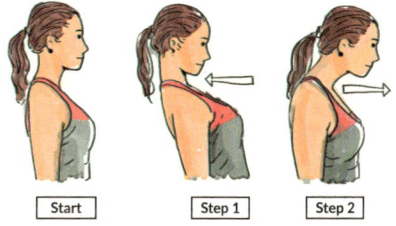

Start   Step 1   Step 2

Duration:

(Goal: 30 sec, alternating)

4. Child's Pose

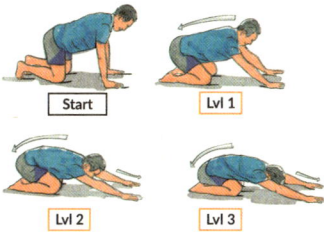

Start   Lvl 1
Lvl 2   Lvl 3

Duration:

(Goal: 60 sec)   Level:

5. Cat-Cow

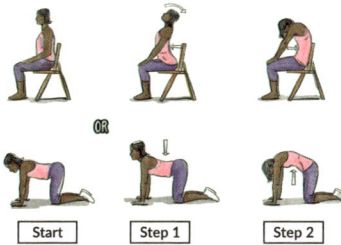

OR

Start   Step 1   Step 2

Duration:

(Goal: 30 sec, alternating)

6. Seated Spinal Twist

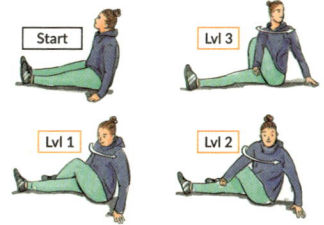

Start   Lvl 3
Lvl 1   Lvl 2

Duration:

(Goal: 15 sec each side)   Level:

7. Leaning Long Arm Shoulder Stretch

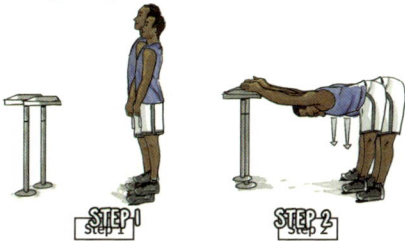

STEP 1   STEP 2

Duration: *(Goal: 30 sec)*

8. Floor Angel

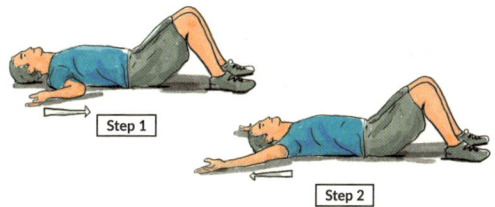

Step 1

Step 2

Duration: *(Goal: 30 sec, alternating)*

9. Behind the Back Elbow to Elbow Grip

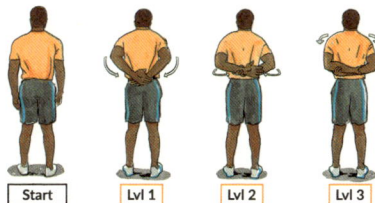

Start   Lvl 1   Lvl 2   Lvl 3   Level:

Duration: *(Goal: 30 sec)*

10. Locust Pose

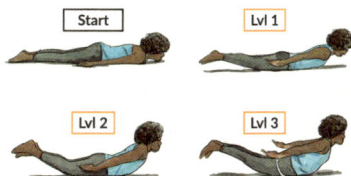

Start   Lvl 1
Lvl 2   Lvl 3

Level:

Duration: *(Goal: 30 sec)*

Day 40: Lower Body

1. Runner's Lunge

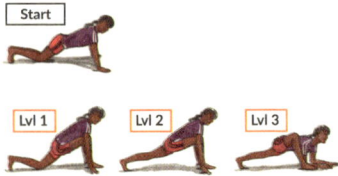

Duration:

(Goal: 30 sec each side) Level:

2. Lying Hip Extension

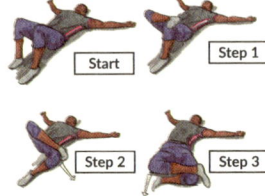

Duration:

(Goal: 30 sec each side)

3. Butterfly

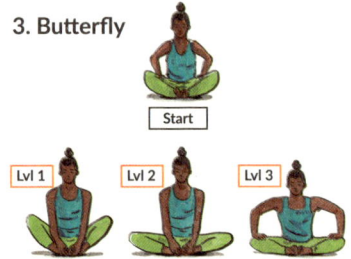

Duration:

(Goal: 30 sec) Level:

4. Scorpion Pose

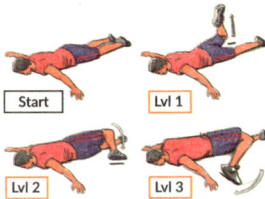

Duration:

(Goal: 30 sec each side) Level:

5. Happy Baby Pose

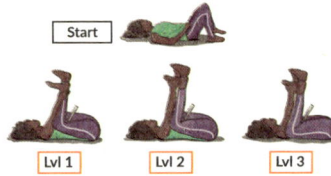

Duration:

(Goal: 30 sec) Level:

6. Pigeon Stretch

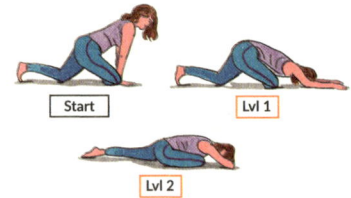

Duration:

(Goal: 30 sec each side) Level:

7. Figure 4

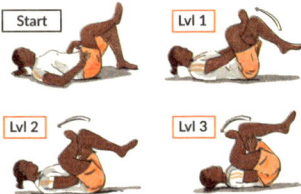

Duration:

(Goal: 30 sec each side) Level:

8. Halfway Center Split

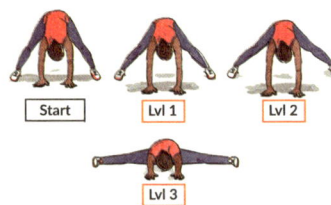

Duration:

(Goal: 30 sec) Level:

9. Lying Hamstring Extension

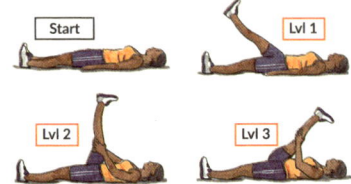

Duration:

(Goal: 30 sec each side) Level:

10. Seated Forward Fold Hamstring Stretch

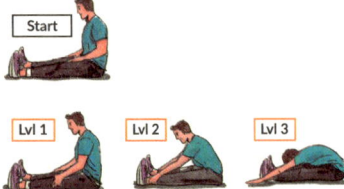

Duration:

(Goal: 30 sec) Level:

11. Lying Quad Stretch

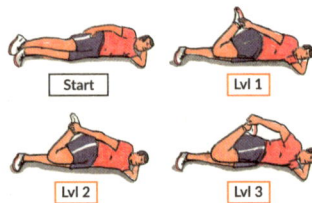

Duration:

(Goal: 30 sec each side) Level:

12. Standing Wall Calf Stretch w/ Achilles Focus

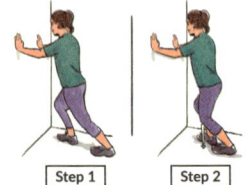

Duration:

(Goal: 15 sec each side)

Daily Reflection

Benefits I'm Experiencing:

Feel
Lighter

More Freedom
of Movement

Improved
Mental Clarity

Less
Pain

Less
Stressed

Improved
Posture

Notes On My Body:

What's the actual real-life difference between days you stretch vs. days you don't stretch? It could be something as simple as feeling accomplished for getting something done that you know is important.

Day 41: Dynamic Warm-Up

Full Session Exercise Guide:
habitnest.com/pages/stretching-day-41

1. Standing Hamstring Scoop

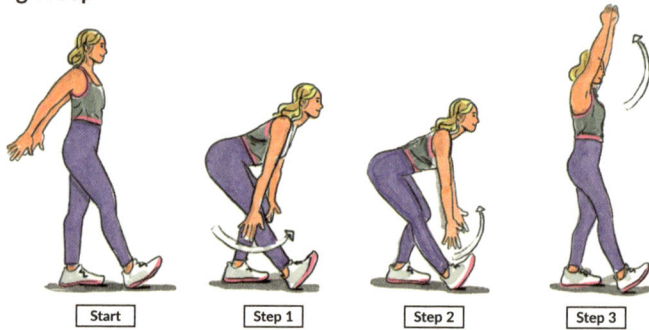

| Start | Step 1 | Step 2 | Step 3 |

Reps: .... *(Goal: 10-20 each side)*

2. Good Morning

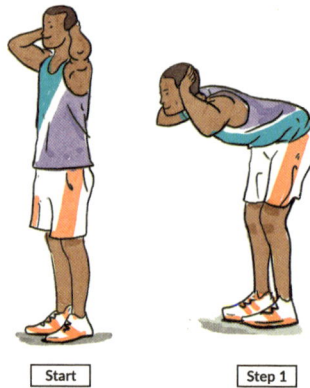

| Start | Step 1 |

Reps: .... *(Goal: 15-20)*

3. Pike Push-Up

Lvl 1

Lvl 2

Level:

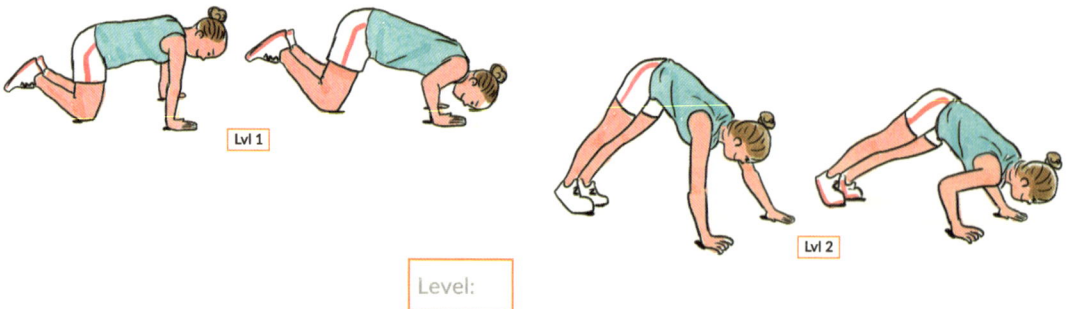

Reps: .... *(Goal: 15-25)*

Day 41: Upper Body

1. Up & Down Neck Tilt

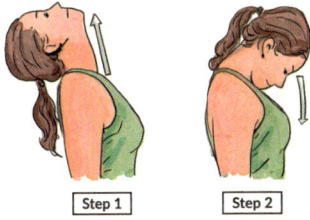

Step 1   Step 2

Duration:
....
(Goal: 30 sec, alternating)

2. Side Neck Tilt

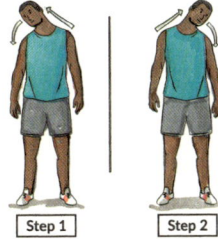

Step 1   Step 2

Duration:
....
(Goal: 15 sec each side)

3. Forward & Backward Neck Tilt

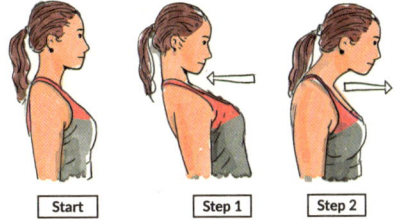

Start   Step 1   Step 2

Duration:
....
(Goal: 30 sec, alternating)

4. Child's Pose

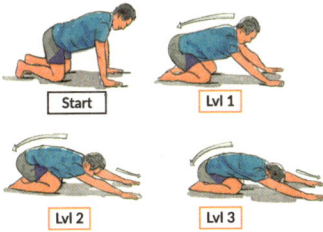

Start   Lvl 1
Lvl 2   Lvl 3

Duration:
....
(Goal: 60 sec)   Level:

5. Cat-Cow

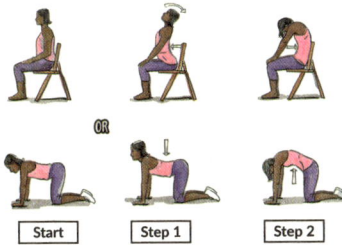

OR

Start   Step 1   Step 2

Duration:
....
(Goal: 30 sec, alternating)

6. Seated Spinal Twist

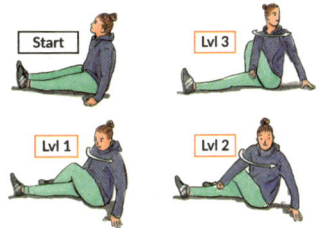

Start   Lvl 3
Lvl 1   Lvl 2

Duration:
....
(Goal: 15 sec each side)   Level:

7. Leaning Long Arm Shoulder Stretch

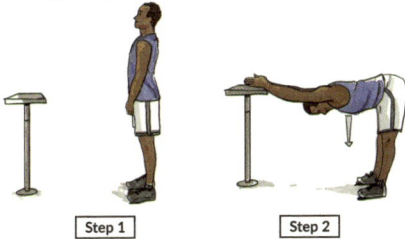

Step 1   Step 2

Duration:
....   *(Goal: 30 sec)*

8. Floor Angel

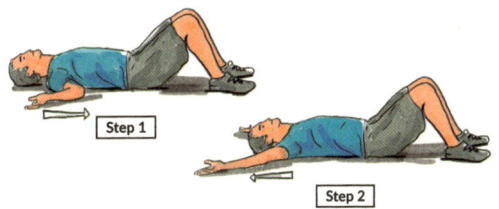

Step 1   Step 2

Duration:
....   *(Goal: 30 sec, alternating)*

9. Behind the Back Elbow to Elbow Grip

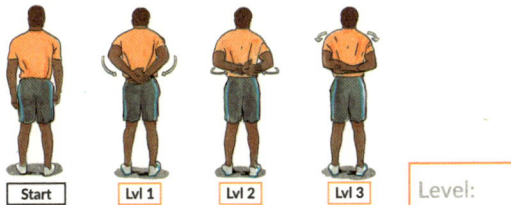

Start   Lvl 1   Lvl 2   Lvl 3   Level:

Duration:
....   *(Goal: 30 sec)*

10. Locust Pose

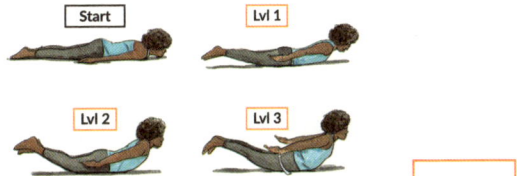

Start   Lvl 1
Lvl 2   Lvl 3

Level:

Duration:
....   *(Goal: 30 sec)*

Day 41: Lower Body

1. Runner's Lunge

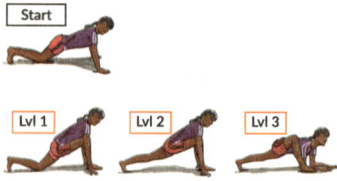

Duration:
....

(Goal: 30 sec each side) Level:

2. Lying Hip Extension

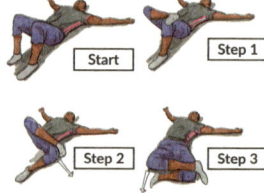

Duration:
....

(Goal: 30 sec each side)

3. Butterfly

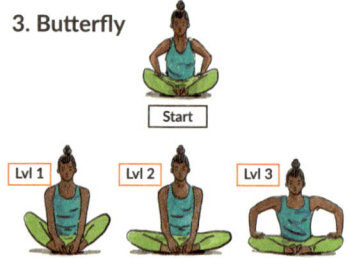

Duration:
....

(Goal: 30 sec) Level:

4. Scorpion Pose

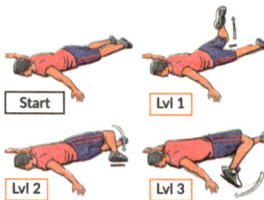

Duration:
....

(Goal: 30 sec each side) Level:

5. Happy Baby Pose

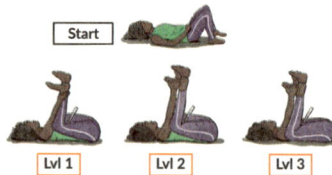

Duration:
....

(Goal: 30 sec) Level:

6. Pigeon Stretch

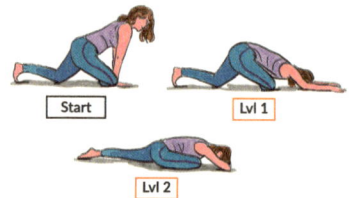

Duration:
....

(Goal: 30 sec each side) Level:

7. Figure 4

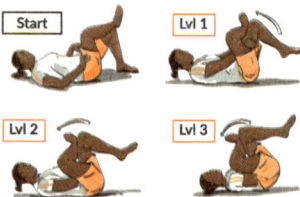

Duration:
....

(Goal: 30 sec each side) Level:

8. Halfway Center Split

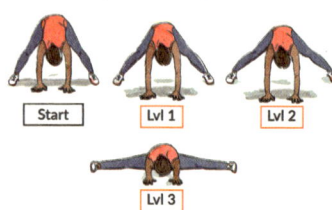

Duration:
....

(Goal: 30 sec) Level:

9. Lying Hamstring Extension

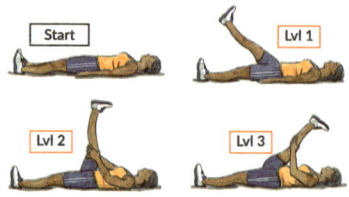

Duration:
....

(Goal: 30 sec each side) Level:

10. Seated Forward Fold Hamstring Stretch

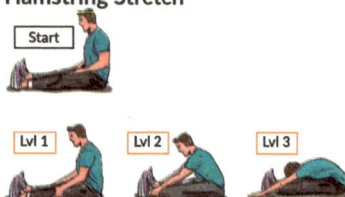

Duration:
....

(Goal: 30 sec) Level:

11. Lying Quad Stretch

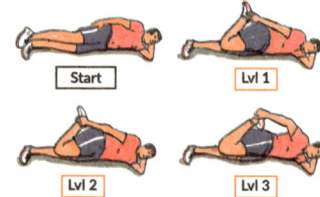

Duration:
....

(Goal: 30 sec each side) Level:

12. Standing Wall Calf Stretch w/ Achilles Focus

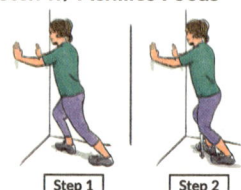

Duration:
....

(Goal: 15 sec each side)

Daily Reflection

Benefits I'm Experiencing:

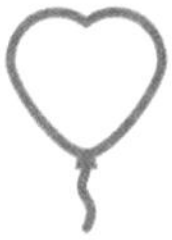

Feel
Lighter

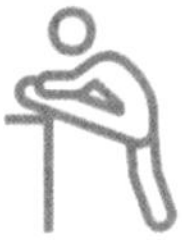

More Freedom
of Movement

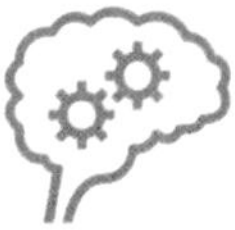

Improved
Mental Clarity

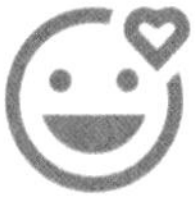

Less
Pain

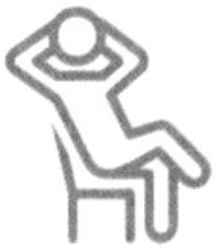

Less
Stressed

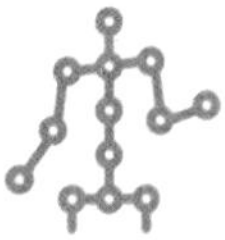

Improved
Posture

Notes On My Body:

1. Knee Hug

Start   Step 1   Step 2

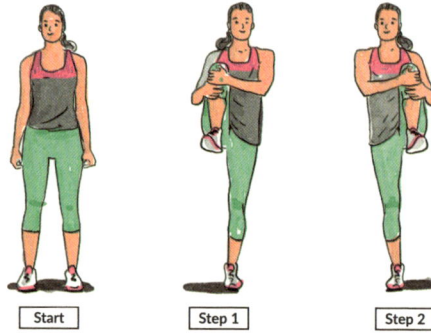

Reps: *(Goal: 10-15 each side)*

2. Low Lunge w/ Elbow Twist

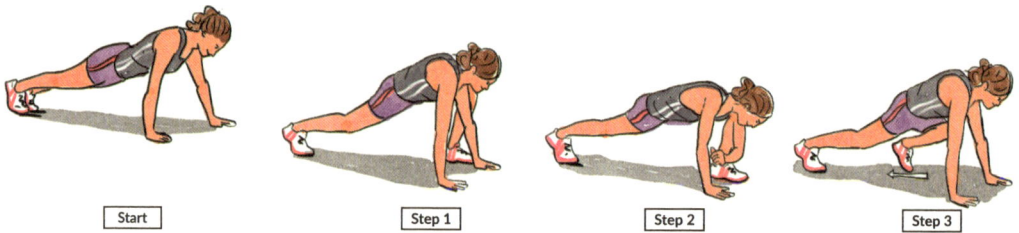

Start   Step 1   Step 2   Step 3

Reps: *(Goal: 10-15 in each direction)*

3. Y Raise

Step 1   Step 2

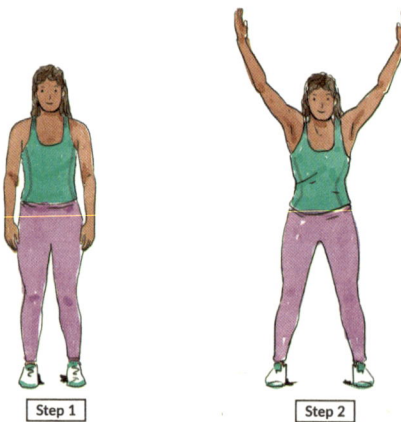

Reps: *(Goal: 15-25)*

Day 42: Upper Body

1. Up & Down Neck Tilt

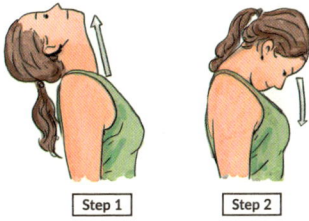

Step 1   Step 2

Duration:

(Goal: 30 sec, alternating)

2. Side Neck Tilt

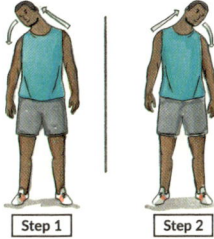

Step 1   Step 2

Duration:

(Goal: 15 sec each side)

3. Forward & Backward Neck Tilt

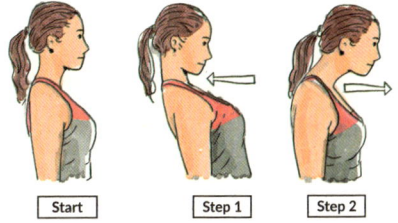

Start   Step 1   Step 2

Duration:

(Goal: 30 sec, alternating)

4. Child's Pose

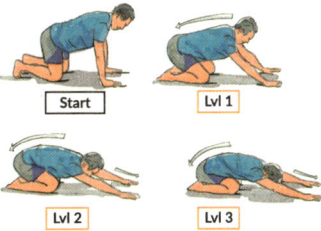

Start   Lvl 1   Lvl 2   Lvl 3

Duration:

(Goal: 60 sec)   Level:

5. Cat-Cow

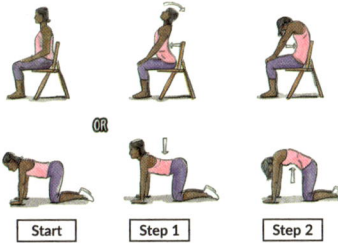

OR

Start   Step 1   Step 2

Duration:

(Goal: 30 sec, alternating)

6. Seated Spinal Twist

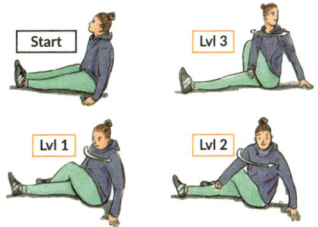

Start   Lvl 3   Lvl 1   Lvl 2

Duration:

(Goal: 15 sec each side)   Level:

7. Leaning Long Arm Shoulder Stretch

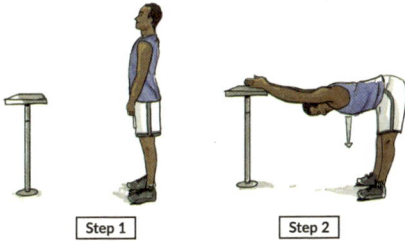

Step 1   Step 2

Duration: *(Goal: 30 sec)*

8. Floor Angel

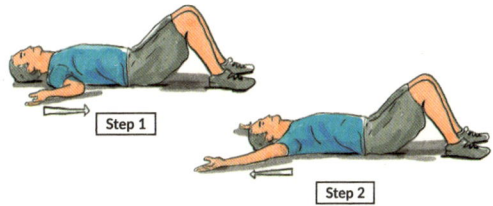

Step 1   Step 2

Duration: *(Goal: 30 sec, alternating)*

9. Behind the Back Elbow to Elbow Grip

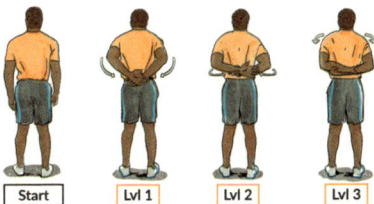

Start   Lvl 1   Lvl 2   Lvl 3   Level:

Duration: *(Goal: 30 sec)*

10. Locust Pose

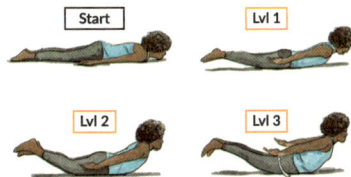

Start   Lvl 1   Lvl 2   Lvl 3   Level:

Duration: *(Goal: 30 sec)*

Day 42: Lower Body

1. Runner's Lunge

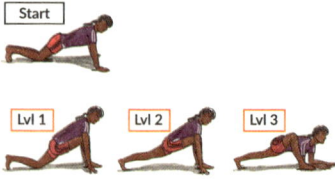

Duration:

(Goal: 30 sec each side)   Level:

2. Lying Hip Extension

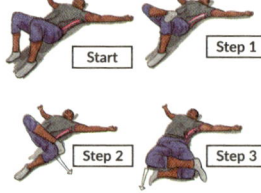

Duration:

(Goal: 30 sec each side)

3. Butterfly

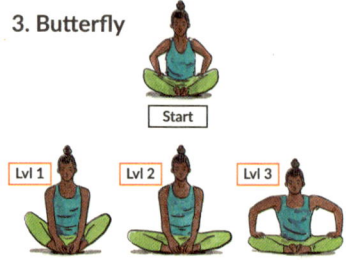

Duration:

(Goal: 30 sec)   Level:

4. Scorpion Pose

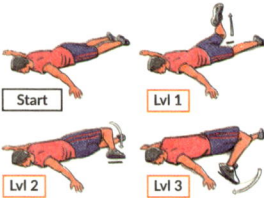

Duration:

(Goal: 30 sec each side)   Level:

5. Happy Baby Pose

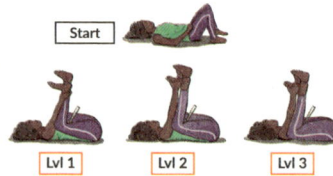

Duration:

(Goal: 30 sec)   Level:

6. Pigeon Stretch

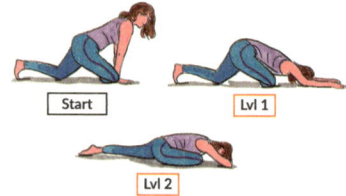

Duration:

(Goal: 30 sec each side)   Level:

7. Figure 4

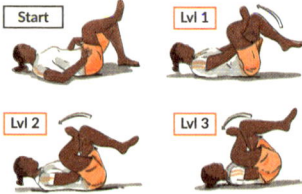

Duration:

(Goal: 30 sec each side)   Level:

8. Halfway Center Split

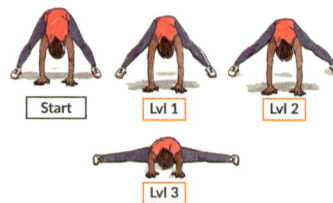

Duration:

(Goal: 30 sec)   Level:

9. Lying Hamstring Extension

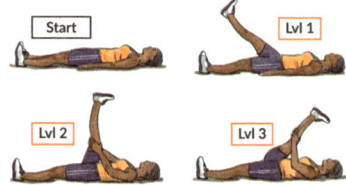

Duration:

(Goal: 30 sec each side)   Level:

10. Seated Forward Fold Hamstring Stretch

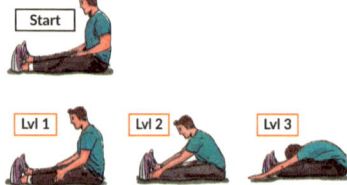

Duration:

(Goal: 30 sec)   Level:

11. Lying Quad Stretch

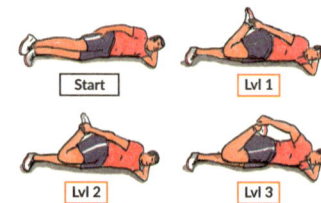

Duration:

(Goal: 30 sec each side)   Level:

12. Standing Wall Calf Stretch w/ Achilles Focus

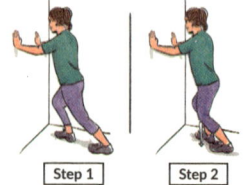

Duration:

(Goal: 15 sec each side)

Daily Reflection

Benefits I'm Experiencing:

Feel Lighter	More Freedom of Movement	Improved Mental Clarity
Less Pain	Less Stressed	Improved Posture

Notes On My Body:

Day 43: Dynamic Warm-Up

Full Session Exercise Guide:
habitnest.com/pages/stretching-day-43

1. World's Greatest Stretch

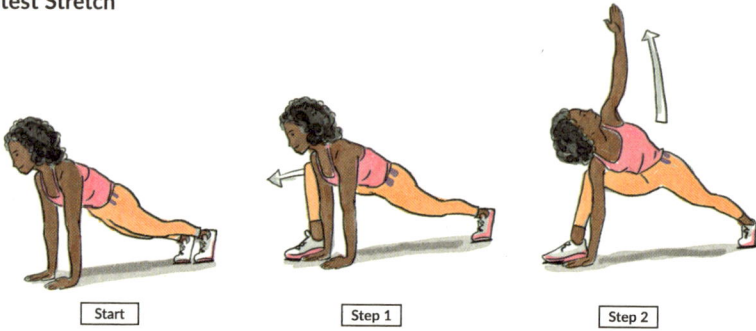

Start

Step 1

Step 2

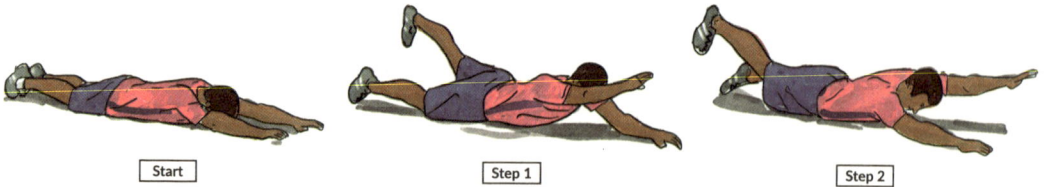

Reps: _(Goal: 10-20)_

2. Air Squat to Calf Raise

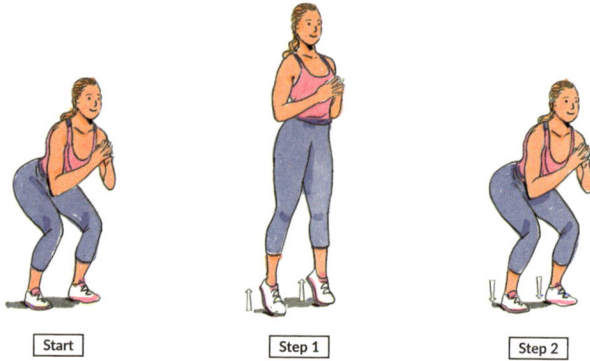

Start

Step 1

Step 2

Reps: _(Goal: 20-30)_

3. Aquaman

Start

Step 1

Step 2

Reps: _(Goal: 10-20)_

Day 43: Upper Body

1. Lateral Side to Side Neck Rotation

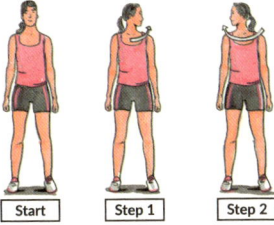

Start | Step 1 | Step 2

Duration:

(Goal: 30 sec, alternating)

2. Side Neck Stretch w/ Upside Down Palm on Wall

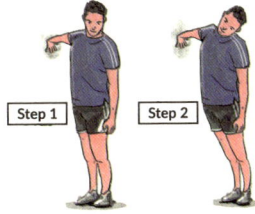

Step 1 | Step 2

Duration:

(Goal: 15 sec each side)

3. Levator Scap Neck Stretch

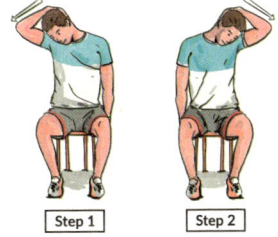

Step 1 | Step 2

Duration:

(Goal: 15 sec each side)

4. Sphinx/Cobra

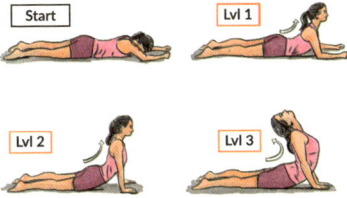

Start | Lvl 1 | Lvl 2 | Lvl 3

Duration:

(Goal: 30 sec)

Level:

5. Seated Forward Curl

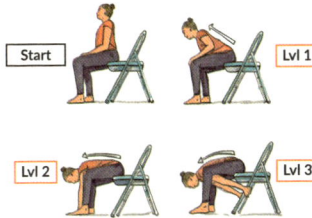

Start | Lvl 1 | Lvl 2 | Lvl 3

Duration:

(Goal: 30 sec)

Level:

6. Wall Lat Stretch

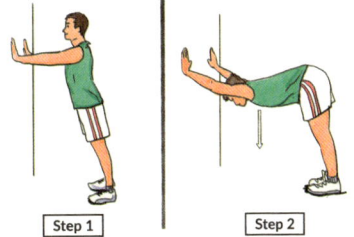

Step 1 | Step 2

Duration:

(Goal: 15 sec)

7. Static Y Hold

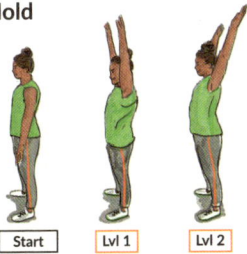

Start | Lvl 1 | Lvl 2

Level:

(Goal: 30 sec)

Duration:

8. Reverse Prayer

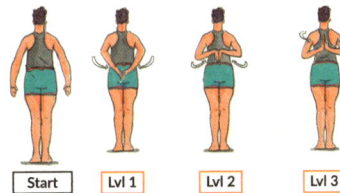

Start | Lvl 1 | Lvl 2 | Lvl 3

Level:

(Goal: 30 sec)

Duration:

9. Elbow Opener

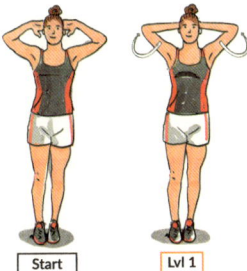

Start | Lvl 1

Duration:

(Goal: 30 sec)

10. Forearm Stretch w/ Hands on Surface

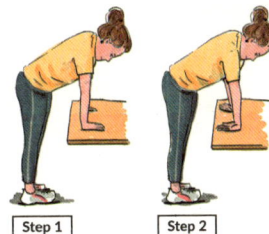

Step 1 | Step 2

Duration:

(Goal: 15 sec each side)

Day 43: Lower Body

1. Frog Pose

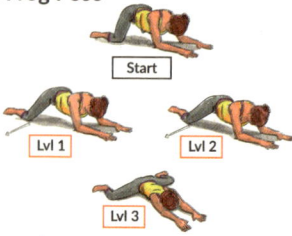

Start
Lvl 1
Lvl 2
Lvl 3

Duration:

(Goal: 60 sec)

Level:

2. Reclining Angle Bound Pose

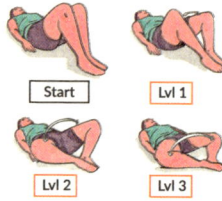

Start
Lvl 1
Lvl 2
Lvl 3

Duration:

(Goal: 30 sec)

Level:

3. Reverse Tabletop

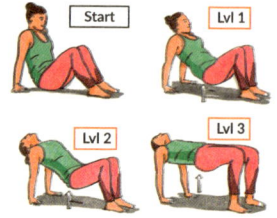

Start
Lvl 1
Lvl 2
Lvl 3

Duration:

(Goal: 30 sec)

Level:

4. Warrior II Pose

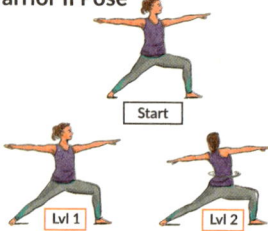

Start
Lvl 1
Lvl 2

Duration:

(Goal: 30 sec each side)

Level:

5. Pry Squat

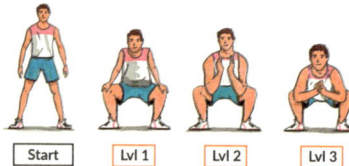

Start
Lvl 1
Lvl 2
Lvl 3

Duration:

(Goal: 30 sec)

Level:

6. Seated Forward Fold Hamstring Stretch

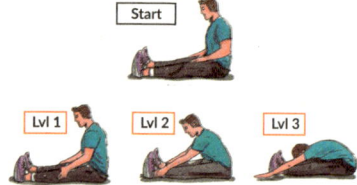

Start
Lvl 1
Lvl 2
Lvl 3

Duration:

(Goal: 30 sec)

Level:

7. Lateral Squat

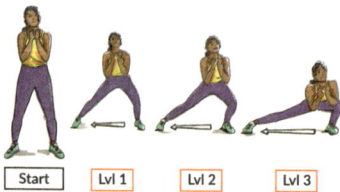

Start
Lvl 1
Lvl 2
Lvl 3

Duration:

(Goal: 30 sec each side)

Level:

8. Lateral Squat w/ Toe Raise

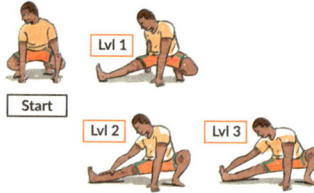

Lvl 1
Start
Lvl 2
Lvl 3

Duration:

(Goal: 30 sec each side)

Level:

9. Wig-Wag

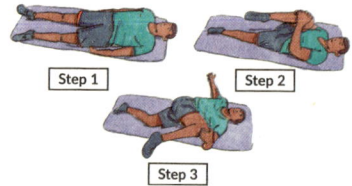

Step 1
Step 2
Step 3

Duration:

(Goal: 30 sec each side)

10. Knee to Chest Stretch

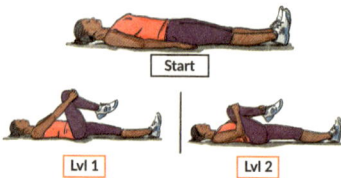

Start
Lvl 1
Lvl 2

Duration:

(Goal: 30 sec each side)

Level:

11. Prone Quad Stretch

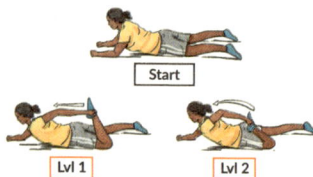

Start
Lvl 1
Lvl 2

Duration:

(Goal: 30 sec each side)

Level:

12. Standing Wall Calf Stretch

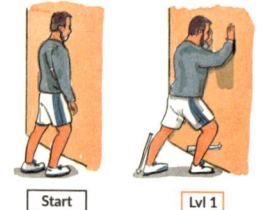

Start
Lvl 1

Duration:

(Goal: 15 sec each side)

Daily Reflection

Benefits I'm Experiencing:

Feel
Lighter

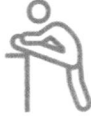

More Freedom
of Movement

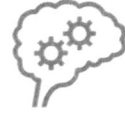

Improved
Mental Clarity

Less
Pain

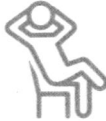

Less
Stressed

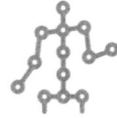

Improved
Posture

Notes On My Body:

Day 44: Dynamic Warm-Up

Full Session Exercise Guide:
habitnest.com/pages/stretching-day-44

1. Inch Worm Walk Out

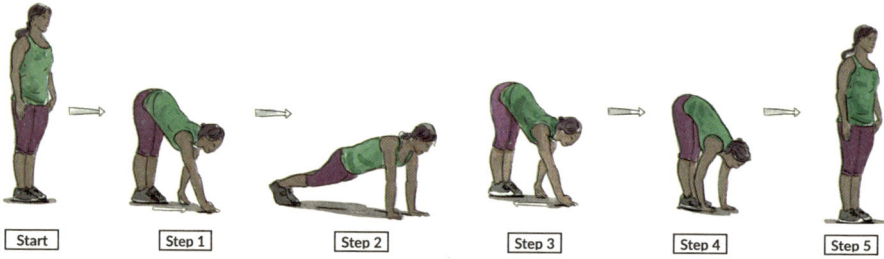

Start | Step 1 | Step 2 | Step 3 | Step 4 | Step 5

Reps: _____ (Goal: 10-20)

2. Plank w/ Shoulder Tap

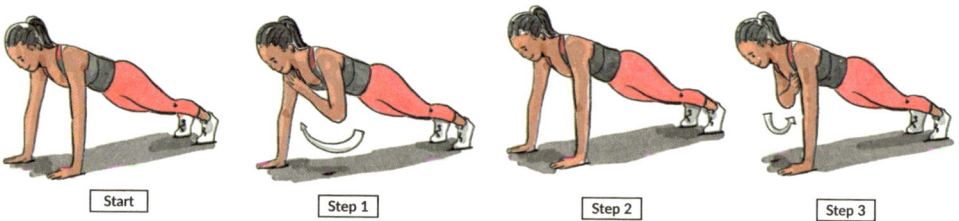

Start | Step 1 | Step 2 | Step 3

Reps: _____ (Goal: 10-20 each side)

3. Rocking Feet w/ Arm Raise

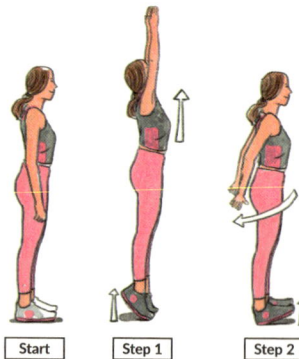

Start | Step 1 | Step 2

Reps: _____ (Goal: 10-20 in each direction)

Day 44: Upper Body

1. Lateral Side to Side Neck Rotation

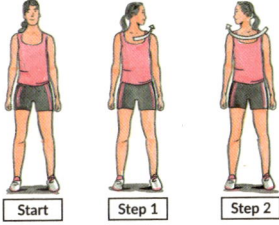

Start | Step 1 | Step 2

Duration:

(Goal: 30 sec, alternating)

2. Side Neck Stretch w/ Upside Down Palm on Wall

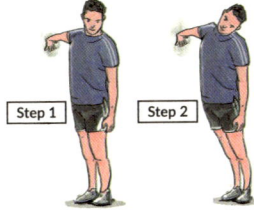

Step 1 | Step 2

Duration:

(Goal: 15 sec each side)

3. Levator Scap Neck Stretch

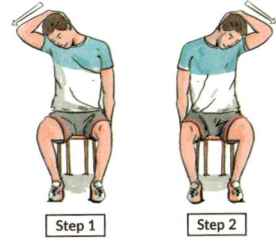

Step 1 | Step 2

Duration:

(Goal: 15 sec each side)

4. Sphinx/Cobra

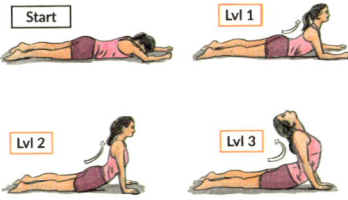

Start | Lvl 1 | Lvl 2 | Lvl 3

Duration:

(Goal: 30 sec)   Level:

5. Seated Forward Curl

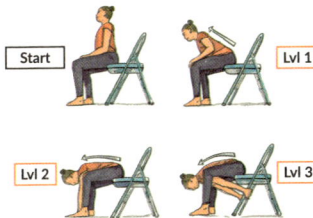

Start | Lvl 1 | Lvl 2 | Lvl 3

Duration:

(Goal: 30 sec)   Level:

6. Wall Lat Stretch

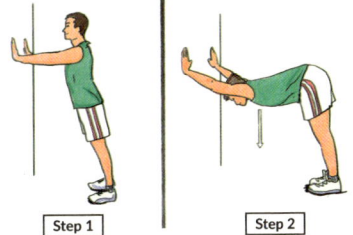

Step 1 | Step 2

Duration:

(Goal: 30 sec)

7. Static Y Hold

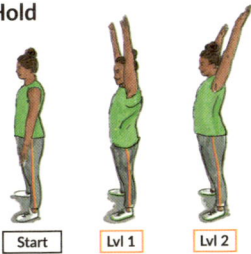

Start | Lvl 1 | Lvl 2

Level:

Duration:

(Goal: 30 sec)

8. Reverse Prayer

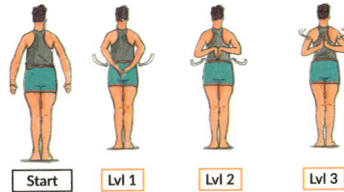

Start | Lvl 1 | Lvl 2 | Lvl 3

Level:

Duration:

(Goal: 30 sec)

9. Elbow Opener

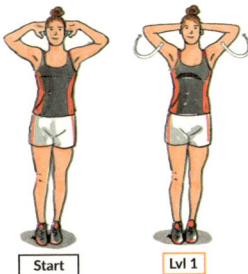

Start | Lvl 1

Duration:

(Goal: 30 sec)

10. Forearm Stretch w/ Hands on Surface

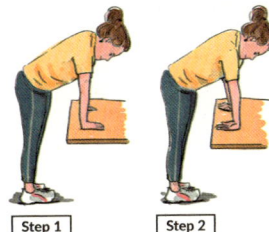

Step 1 | Step 2

Duration:

(Goal: 15 sec each side)

Day 44: Lower Body

1. Frog Pose
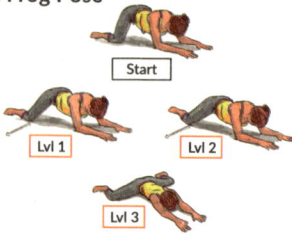

Duration:

(Goal: 60 sec)

Level:

2. Reclining Angle Bound Pose
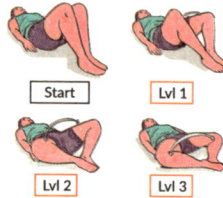

Duration:

(Goal: 30 sec)

Level:

3. Reverse Tabletop
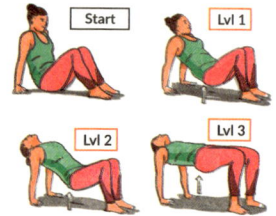

Duration:

(Goal: 30 sec)

Level:

4. Warrior II Pose
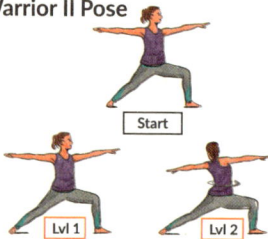

Duration:

(Goal: 30 sec each side)

Level:

5. Pry Squat
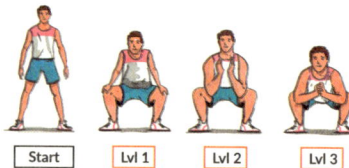

Duration:

(Goal: 30 sec)

Level:

6. Seated Forward Fold Hamstring Stretch
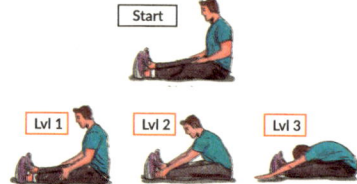

Duration:

(Goal: 30 sec)

Level:

7. Lateral Squat
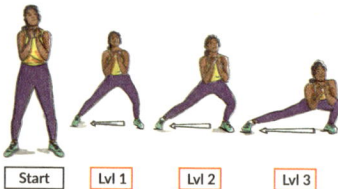

Duration:

(Goal: 30 sec each side)

Level:

8. Lateral Squat w/ Toe Raise
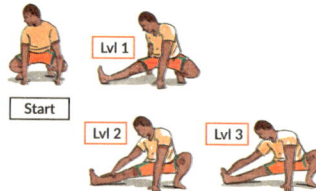

Duration:

(Goal: 30 sec each side)

Level:

9. Wig-Wag
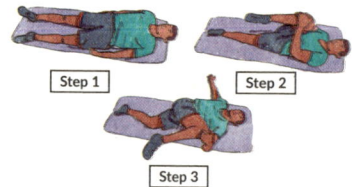

Duration:

(Goal: 30 sec each side)

10. Knee to Chest Stretch
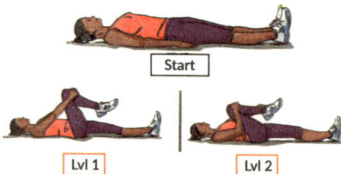

Duration:

(Goal: 30 sec each side)

Level:

11. Prone Quad Stretch
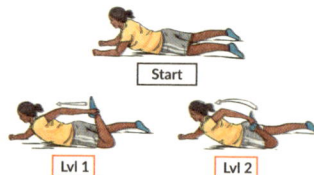

Duration:

(Goal: 30 sec each side)

Level:

12. Standing Wall Calf Stretch
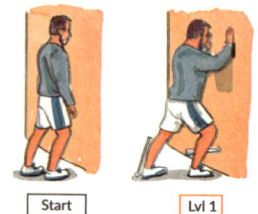

Duration:

(Goal: 15 sec each side)

Daily Reflection

Benefits I'm Experiencing:

Feel Lighter	More Freedom of Movement	Improved Mental Clarity
Less Pain	Less Stressed	Improved Posture

Notes On My Body:

....

....

....

....

....

....

....

....

Do you notice your body starting to become more balanced with regards to asymmetries in your flexibility? What other changes have you noted in your flexibility, mobility, and range of motion?

Day 45: Dynamic Warm-Up

Full Session Exercise Guide:
habitnest.com/pages/stretching-day-45

1. World's Greatest Stretch

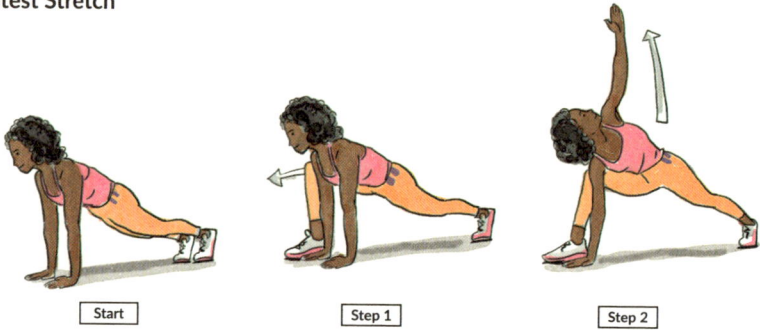

Start | Step 1 | Step 2

Reps: _____ (Goal: 10-20)

2. Good Morning

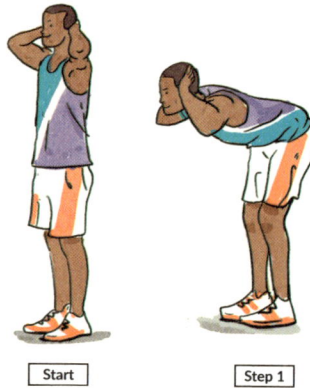

Start | Step 1

Reps: _____ (Goal: 15-20)

3. Standing Hip Circles

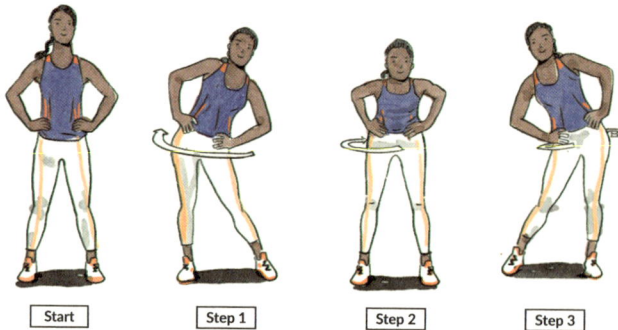

Start | Step 1 | Step 2 | Step 3

Reps: _____ (Goal: 10-15 in each direction)

Day 45: Upper Body

1. Lateral Side to Side Neck Rotation

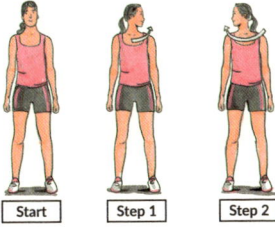

Start | Step 1 | Step 2

Duration:

(Goal: 30 sec, alternating)

2. Side Neck Stretch w/ Upside Down Palm on Wall

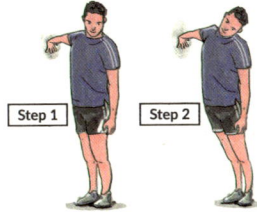

Step 1 | Step 2

Duration:

(Goal: 15 sec each side)

3. Levator Scap Neck Stretch

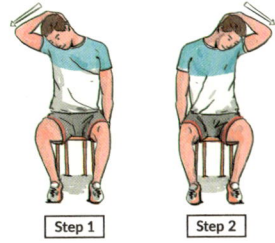

Step 1 | Step 2

Duration:

(Goal: 15 sec each side)

4. Sphinx/Cobra

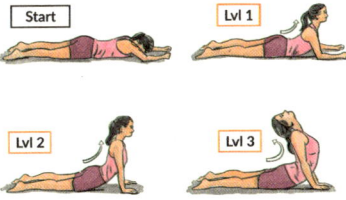

Start | Lvl 1 | Lvl 2 | Lvl 3

Duration:

(Goal: 30 sec)

Level:

5. Seated Forward Curl

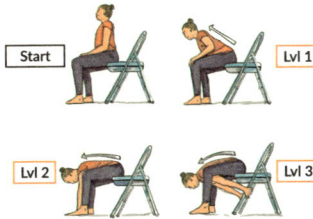

Start | Lvl 1 | Lvl 2 | Lvl 3

Duration:

(Goal: 30 sec)

Level:

6. Wall Lat Stretch

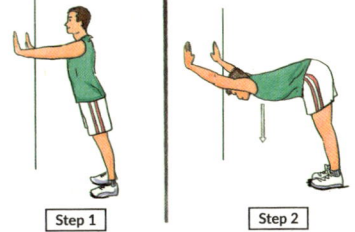

Step 1 | Step 2

Duration:

(Goal: 30 sec)

7. Static Y Hold

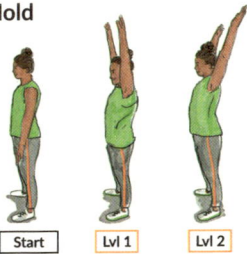

Start | Lvl 1 | Lvl 2

Level:

(Goal: 30 sec)

Duration:

8. Reverse Prayer

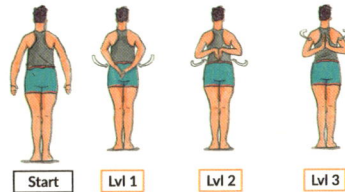

Start | Lvl 1 | Lvl 2 | Lvl 3

Level:

(Goal: 30 sec)

Duration:

9. Elbow Opener

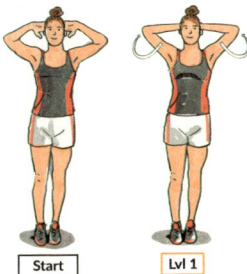

Start | Lvl 1

Duration:

(Goal: 30 sec)

10. Forearm Stretch w/ Hands on Surface

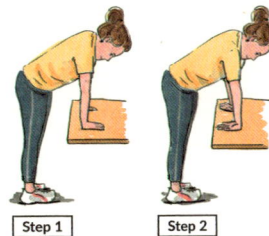

Step 1 | Step 2

Duration:

(Goal: 15 sec each side)

Day 45: Lower Body

1. Frog Pose

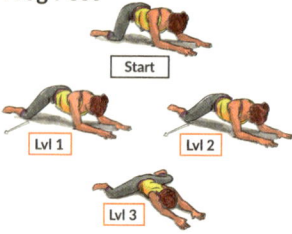

Start
Lvl 1
Lvl 2
Lvl 3

Duration:

(Goal: 60 sec)

Level:

2. Reclining Angle Bound Pose

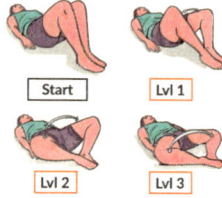

Start
Lvl 1
Lvl 2
Lvl 3

Duration:

(Goal: 30 sec)

Level:

3. Reverse Tabletop

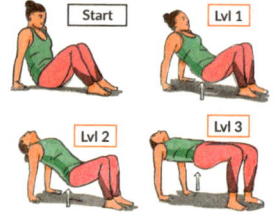

Start
Lvl 1
Lvl 2
Lvl 3

Duration:

(Goal: 30 sec)

Level:

4. Warrior II Pose

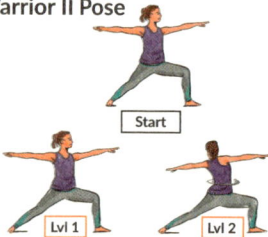

Start
Lvl 1
Lvl 2

Duration:

(Goal: 30 sec each side)

Level:

5. Pry Squat

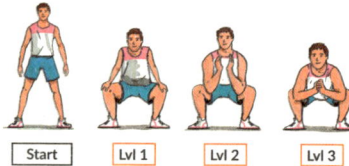

Start
Lvl 1
Lvl 2
Lvl 3

Duration:

(Goal: 30 sec)

Level:

6. Seated Forward Fold Hamstring Stretch

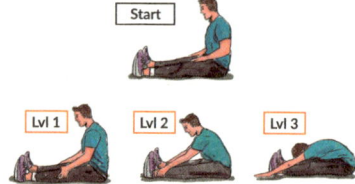

Start
Lvl 1
Lvl 2
Lvl 3

Duration:

(Goal: 30 sec)

Level:

7. Lateral Squat

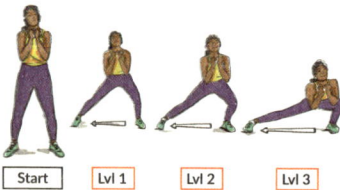

Start
Lvl 1
Lvl 2
Lvl 3

Duration:

(Goal: 30 sec each side)

Level:

8. Lateral Squat w/ Toe Raise

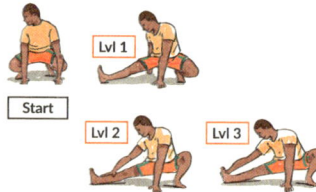

Lvl 1
Start
Lvl 2
Lvl 3

Duration:

(Goal: 30 sec each side)

Level:

9. Wig-Wag

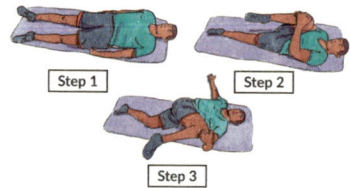

Step 1
Step 2
Step 3

Duration:

(Goal: 30 sec each side)

10. Knee to Chest Stretch

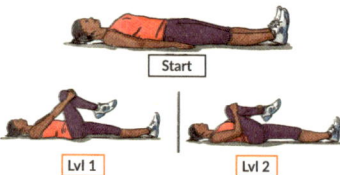

Start
Lvl 1
Lvl 2

Duration:

(Goal: 30 sec each side)

Level:

11. Prone Quad Stretch

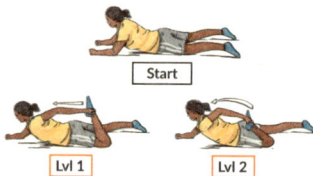

Start
Lvl 1
Lvl 2

Duration:

(Goal: 30 sec each side)

Level:

12. Standing Wall Calf Stretch

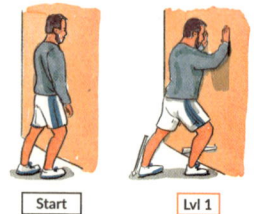

Start
Lvl 1

Duration:

(Goal: 15 sec each side)

Daily Reflection

Benefits I'm Experiencing:

Feel
Lighter

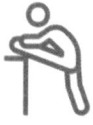

More Freedom
of Movement

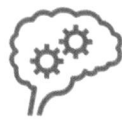

Improved
Mental Clarity

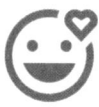

Less
Pain

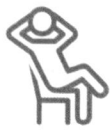

Less
Stressed

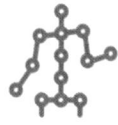

Improved
Posture

Notes On My Body:

Day 46: Dynamic Warm-Up

Full Session Exercise Guide:
habitnest.com/pages/stretching-day-46

1. Inch Worm Walk Out

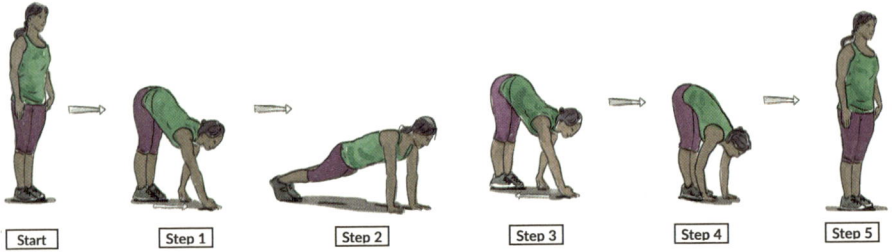

Start   Step 1   Step 2   Step 3   Step 4   Step 5

Reps: .... *(Goal: 10-20)*

2. Air Squat to Calf Raise

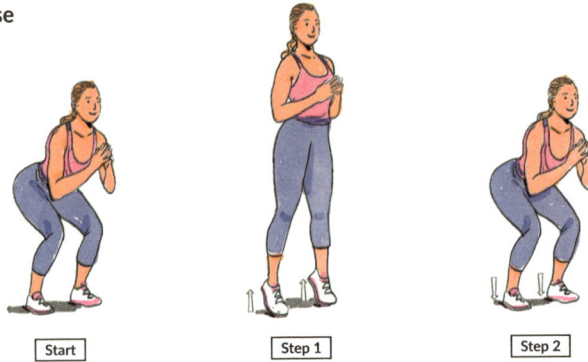

Start   Step 1   Step 2

Reps: .... *(Goal: 20-30)*

3. Push-Up

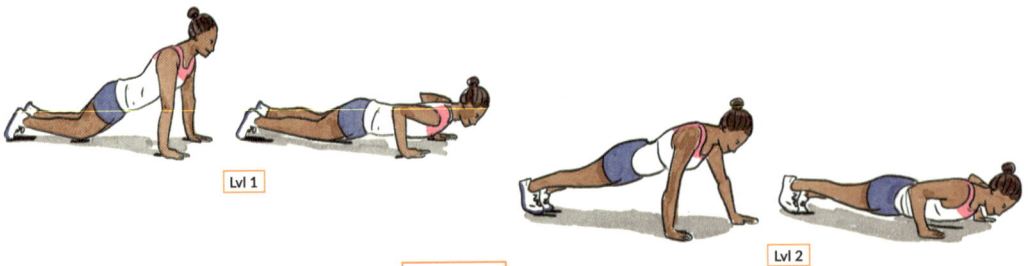

Lvl 1   Lvl 2

Level:

Reps: .... *(Goal: 15-25)*

Day 46: Upper Body

1. Lateral Side to Side Neck Rotation

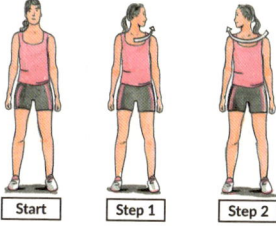

Start | Step 1 | Step 2

Duration:

(Goal: 30 sec, alternating)

2. Side Neck Stretch w/ Upside Down Palm on Wall

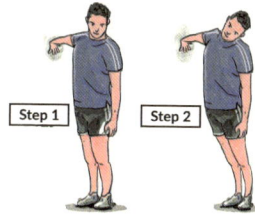

Step 1 | Step 2

Duration:

(Goal: 15 sec each side)

3. Levator Scap Neck Stretch

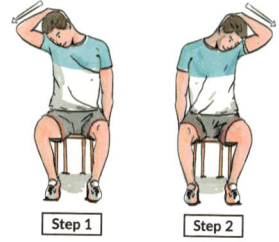

Step 1 | Step 2

Duration:

(Goal: 15 sec each side)

4. Sphinx/Cobra

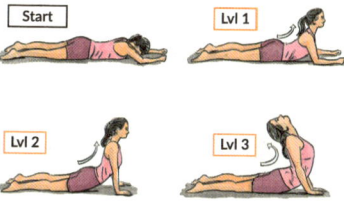

Start | Lvl 1
Lvl 2 | Lvl 3

Duration:

(Goal: 30 sec)

Level:

5. Seated Forward Curl

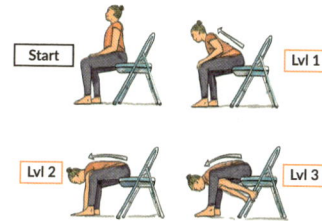

Start | Lvl 1
Lvl 2 | Lvl 3

Duration:

(Goal: 30 sec)

Level:

6. Wall Lat Stretch

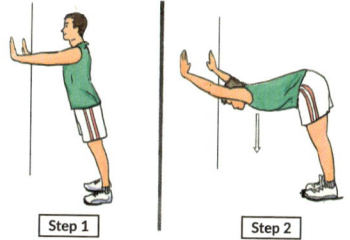

Step 1 | Step 2

Duration:

(Goal: 30 sec)

7. Static Y Hold

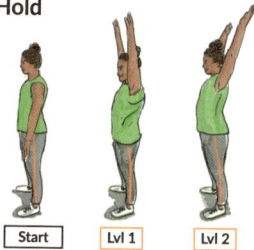

Start | Lvl 1 | Lvl 2

Level:

Duration:

(Goal: 30 sec)

8. Reverse Prayer

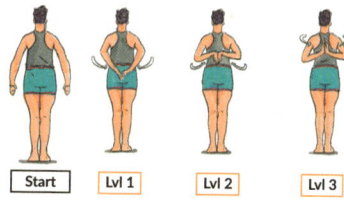

Start | Lvl 1 | Lvl 2 | Lvl 3

Level:

Duration:

(Goal: 30 sec)

9. Elbow Opener

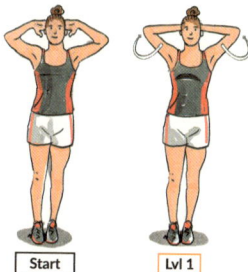

Start | Lvl 1

Duration:

(Goal: 30 sec)

10. Forearm Stretch w/ Hands on Surface

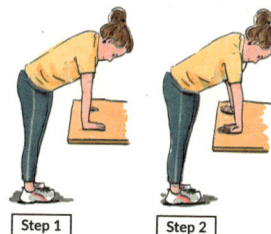

Step 1 | Step 2

Duration:

(Goal: 15 sec each side)

Day 46: Lower Body

1. Frog Pose

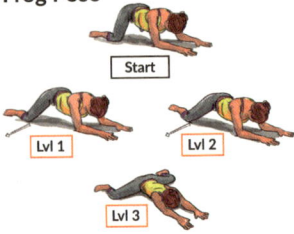

Start
Lvl 1
Lvl 2
Lvl 3

Duration:
....

(Goal: 60 sec)
Level:

2. Reclining Angle Bound Pose

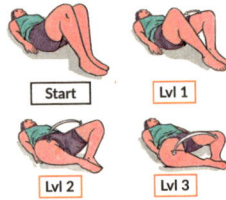

Start
Lvl 1
Lvl 2
Lvl 3

Duration:
....

(Goal: 30 sec)
Level:

3. Reverse Tabletop

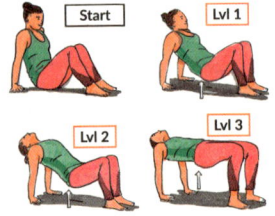

Start
Lvl 1
Lvl 2
Lvl 3

Duration:
....

(Goal: 30 sec)
Level:

4. Warrior II Pose

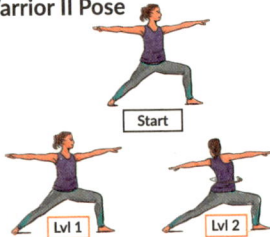

Start
Lvl 1
Lvl 2

Duration:
....

(Goal: 30 sec each side)
Level:

5. Pry Squat

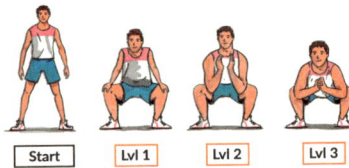

Start
Lvl 1
Lvl 2
Lvl 3

Duration:
....

(Goal: 30 sec)
Level:

6. Seated Forward Fold Hamstring Stretch

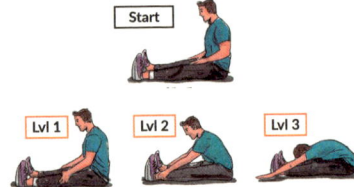

Start
Lvl 1
Lvl 2
Lvl 3

Duration:
....

(Goal: 30 sec)
Level:

7. Lateral Squat

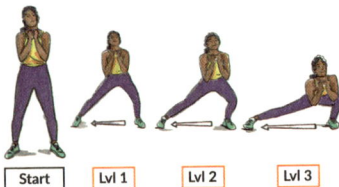

Start
Lvl 1
Lvl 2
Lvl 3

Duration:
....

(Goal: 30 sec each side)
Level:

8. Lateral Squat w/ Toe Raise

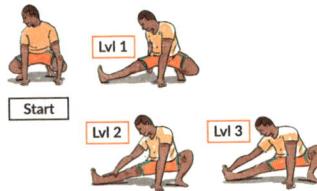

Lvl 1
Start
Lvl 2
Lvl 3

Duration:
....

(Goal: 30 sec each side)
Level:

9. Wig-Wag

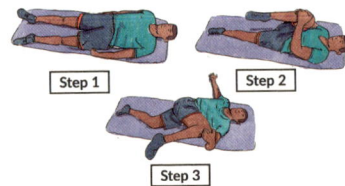

Step 1
Step 2
Step 3

Duration:
....

(Goal: 30 sec each side)

10. Knee to Chest Stretch

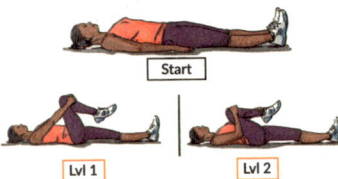

Start
Lvl 1
Lvl 2

Duration:
....

(Goal: 30 sec each side)
Level:

11. Prone Quad Stretch

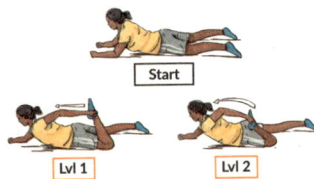

Start
Lvl 1
Lvl 2

Duration:
....

(Goal: 30 sec each side)
Level:

12. Standing Wall Calf Stretch

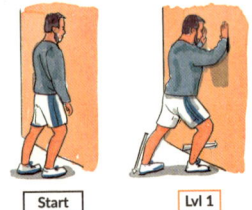

Start
Lvl 1

Duration:
....

(Goal: 15 sec each side)

Daily Reflection

Benefits I'm Experiencing:

Feel
Lighter

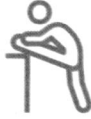

More Freedom
of Movement

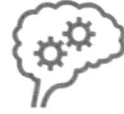

Improved
Mental Clarity

Less
Pain

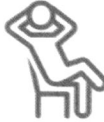

Less
Stressed

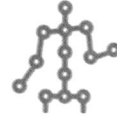

Improved
Posture

Notes On My Body:

Day 47: Dynamic Warm-Up

Full Session Exercise Guide:
habitnest.com/pages/stretching-day-47

1. Pike Push-Up

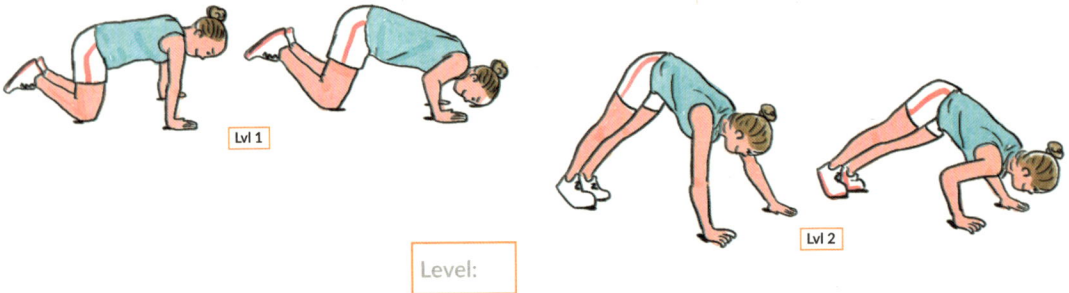

Lvl 1

Lvl 2

Level:

Reps: *(Goal: 15-25)*

2. Clam Opener w/ Side Plank

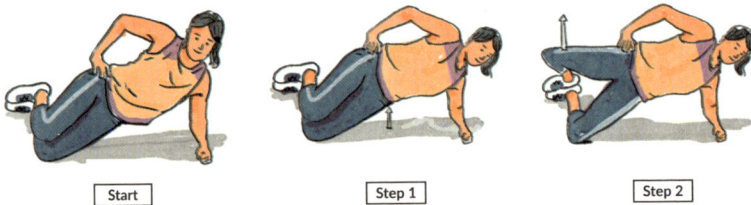

Start

Step 1

Step 2

Reps: *(Goal: 10-15 each side)*

3. Towel Snatch

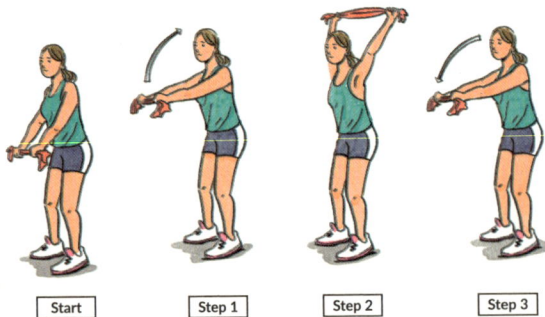

Start

Step 1

Step 2

Step 3

Reps: *(Goal: 10-20)*

Day 47: Upper Body

1. Lateral Side to Side Neck Rotation

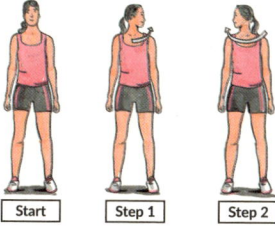

Start   Step 1   Step 2

Duration:

(Goal: 30 sec, alternating)

2. Side Neck Stretch w/ Upside Down Palm on Wall

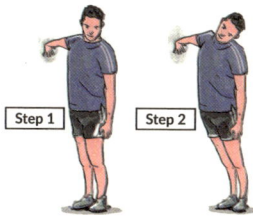

Step 1   Step 2

Duration:

(Goal: 15 sec each side)

3. Levator Scap Neck Stretch

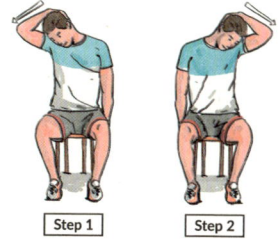

Step 1   Step 2

Duration:

(Goal: 15 sec each side)

4. Sphinx/Cobra

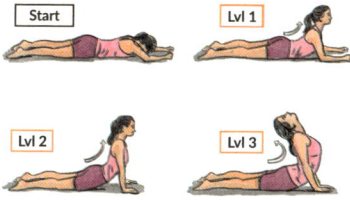

Start   Lvl 1

Lvl 2   Lvl 3

Duration:

(Goal: 30 sec)   Level:

5. Seated Forward Curl

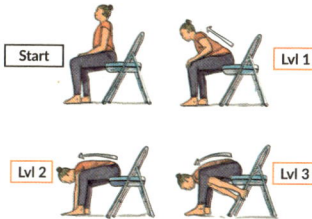

Start   Lvl 1

Lvl 2   Lvl 3

Duration:

(Goal: 30 sec)   Level:

6. Wall Lat Stretch

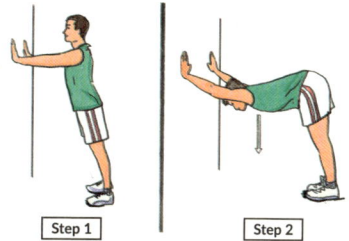

Step 1   Step 2

Duration:

(Goal: 30 sec)

7. Static Y Hold

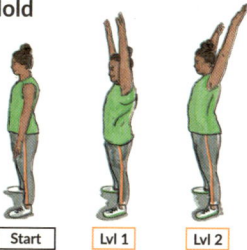

Start   Lvl 1   Lvl 2

Level:

Duration:

(Goal: 30 sec)

8. Reverse Prayer

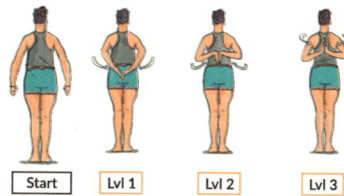

Start   Lvl 1   Lvl 2   Lvl 3

Level:

Duration:

(Goal: 30 sec)

9. Elbow Opener

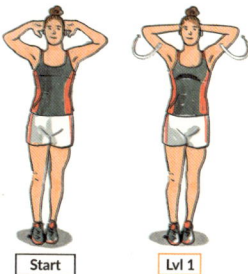

Start   Lvl 1

Duration:

(Goal: 30 sec)

10. Forearm Stretch w/ Hands on Surface

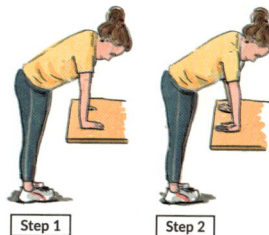

Step 1   Step 2

Duration:

(Goal: 15 sec each side)

Day 47: Lower Body

1. Frog Pose

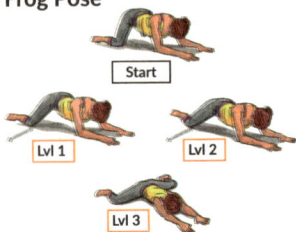
Start
Lvl 1   Lvl 2
Lvl 3

Duration:

(Goal: 60 sec)   Level:

2. Reclining Angle Bound Pose

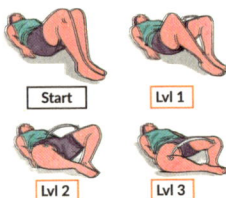
Start   Lvl 1
Lvl 2   Lvl 3

Duration:

(Goal: 30 sec)   Level:

3. Reverse Tabletop

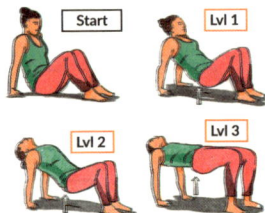
Start   Lvl 1
Lvl 2   Lvl 3

Duration:

(Goal: 30 sec)   Level:

4. Warrior II Pose

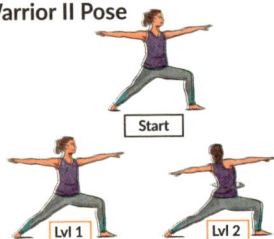
Start
Lvl 1   Lvl 2

Duration:

(Goal: 30 sec each side)   Level:

5. Pry Squat

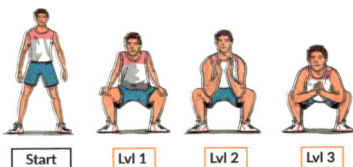
Start   Lvl 1   Lvl 2   Lvl 3

Duration:

(Goal: 30 sec)   Level:

6. Seated Forward Fold Hamstring Stretch

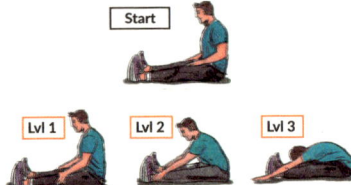
Start
Lvl 1   Lvl 2   Lvl 3

Duration:

(Goal: 30 sec)   Level:

7. Lateral Squat

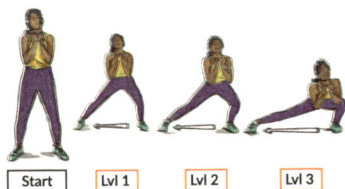
Start   Lvl 1   Lvl 2   Lvl 3

Duration:

(Goal: 30 sec each side)   Level:

8. Lateral Squat w/ Toe Raise

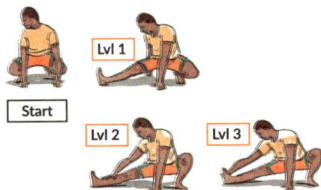
Lvl 1
Start
Lvl 2   Lvl 3

Duration:

(Goal: 30 sec each side)   Level:

9. Wig-Wag

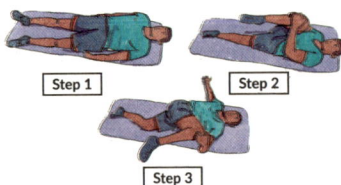
Step 1   Step 2
Step 3

Duration:

(Goal: 30 sec each side)

10. Knee to Chest Stretch

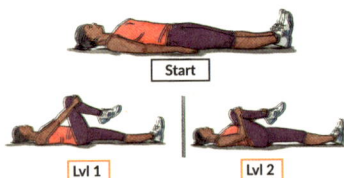
Start
Lvl 1   Lvl 2

Duration:

(Goal: 30 sec each side)   Level:

11. Prone Quad Stretch

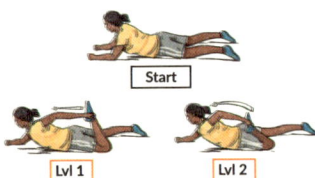
Start
Lvl 1   Lvl 2

Duration:

(Goal: 30 sec each side)   Level:

12. Standing Wall Calf Stretch

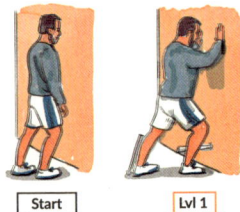
Start   Lvl 1

Duration:

(Goal: 15 sec each side)

236

Daily Reflection

Benefits I'm Experiencing:

Feel
Lighter

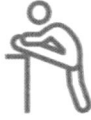

More Freedom
of Movement

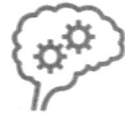

Improved
Mental Clarity

Less
Pain

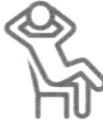

Less
Stressed

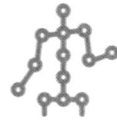

Improved
Posture

Notes On My Body:

How does your body feel immediately after you stretch?
How do you feel mentally and emotionally?

Day 48: Dynamic Warm-Up

Full Session Exercise Guide:
habitnest.com/pages/stretching-day-48

1. World's Greatest Stretch

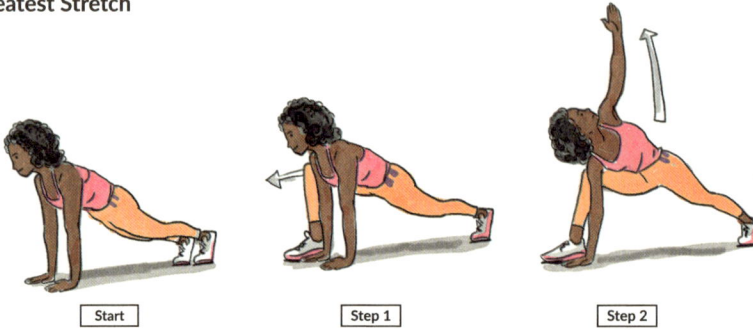

Start

Step 1

Step 2

Reps: *(Goal: 10-20)*

2. Split Squat

Step 1

Step 2

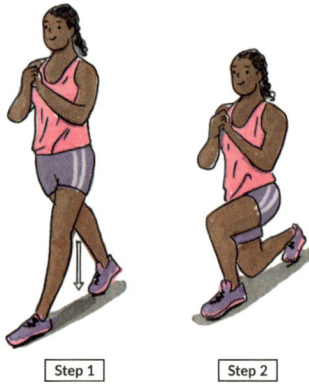

Reps: *(Goal: 15-20 each side)*

3. Bird-Dog

Start

Step 1

Step 2

Step 3

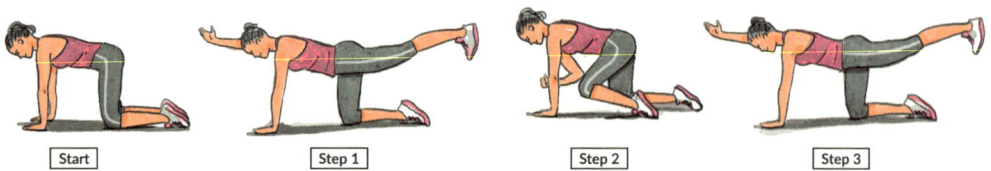

Reps: *(Goal: 10-15 each side)*

Day 48: Upper Body

1. Lateral Side to Side Neck Rotation

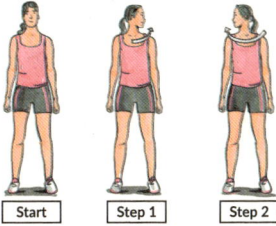

Start | Step 1 | Step 2

Duration:

(Goal: 30 sec, alternating)

2. Side Neck Stretch w/ Upside Down Palm on Wall

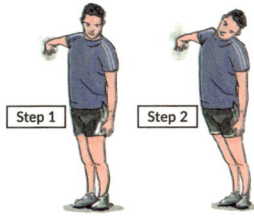

Step 1 | Step 2

Duration:

(Goal: 15 sec each side)

3. Levator Scap Neck Stretch

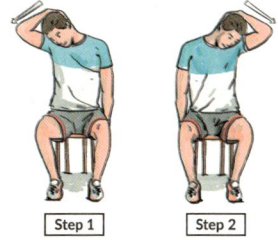

Step 1 | Step 2

Duration:

(Goal: 15 sec each side)

4. Sphinx/Cobra

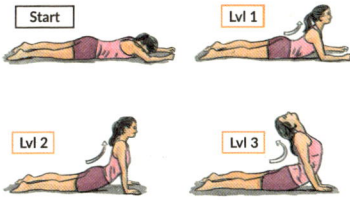

Start | Lvl 1 | Lvl 2 | Lvl 3

Duration:

(Goal: 30 sec)

Level:

5. Seated Forward Curl

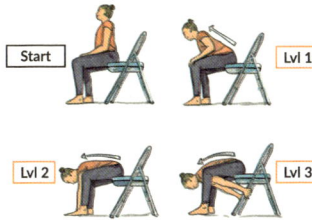

Start | Lvl 1 | Lvl 2 | Lvl 3

Duration:

(Goal: 30 sec)

Level:

6. Wall Lat Stretch

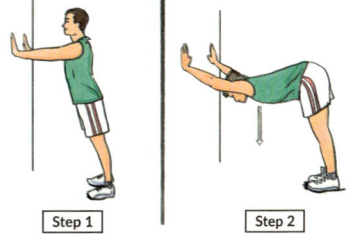

Step 1 | Step 2

Duration:

(Goal: 30 sec)

7. Static Y Hold

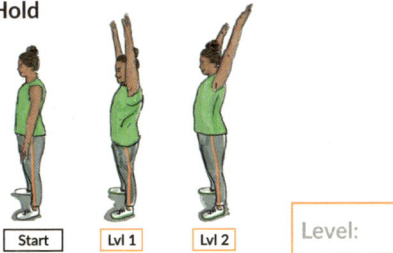

Start | Lvl 1 | Lvl 2

Level:

Duration:

(Goal: 30 sec)

8. Reverse Prayer

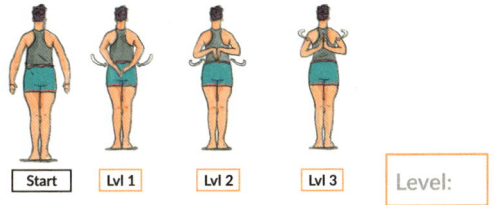

Start | Lvl 1 | Lvl 2 | Lvl 3

Level:

Duration:

(Goal: 30 sec)

9. Elbow Opener

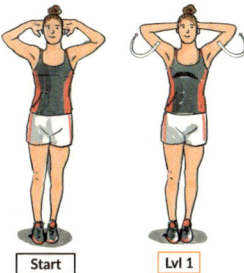

Start | Lvl 1

Duration:

(Goal: 30 sec)

10. Forearm Stretch w/ Hands on Surface

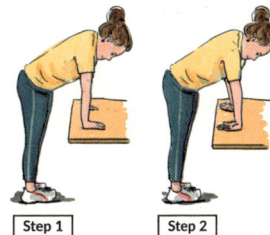

Step 1 | Step 2

Duration:

(Goal: 15 sec each side)

Day 48: Lower Body

1. Frog Pose

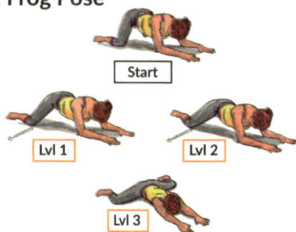

Duration:
....

(Goal: 60 sec)

Level:

2. Reclining Angle Bound Pose

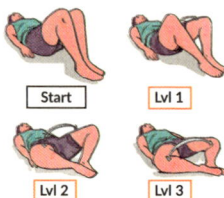

Duration:
....

(Goal: 30 sec)

Level:

3. Reverse Tabletop

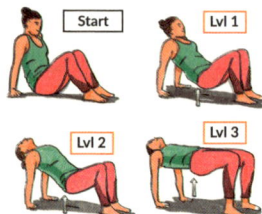

Duration:
....

(Goal: 30 sec)

Level:

4. Warrior II Pose

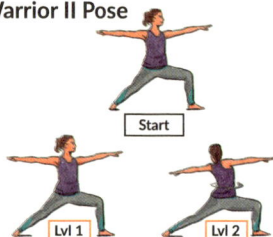

Duration:
....

(Goal: 30 sec each side)

Level:

5. Pry Squat

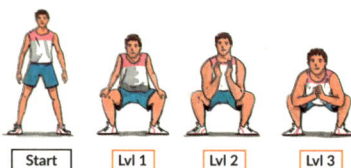

Duration:
....

(Goal: 30 sec)

Level:

6. Seated Forward Fold Hamstring Stretch

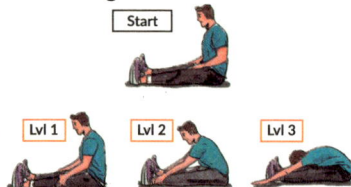

Duration:
....

(Goal: 30 sec)

Level:

7. Lateral Squat

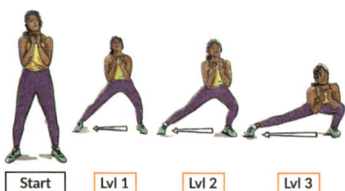

Duration:
....

(Goal: 30 sec each side)

Level:

8. Lateral Squat w/ Toe Raise

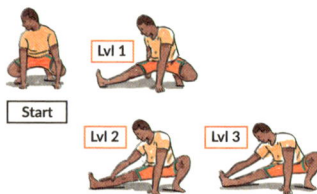

Duration:
....

(Goal: 30 sec each side)

Level:

9. Wig-Wag

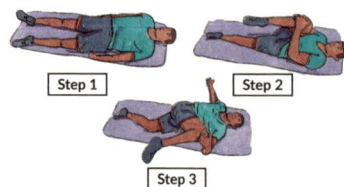

Duration:
....

(Goal: 30 sec each side)

10. Knee to Chest Stretch

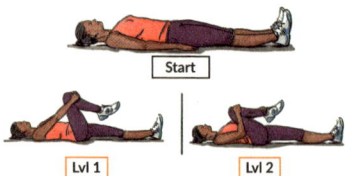

Duration:
....

(Goal: 30 sec each side)

Level:

11. Prone Quad Stretch

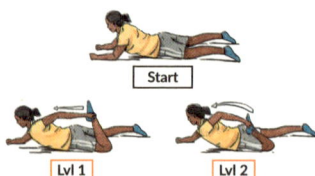

Duration:
....

(Goal: 30 sec each side)

Level:

12. Standing Wall Calf Stretch

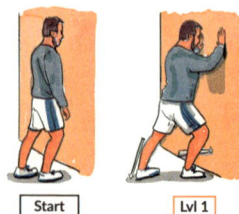

Duration:
....

(Goal: 15 sec each side)

Level:

Daily Reflection

Benefits I'm Experiencing:

Feel
Lighter

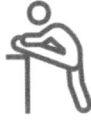

More Freedom
of Movement

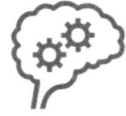

Improved
Mental Clarity

Less
Pain

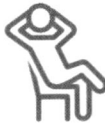

Less
Stressed

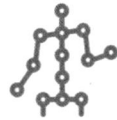

Improved
Posture

Notes On My Body:

....

....

....

....

....

....

....

....

Day 49: Dynamic Warm-Up

Full Session Exercise Guide:
habitnest.com/pages/stretching-day-49

1. Plank w/ Shoulder Tap

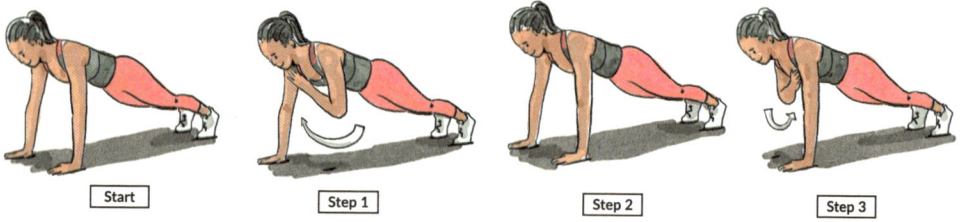

| Start | Step 1 | Step 2 | Step 3 |

Reps: .... *(Goal: 10-20 each side)*

2. Side Plank w/ Twist

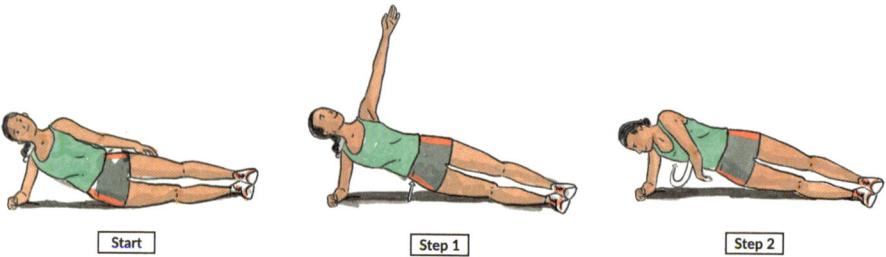

| Start | Step 1 | Step 2 |

Reps: .... *(Goal: 10-15 each side)*

3. Good Morning

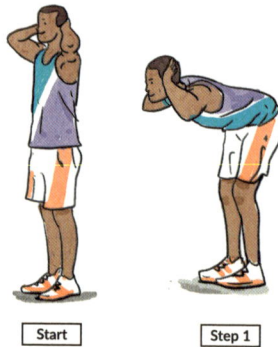

| Start | Step 1 |

Reps: .... *(Goal: 15-20)*

Day 49: Upper Body

1. Lateral Side to Side Neck Rotation

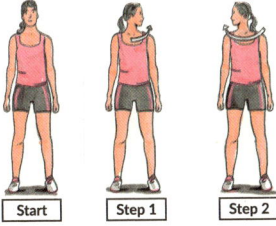

Start | Step 1 | Step 2

Duration:

(Goal: 30 sec, alternating)

2. Side Neck Stretch w/ Upside Down Palm on Wall

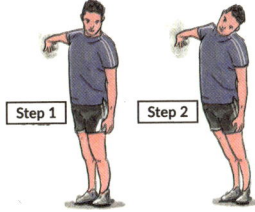

Step 1 | Step 2

Duration:

(Goal: 15 sec each side)

3. Levator Scap Neck Stretch

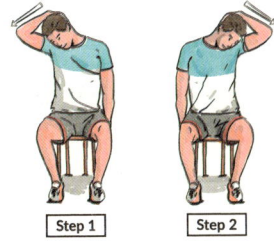

Step 1 | Step 2

Duration:

(Goal: 15 sec each side)

4. Sphinx/Cobra

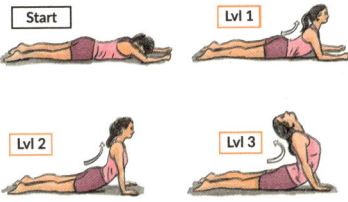

Start | Lvl 1 | Lvl 2 | Lvl 3

Duration:

(Goal: 30 sec)   Level:

5. Seated Forward Curl

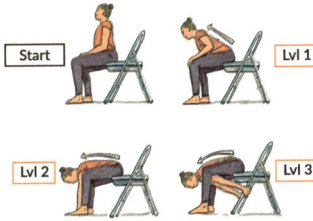

Start | Lvl 1 | Lvl 2 | Lvl 3

Duration:

(Goal: 30 sec)   Level:

6. Wall Lat Stretch

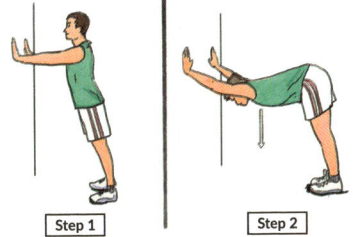

Step 1 | Step 2

Duration:

(Goal: 30 sec)

7. Static Y Hold

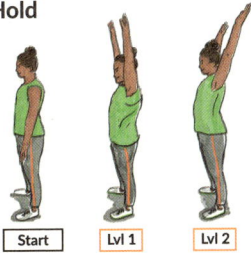

Start | Lvl 1 | Lvl 2

Level:

Duration:

(Goal: 30 sec)

8. Reverse Prayer

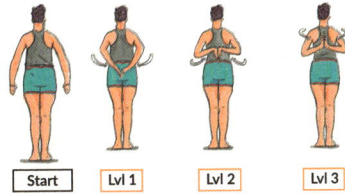

Start | Lvl 1 | Lvl 2 | Lvl 3

Level:

Duration:

(Goal: 30 sec)

9. Elbow Opener

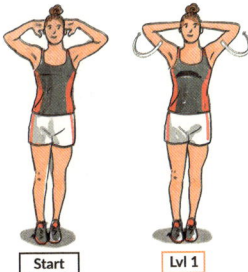

Start | Lvl 1

Duration:

(Goal: 30 sec)

10. Forearm Stretch w/ Hands on Surface

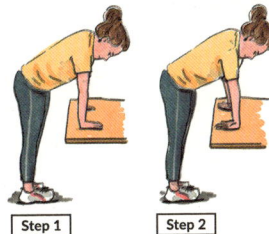

Step 1 | Step 2

Duration:

(Goal: 15 sec each side)

Day 49: Lower Body

1. Frog Pose

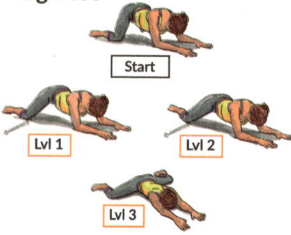

Duration:

....

(Goal: 60 sec)

Level:

2. Reclining Angle Bound Pose

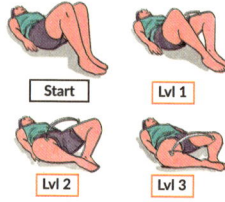

Duration:

....

(Goal: 30 sec)

Level:

3. Reverse Tabletop

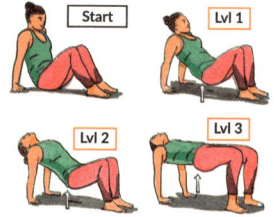

Duration:

....

(Goal: 30 sec)

Level:

4. Warrior II Pose

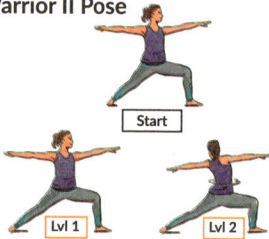

Duration:

....

(Goal: 30 sec each side)

Level:

5. Pry Squat

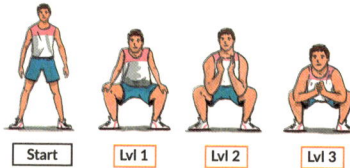

Duration:

....

(Goal: 30 sec)

Level:

6. Seated Forward Fold Hamstring Stretch

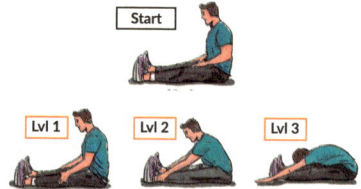

Duration:

....

(Goal: 30 sec)

Level:

7. Lateral Squat

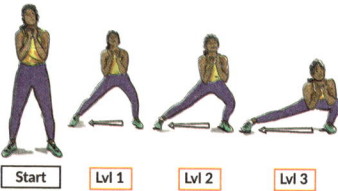

Duration:

....

(Goal: 30 sec each side)

Level:

8. Lateral Squat w/ Toe Raise

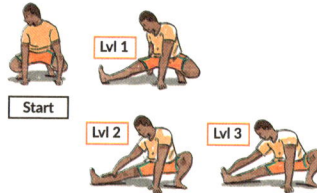

Duration:

....

(Goal: 30 sec each side)

Level:

9. Wig-Wag

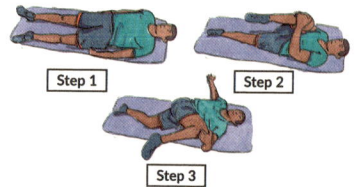

Duration:

....

(Goal: 30 sec each side)

10. Knee to Chest Stretch

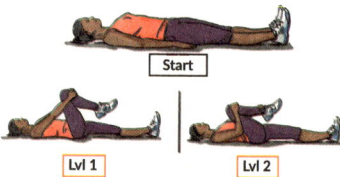

Duration:

....

(Goal: 30 sec each side)

Level:

11. Prone Quad Stretch

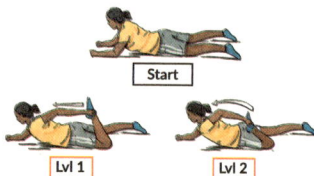

Duration:

....

(Goal: 30 sec each side)

Level:

12. Standing Wall Calf Stretch

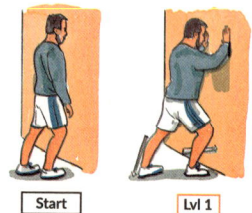

Duration:

....

(Goal: 15 sec each side)

Daily Reflection

Benefits I'm Experiencing:

Feel
Lighter

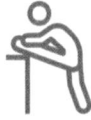

More Freedom
of Movement

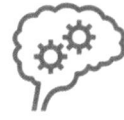

Improved
Mental Clarity

Less
Pain

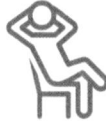

Less
Stressed

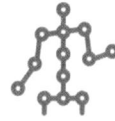

Improved
Posture

Notes On My Body:

Day 50: Dynamic Warm-Up

1. Rocking Feet w/ Arm Raise

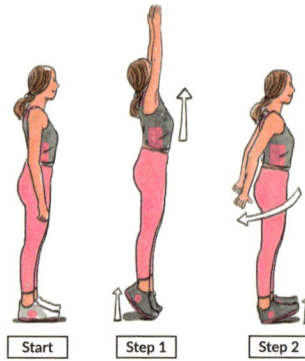

| Start | Step 1 | Step 2 |

Reps: _____ *(Goal: 15-20 in each direction)*

2. Plank

Lvl 1

Lvl 2

Start

Level: _____

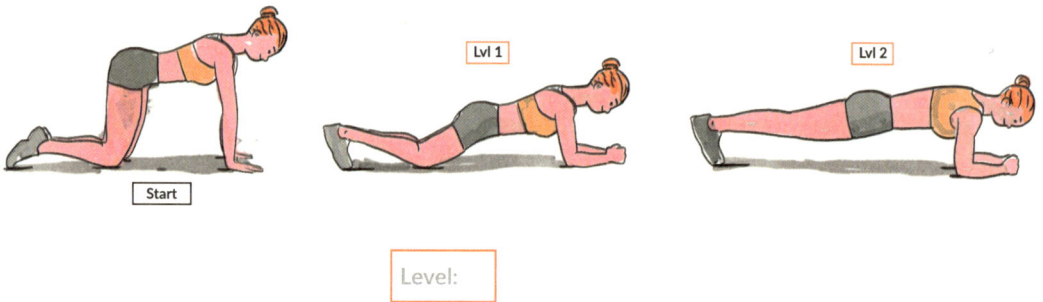

Reps: _____ *(Goal: 30-60 sec)*

3. Glute Bridge

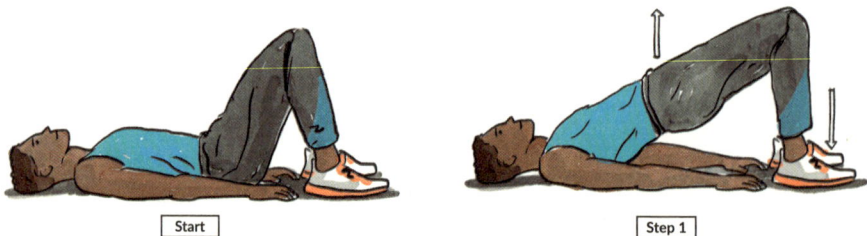

Start

Step 1

Reps: _____ *(Goal: 20-30)*

Day 50: Upper Body

1. Up & Down Neck Tilt

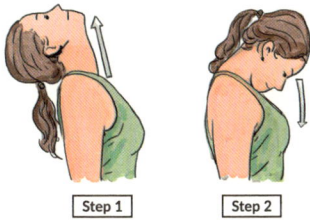

Step 1   Step 2

Duration:

(Goal: 30 sec, alternating)

2. Side Neck Tilt

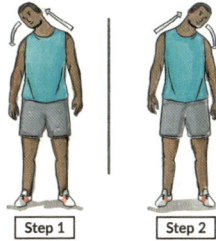

Step 1   Step 2

Duration:

(Goal: 15 sec each side)

3. Forward & Backward Neck Tilt

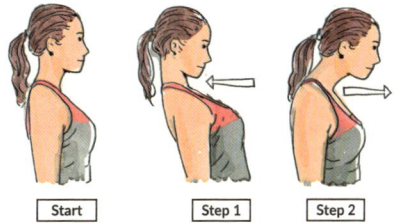

Start   Step 1   Step 2

Duration:

(Goal: 30 sec, alternating)

4. Child's Pose

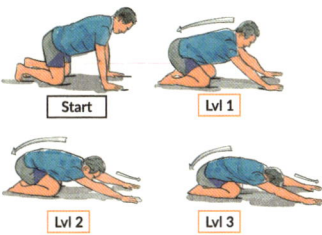

Start   Lvl 1   Lvl 2   Lvl 3

Duration:

(Goal: 60 sec)   Level:

5. Cat-Cow

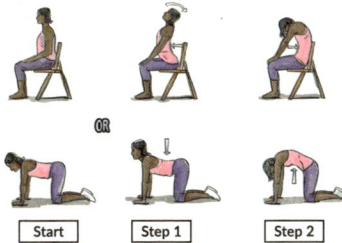

OR

Start   Step 1   Step 2

Duration:

(Goal: 30 sec, alternating)

6. Seated Spinal Twist

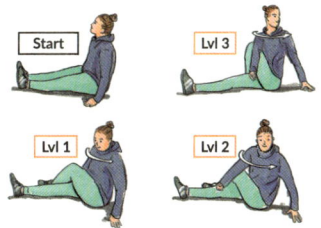

Start   Lvl 3   Lvl 1   Lvl 2

Duration:

(Goal: 15 sec each side)   Level:

7. Standing Oblique Stretch

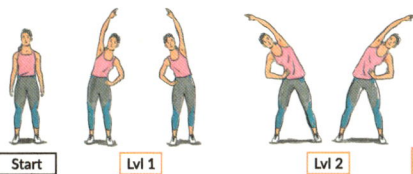

Start   Lvl 1   Lvl 2   Level:

Duration: *(Goal: 15 sec each side)*

8. Open Book Chest Stretch

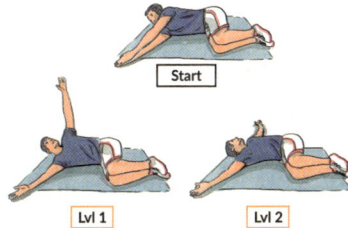

Start   Lvl 1   Lvl 2   Level:

Duration: *(Goal: 30 sec each side)*

9. Cross Arm Shoulder Stretch

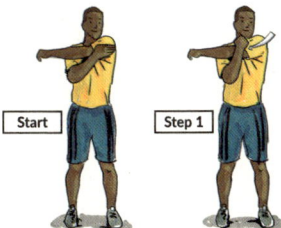

Start   Step 1

Duration: *(Goal: 15 sec each side)*

10. Sphinx/Cobra

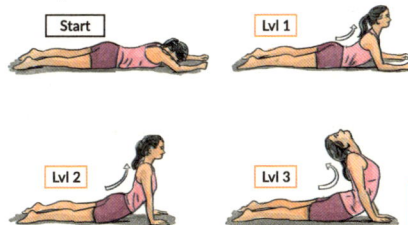

Start   Lvl 1   Lvl 2   Lvl 3   Level:

Duration: *(Goal: 30 sec)*

247

Day 50: Lower Body

1. Runner's Lunge

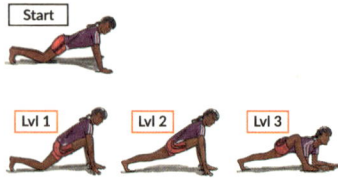

Duration:

(Goal: 30 sec each side) Level:

2. Butterfly

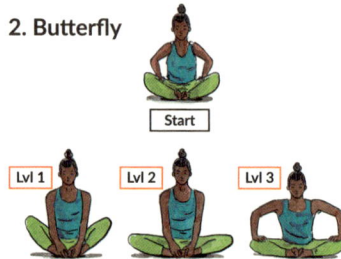

Duration:

(Goal: 30 sec) Level:

3. Scorpion Pose

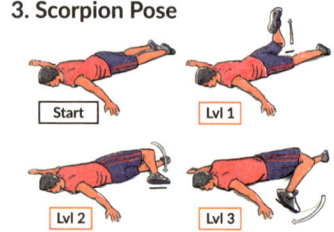

Duration:

(Goal: 30 sec each side) Level:

4. Lying Hip Extension

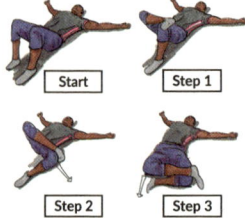

Duration:

(Goal: 30 sec each side)

5. Happy Baby Pose

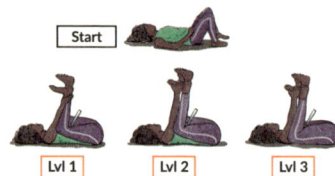

Duration:

(Goal: 30 sec) Level:

6. Pigeon Stretch

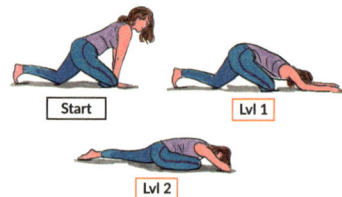

Duration:

(Goal: 30 sec each side) Level:

7. Figure 4

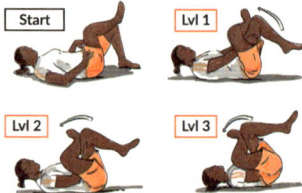

Duration:

(Goal: 30 sec each side) Level:

8. Halfway Center Split

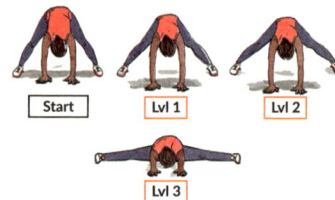

Duration:

(Goal: 30 sec) Level:

9. Seated Single Leg Hamstring Stretch

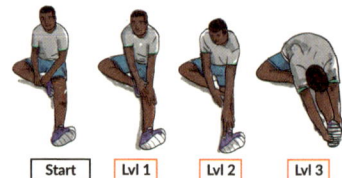

Duration:

(Goal: 30 sec each side) Level:

10. Extended Triangle Pose

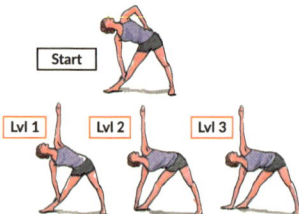

Duration:

(Goal: 30 sec each side) Level:

11. Standing Quad Stretch

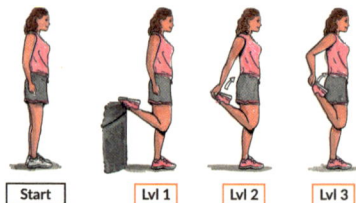

Duration:

(Goal: 30 sec each side) Level:

12. Hanging Calf Stretch

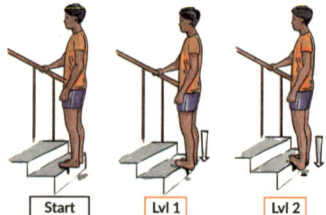

Duration:

(Goal: 30 sec) Level:

Daily Reflection

Benefits I'm Experiencing:

Feel
Lighter

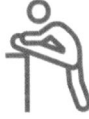

More Freedom
of Movement

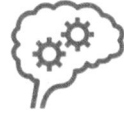

Improved
Mental Clarity

Less
Pain

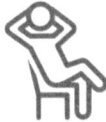

Less
Stressed

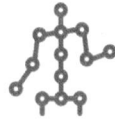

Improved
Posture

Notes On My Body:

Day 51: Dynamic Warm-Up

Full Session Exercise Guide:
habitnest.com/pages/stretching-day-51

1. Clam Opener w/ Side Plank

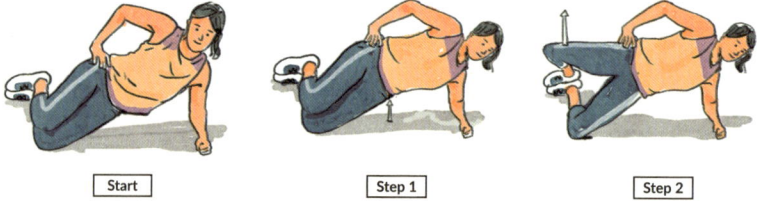

Start

Step 1

Step 2

Reps: _____ (Goal: 10-15 each side)

2. Aquaman

Start

Step 1

Step 2

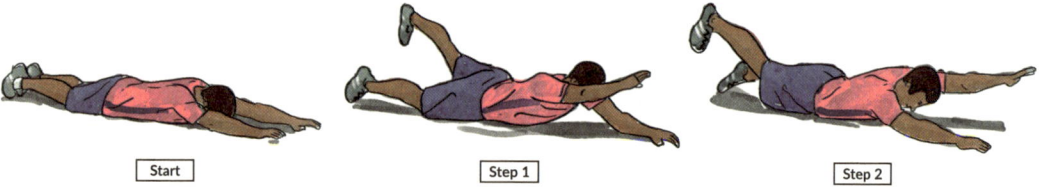

Reps: _____ (Goal: 10-20)

3. Roundhouse Kick to Squat

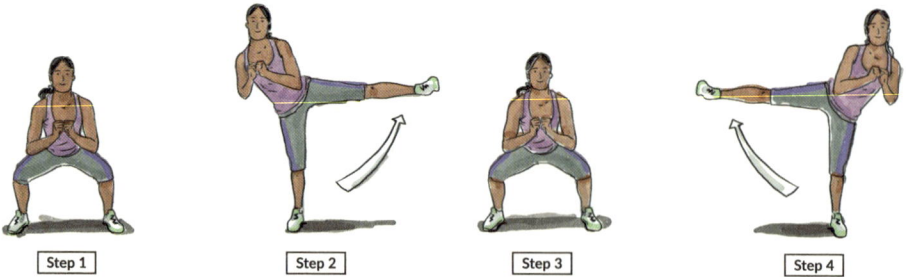

Step 1

Step 2

Step 3

Step 4

Reps: _____ (Goal: 10-15 each side)

Day 51: Upper Body

1. Up & Down Neck Tilt

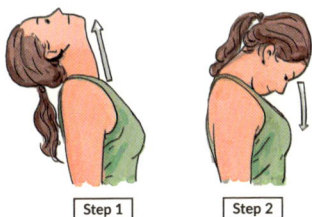

Step 1   Step 2

Duration:
....

(Goal: 30 sec, alternating)

2. Side Neck Tilt

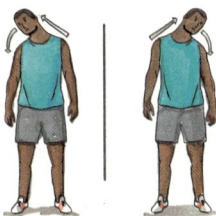

Step 1   Step 2

Duration:
....

(Goal: 15 sec each side)

3. Forward & Backward Neck Tilt

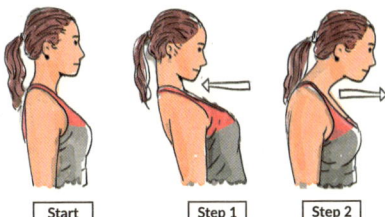

Start   Step 1   Step 2

Duration:
....

(Goal: 30 sec, alternating)

4. Child's Pose

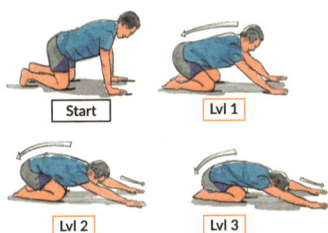

Start   Lvl 1
Lvl 2   Lvl 3

Duration:
....

(Goal: 60 sec)   Level:

5. Cat-Cow

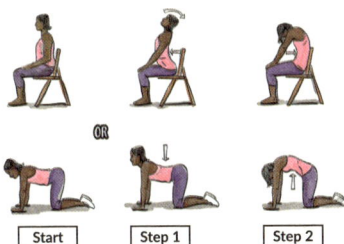

OR

Start   Step 1   Step 2

Duration:
....

(Goal: 30 sec, alternating)

6. Seated Spinal Twist

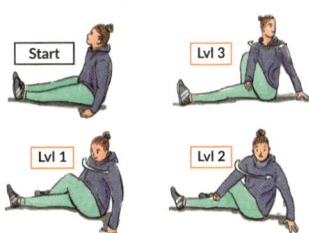

Start   Lvl 3
Lvl 1   Lvl 2

Duration:
....

(Goal: 15 sec each side)   Level:

7. Standing Oblique Stretch

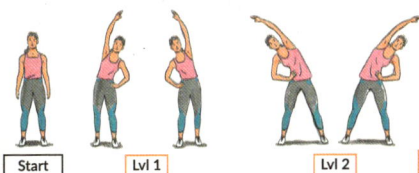

Start   Lvl 1   Lvl 2

Level:

Duration:
....

(Goal: 15 sec each side)

8. Open Book Chest Stretch

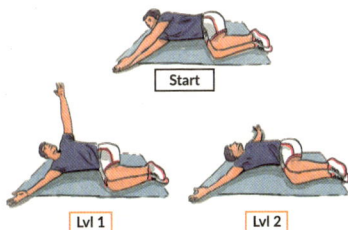

Start

Lvl 1   Lvl 2

Level:

Duration:
....

(Goal: 30 sec each side)

9. Cross Arm Shoulder Stretch

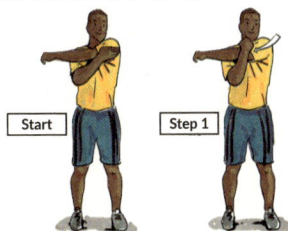

Start   Step 1

Duration:
....

(Goal: 15 sec each side)

10. Sphinx/Cobra

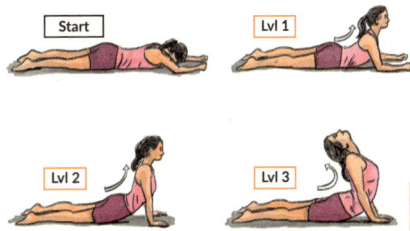

Start   Lvl 1
Lvl 2   Lvl 3

Level:

Duration:
....

(Goal: 30 sec)

Day 51: Lower Body

1. Runner's Lunge

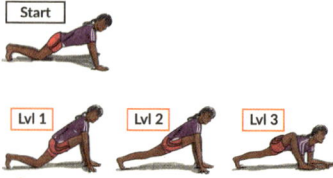

Start

Lvl 1   Lvl 2   Lvl 3

Duration:

(Goal: 30 sec each side)   Level:

2. Butterfly

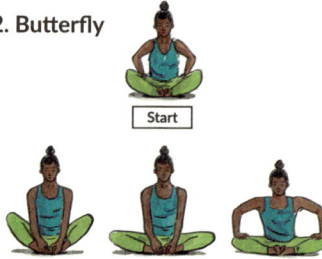

Start

Duration:

(Goal: 30 sec)   Level:

3. Scorpion Pose

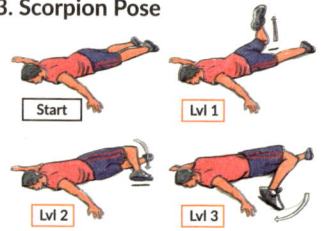

Start   Lvl 1

Lvl 2   Lvl 3

Duration:

(Goal: 30 sec each side)   Level:

4. Lying Hip Extension

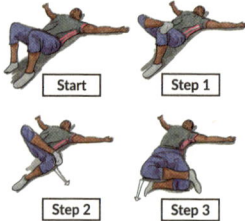

Start   Step 1

Step 2   Step 3

Duration:

(Goal: 30 sec each side)

5. Happy Baby Pose

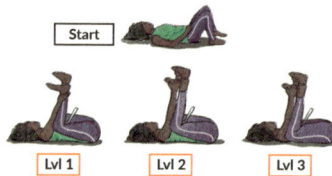

Start

Lvl 1   Lvl 2   Lvl 3

Duration:

(Goal: 30 sec)   Level:

6. Pigeon Stretch

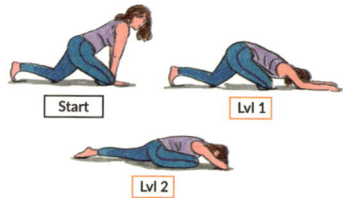

Start   Lvl 1

Lvl 2

Duration:

(Goal: 30 sec each side)   Level:

7. Figure 4

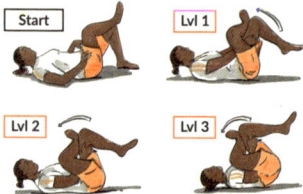

Start   Lvl 1

Lvl 2   Lvl 3

Duration:

(Goal: 30 sec each side)   Level:

8. Halfway Center Split

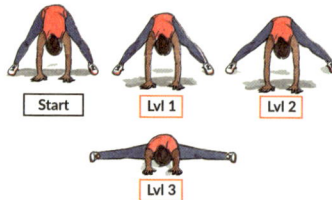

Start   Lvl 1   Lvl 2

Lvl 3

Duration:

(Goal: 30 sec)   Level:

9. Seated Single Leg Hamstring Stretch

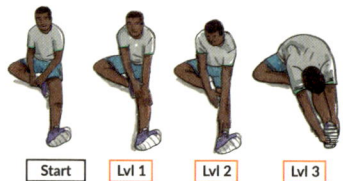

Start   Lvl 1   Lvl 2   Lvl 3

Duration:

(Goal: 30 sec each side)   Level:

10. Extended Triangle Pose

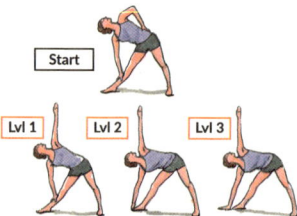

Start

Lvl 1   Lvl 2   Lvl 3

Duration:

(Goal: 30 sec each side)   Level:

11. Standing Quad Stretch

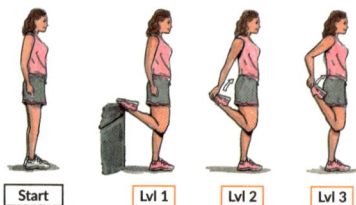

Start   Lvl 1   Lvl 2   Lvl 3

Duration:

(Goal: 30 sec each side)   Level:

12. Hanging Calf Stretch

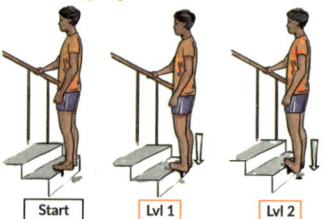

Start   Lvl 1   Lvl 2

Duration:

(Goal: 30 sec)   Level:

Daily Reflection

Benefits I'm Experiencing:

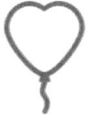

Feel
Lighter

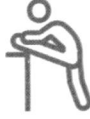

More Freedom
of Movement

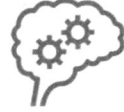

Improved
Mental Clarity

Less
Pain

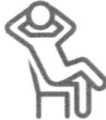

Less
Stressed

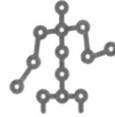

Improved
Posture

Notes On My Body:

Day 52: Dynamic Warm-Up

Full Session Exercise Guide:
habitnest.com/pages/stretching-day-52

1. World's Greatest Stretch

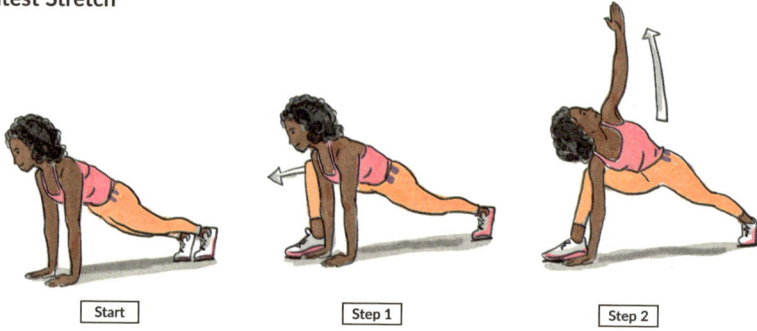

Start	Step 1	Step 2

Reps: _____ (Goal: 10-20)

2. Bird-Dog

Start	Step 1	Step 2	Step 3

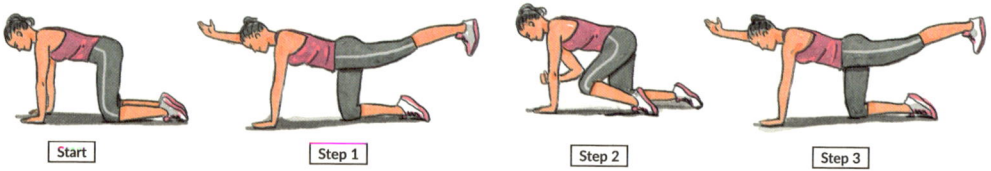

Reps: _____ (Goal: 10-15 each side)

3. Speed Skater Arms

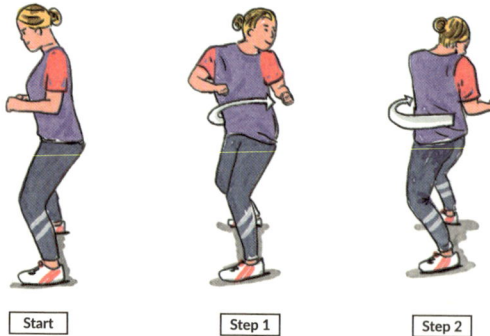

Start	Step 1	Step 2

Reps: _____ (Goal: 25-30)

Day 52: Upper Body

1. Up & Down Neck Tilt

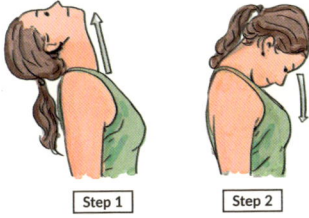

Step 1   Step 2

Duration:
....

(Goal: 30 sec, alternating)

2. Side Neck Tilt

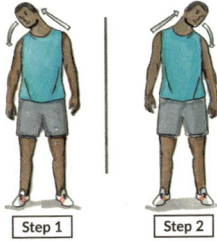

Step 1   Step 2

Duration:
....

(Goal: 15 sec each side)

3. Forward & Backward Neck Tilt

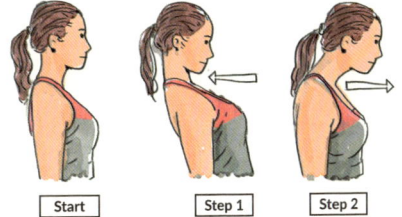

Start   Step 1   Step 2

Duration:
....

(Goal: 30 sec, alternating)

4. Child's Pose

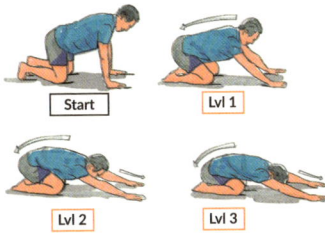

Start   Lvl 1

Lvl 2   Lvl 3

Duration:
....

(Goal: 60 sec)   Level:

5. Cat-Cow

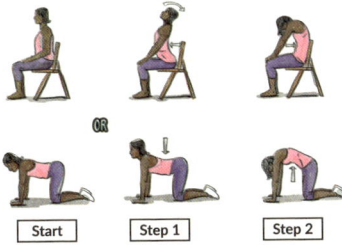

OR

Start   Step 1   Step 2

Duration:
....

(Goal: 30 sec, alternating)

6. Seated Spinal Twist

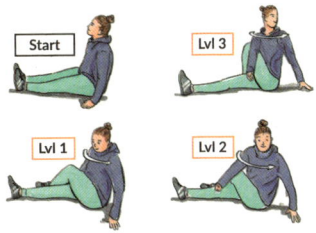

Start   Lvl 3

Lvl 1   Lvl 2

Duration:
....

(Goal: 15 sec each side)   Level:

7. Standing Oblique Stretch

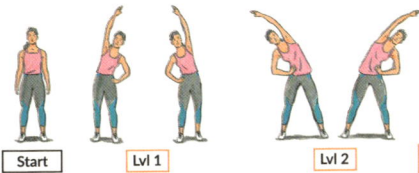

Start   Lvl 1   Lvl 2   Level:

Duration:
....

(Goal: 15 sec each side)

8. Open Book Chest Stretch

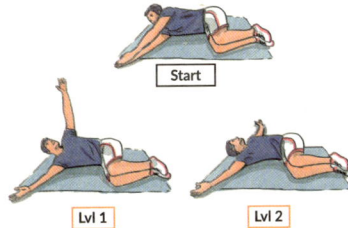

Start

Lvl 1   Lvl 2   Level:

Duration:
....

(Goal: 30 sec each side)

9. Cross Arm Shoulder Stretch

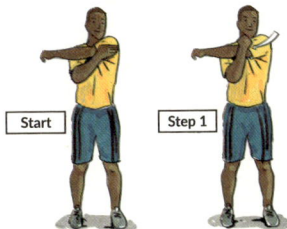

Start   Step 1

Duration:
....

(Goal: 15 sec each side)

10. Sphinx/Cobra

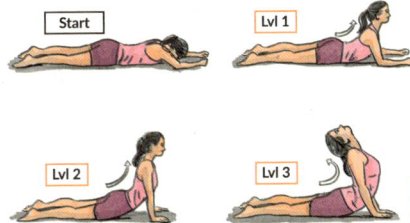

Start   Lvl 1

Lvl 2   Lvl 3   Level:

Duration:
....

(Goal: 30 sec)

Day 52: Lower Body

1. Runner's Lunge

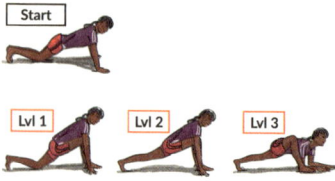

Start
Lvl 1   Lvl 2   Lvl 3

Duration:

(Goal: 30 sec each side)   Level:

2. Butterfly

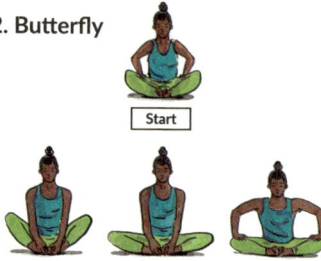

Start

Duration:

(Goal: 30 sec)   Level:

3. Scorpion Pose

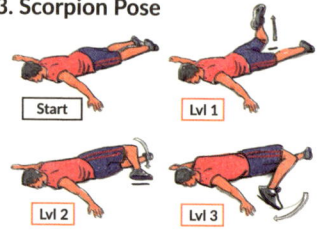

Start   Lvl 1
Lvl 2   Lvl 3

Duration:

(Goal: 30 sec each side)   Level:

4. Lying Hip Extension

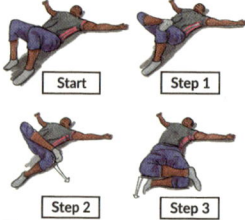

Start   Step 1
Step 2   Step 3

Duration:

(Goal: 30 sec each side)

5. Happy Baby Pose

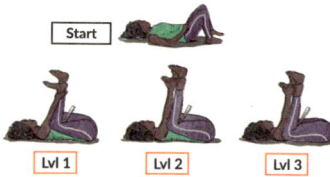

Start
Lvl 1   Lvl 2   Lvl 3

Duration:

(Goal: 30 sec)   Level:

6. Pigeon Stretch

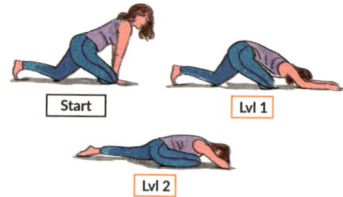

Start   Lvl 1
Lvl 2

Duration:

(Goal: 30 sec each side)   Level:

7. Figure 4

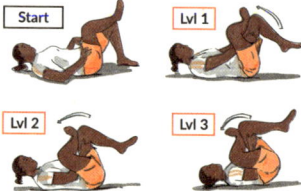

Start   Lvl 1
Lvl 2   Lvl 3

Duration:

(Goal: 30 sec each side)   Level:

8. Halfway Center Split

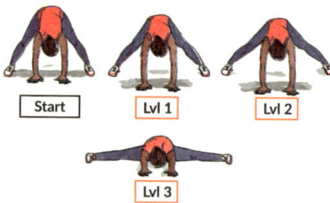

Start   Lvl 1   Lvl 2
Lvl 3

Duration:

(Goal: 30 sec)   Level:

9. Seated Single Leg Hamstring Stretch

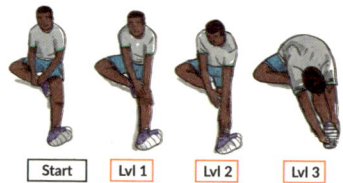

Start   Lvl 1   Lvl 2   Lvl 3

Duration:

(Goal: 30 sec each side)   Level:

10. Extended Triangle Pose

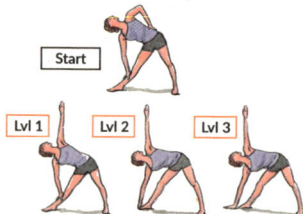

Start
Lvl 1   Lvl 2   Lvl 3

Duration:

(Goal: 30 sec each side)   Level:

11. Standing Quad Stretch

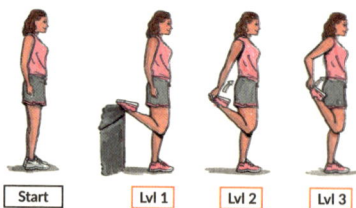

Start   Lvl 1   Lvl 2   Lvl 3

Duration:

(Goal: 30 sec each side)   Level:

12. Hanging Calf Stretch

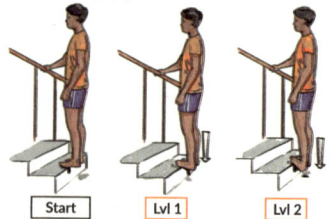

Start   Lvl 1   Lvl 2

Duration:

(Goal: 30 sec)   Level:

Daily Reflection

Benefits I'm Experiencing:

Feel
Lighter

More Freedom
of Movement

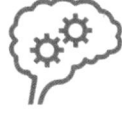

Improved
Mental Clarity

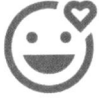

Less
Pain

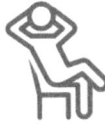

Less
Stressed

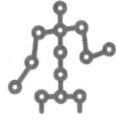

Improved
Posture

Notes On My Body:

Day 53: Dynamic Warm-Up

Full Session Exercise Guide:
habitnest.com/pages/stretching-day-53

1. Inch Worm Walk Out

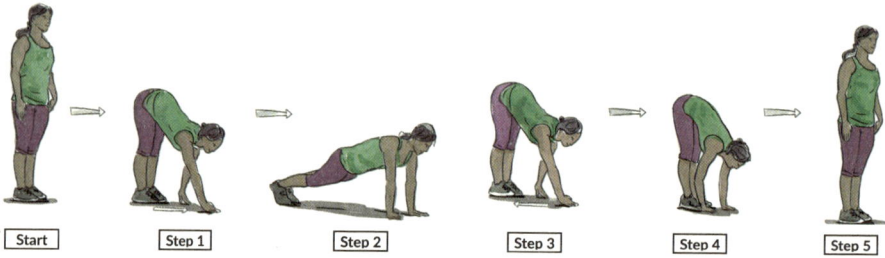

| Start | Step 1 | Step 2 | Step 3 | Step 4 | Step 5 |

Reps: _____ *(Goal: 10-15)*

2. Y Raise

| Step 1 | Step 2 |

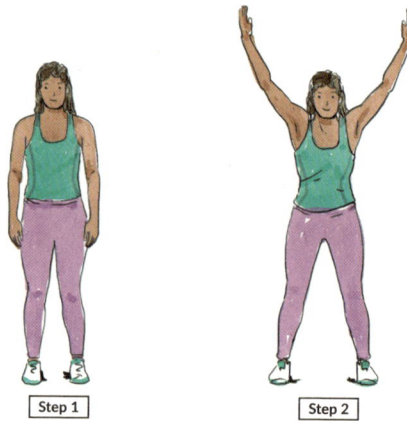

Reps: _____ *(Goal: 15-25)*

3. Low Lunge w/ Elbow Twist

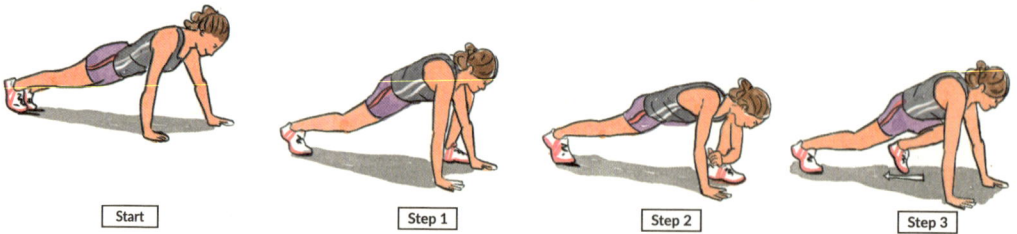

| Start | Step 1 | Step 2 | Step 3 |

Reps: _____ *(Goal: 10-15 each side)*

Day 53: Upper Body

1. Up & Down Neck Tilt

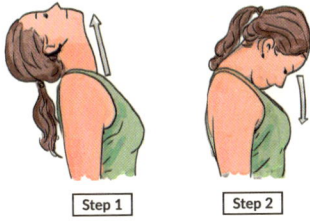

Step 1   Step 2

Duration:
....

(Goal: 30 sec, alternating)

2. Side Neck Tilt

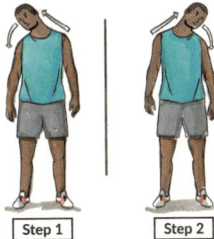

Step 1   Step 2

Duration:
....

(Goal: 15 sec each side)

3. Forward & Backward Neck Tilt

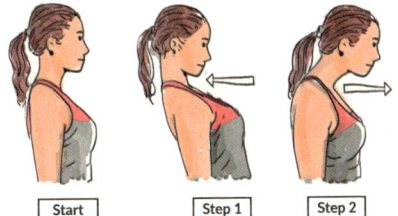

Start   Step 1   Step 2

Duration:
....

(Goal: 30 sec, alternating)

4. Child's Pose

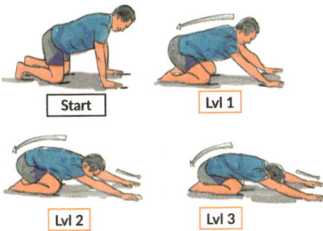

Start   Lvl 1
Lvl 2   Lvl 3

Duration:
....

(Goal: 60 sec) | Level: |

5. Cat-Cow

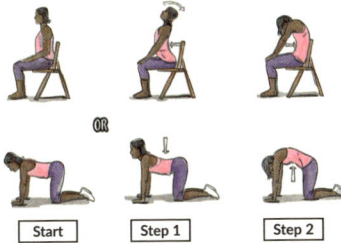

OR

Start   Step 1   Step 2

Duration:
....

(Goal: 30 sec, alternating)

6. Seated Spinal Twist

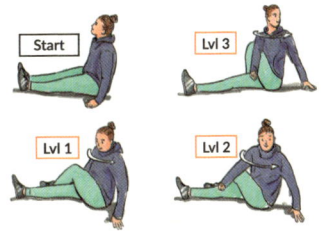

Start   Lvl 3
Lvl 1   Lvl 2

Duration:
....

(Goal: 15 sec each side) | Level: |

7. Standing Oblique Stretch

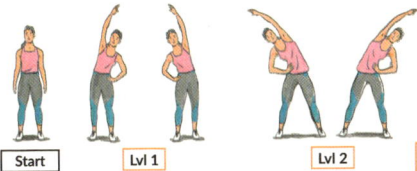

Start   Lvl 1   Lvl 2 | Level: |

Duration:
....   *(Goal: 15 sec each side)*

8. Open Book Chest Stretch

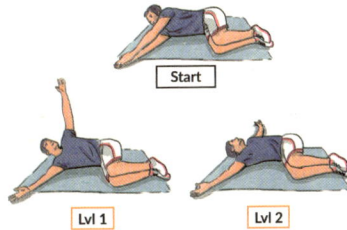

Start

Lvl 1   Lvl 2 | Level: |

Duration:
....   *(Goal: 30 sec each side)*

9. Cross Arm Shoulder Stretch

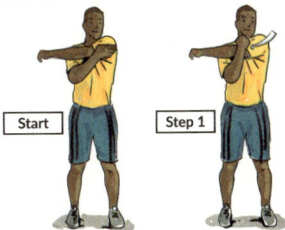

Start   Step 1

Duration:
....   *(Goal: 15 sec each side)*

10. Sphinx/Cobra

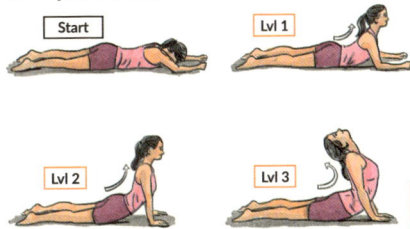

Start   Lvl 1
Lvl 2   Lvl 3 | Level: |

Duration:
....   *(Goal: 30 sec)*

Day 53: Lower Body

1. Runner's Lunge

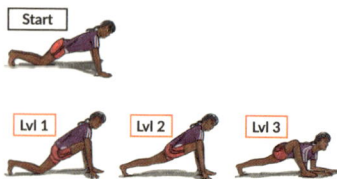

Duration:

(Goal: 30 sec each side)   Level:

2. Butterfly

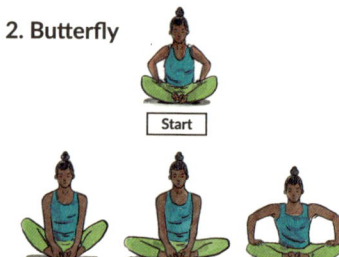

Duration:

(Goal: 30 sec)   Level:

3. Scorpion Pose

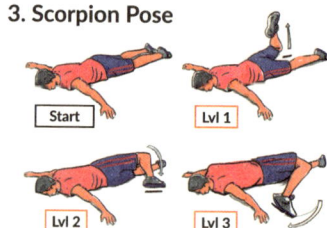

Duration:

(Goal: 30 sec each side)   Level:

4. Lying Hip Extension

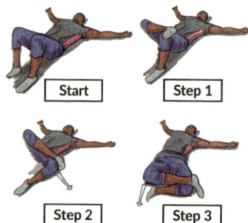

Duration:

(Goal: 30 sec each side)

5. Happy Baby Pose

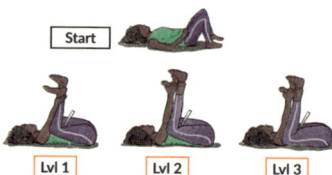

Duration:

(Goal: 30 sec)   Level:

6. Pigeon Stretch

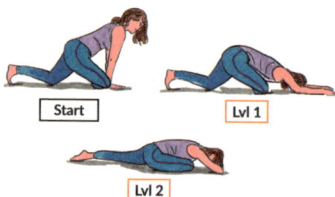

Duration:

(Goal: 30 sec each side)   Level:

7. Figure 4

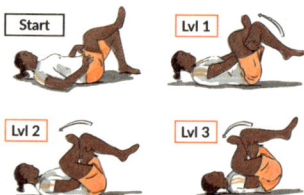

Duration:

(Goal: 30 sec each side)   Level:

8. Halfway Center Split

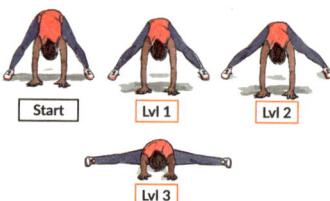

Duration:

(Goal: 30 sec)   Level:

9. Seated Single Leg Hamstring Stretch

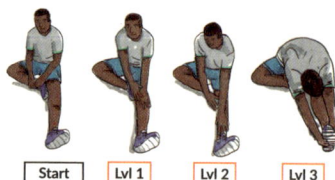

Duration:

(Goal: 30 sec each side)   Level:

10. Extended Triangle Pose

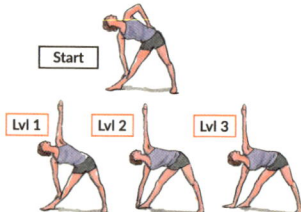

Duration:

(Goal: 30 sec each side)   Level:

11. Standing Quad Stretch

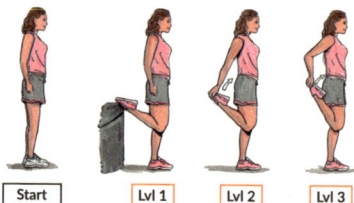

Duration:

(Goal: 30 sec each side)   Level:

12. Hanging Calf Stretch

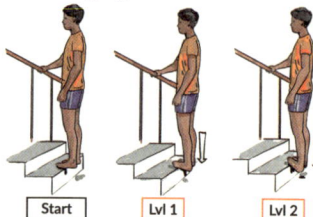

Duration:

(Goal: 30 sec)   Level:

Daily Reflection

Benefits I'm Experiencing:

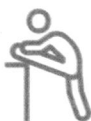

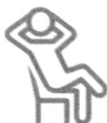

Feel Lighter	More Freedom of Movement	Improved Mental Clarity
Less Pain	Less Stressed	Improved Posture

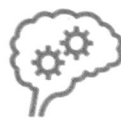

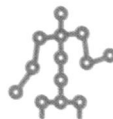

Notes On My Body:

Day 54: Dynamic Warm-Up

1. Walking Jacks (or Jumping Jacks)

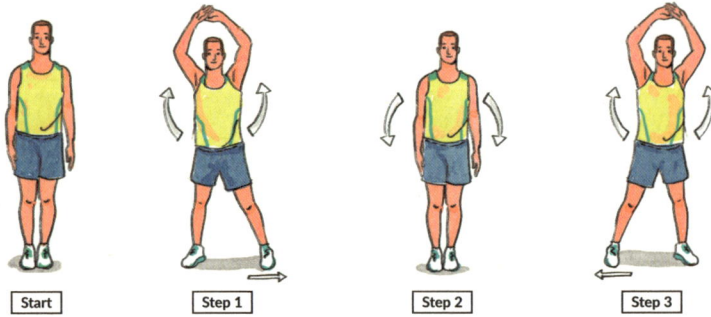

| Start | Step 1 | Step 2 | Step 3 |

Reps: _____ (Goal: 20-30)

2. Plank w/ Shoulder Tap

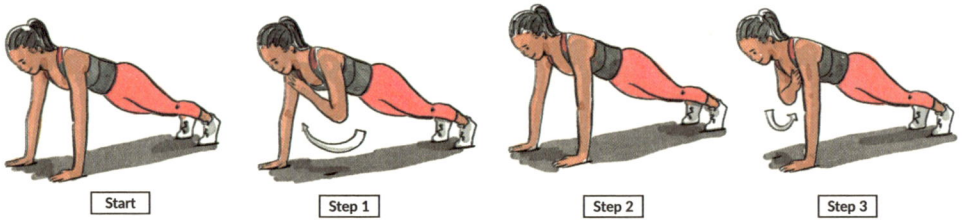

| Start | Step 1 | Step 2 | Step 3 |

Reps: _____ (Goal: 10-20 each side)

3. Standing Hip Circles

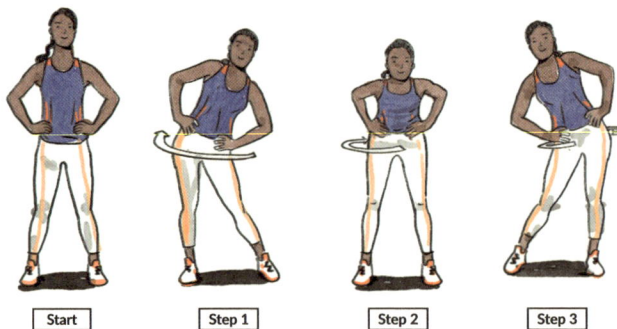

| Start | Step 1 | Step 2 | Step 3 |

Reps: _____ (Goal: 10-15 in each direction)

Day 54: Upper Body

1. Up & Down Neck Tilt

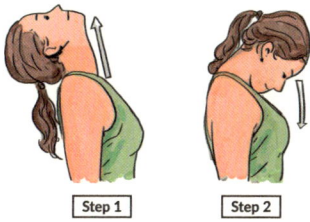

Step 1   Step 2

Duration:

(Goal: 30 sec, alternating)

2. Side Neck Tilt

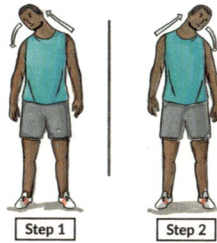

Step 1   Step 2

Duration:

(Goal: 15 sec each side)

3. Forward & Backward Neck Tilt

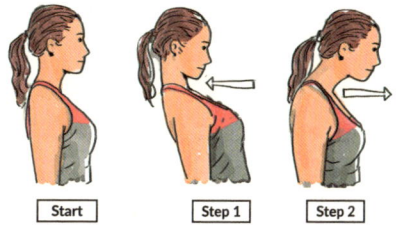

Start   Step 1   Step 2

Duration:

(Goal: 30 sec, alternating)

4. Child's Pose

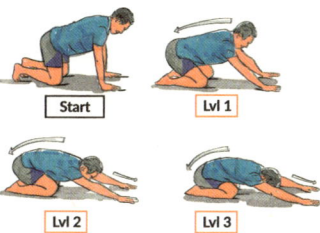

Start   Lvl 1
Lvl 2   Lvl 3

Duration:

(Goal: 60 sec)   Level:

5. Cat-Cow

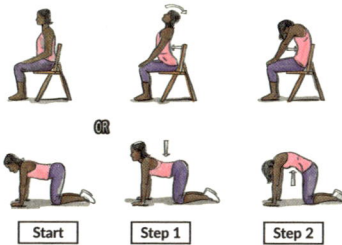

OR

Start   Step 1   Step 2

Duration:

(Goal: 30 sec, alternating)

6. Seated Spinal Twist

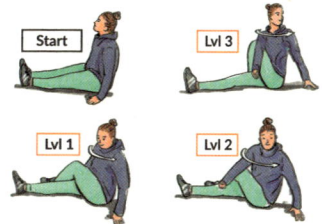

Start   Lvl 3
Lvl 1   Lvl 2

Duration:

(Goal: 15 sec each side)   Level:

7. Standing Oblique Stretch

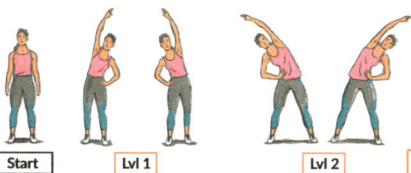

Start   Lvl 1   Lvl 2   Level:

Duration: *(Goal: 15 sec each side)*

8. Open Book Chest Stretch

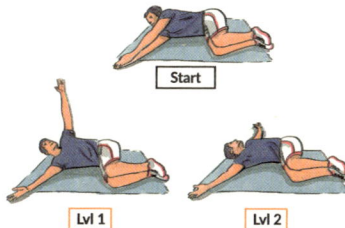

Start
Lvl 1   Lvl 2   Level:

Duration: *(Goal: 30 sec each side)*

9. Cross Arm Shoulder Stretch

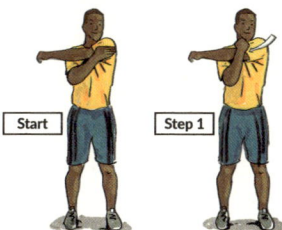

Start   Step 1

Duration: *(Goal: 15 sec each side)*

10. Sphinx/Cobra

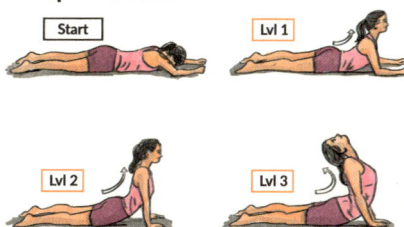

Start   Lvl 1
Lvl 2   Lvl 3   Level:

Duration: *(Goal: 30 sec)*

Day 54: Lower Body

1. Runner's Lunge

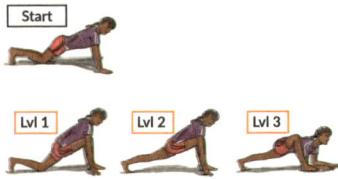

Duration:

(Goal: 30 sec each side)

Level:

2. Butterfly

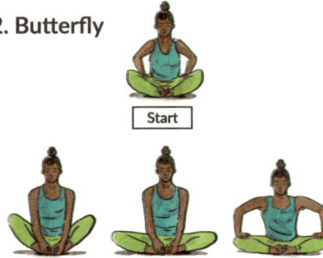

Duration:

(Goal: 30 sec)

Level:

3. Scorpion Pose

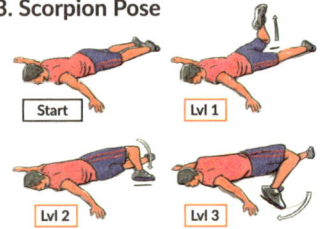

Duration:

(Goal: 30 sec each side)

Level:

4. Lying Hip Extension

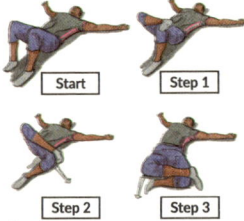

Duration:

(Goal: 30 sec each side)

5. Happy Baby Pose

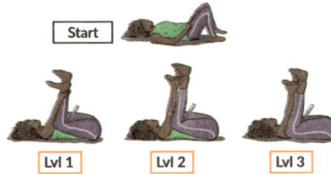

Duration:

(Goal: 30 sec)

Level:

6. Pigeon Stretch

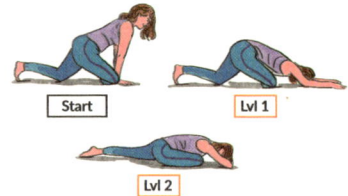

Duration:

(Goal: 30 sec each side)

Level:

7. Figure 4

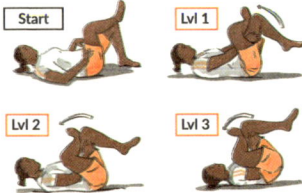

Duration:

(Goal: 30 sec each side)

Level:

8. Halfway Center Split

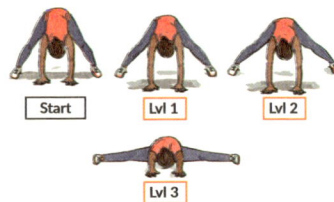

Duration:

(Goal: 30 sec)

Level:

9. Seated Single Leg Hamstring Stretch

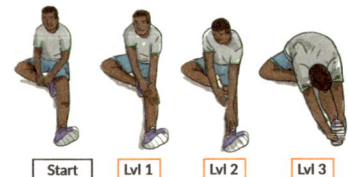

Duration:

(Goal: 30 sec each side)

Level:

10. Extended Triangle Pose

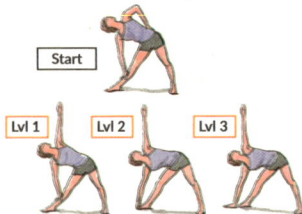

Duration:

(Goal: 30 sec each side)

Level:

11. Standing Quad Stretch

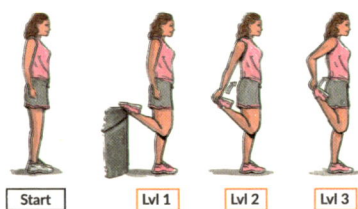

Duration:

(Goal: 30 sec each side)

Level:

12. Hanging Calf Stretch

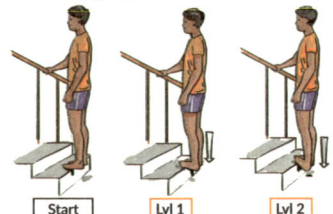

Duration:

(Goal: 30 sec)

Level:

Daily Reflection

Benefits I'm Experiencing:

Feel
Lighter

More Freedom
of Movement

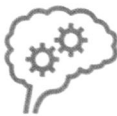

Improved
Mental Clarity

Less
Pain

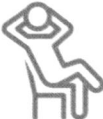

Less
Stressed

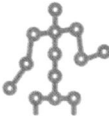

Improved
Posture

Notes On My Body:

Day 55: Dynamic Warm-Up

Full Session Exercise Guide:
habitnest.com/pages/stretching-day-55

1. Standing Hamstring Scoop

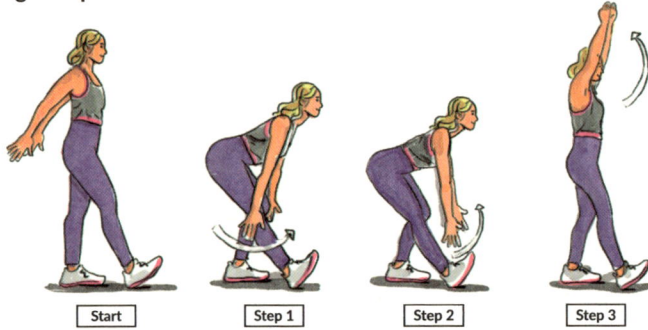

| Start | Step 1 | Step 2 | Step 3 |

Reps: .... *(Goal: 10-20 each side)*

2. Good Morning

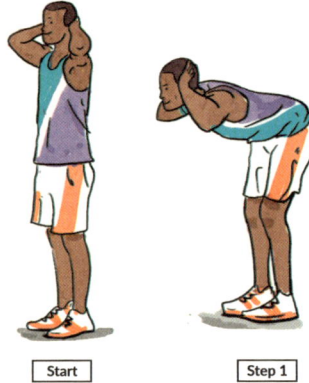

| Start | Step 1 |

Reps: .... *(Goal: 15-20)*

3. Pike Push-Up

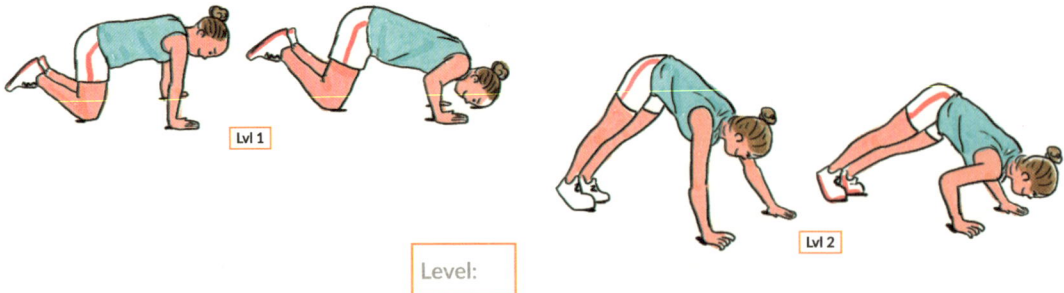

Lvl 1

Lvl 2

Level:

Reps: .... *(Goal: 15-25)*

Day 55: Upper Body

1. Up & Down Neck Tilt

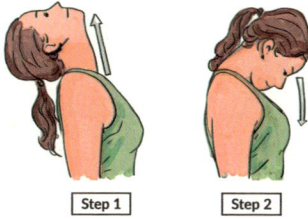

Step 1   Step 2

Duration:
....

(Goal: 30 sec, alternating)

2. Side Neck Tilt

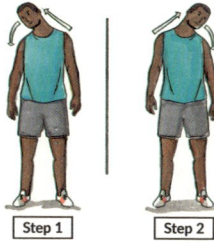

Step 1   Step 2

Duration:
....

(Goal: 15 sec each side)

3. Forward & Backward Neck Tilt

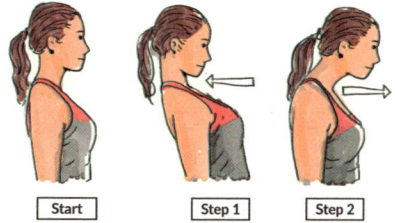

Start   Step 1   Step 2

Duration:
....

(Goal: 30 sec, alternating)

4. Child's Pose

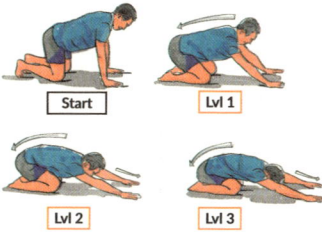

Start   Lvl 1   Lvl 2   Lvl 3

Duration:
....

(Goal: 60 sec)   Level:

5. Cat-Cow

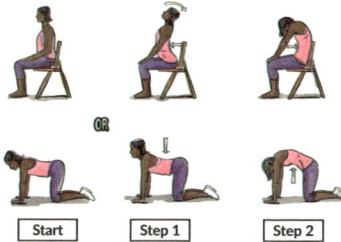

OR

Start   Step 1   Step 2

Duration:
....

(Goal: 30 sec, alternating)

6. Seated Spinal Twist

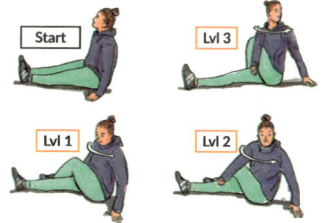

Start   Lvl 3   Lvl 1   Lvl 2

Duration:
....

(Goal: 15 sec each side)   Level:

7. Standing Oblique Stretch

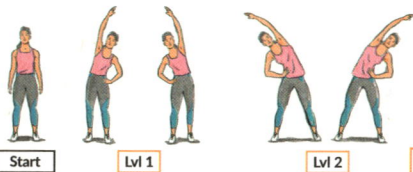

Start   Lvl 1   Lvl 2   Level:

Duration: *(Goal: 15 sec each side)*
....

8. Open Book Chest Stretch

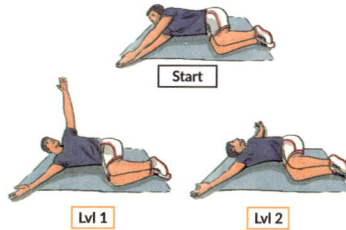

Start   Lvl 1   Lvl 2   Level:

Duration: *(Goal: 30 sec each side)*
....

9. Cross Arm Shoulder Stretch

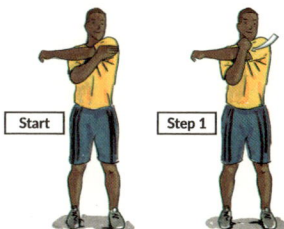

Start   Step 1

Duration: *(Goal: 15 sec each side)*
....

10. Sphinx/Cobra

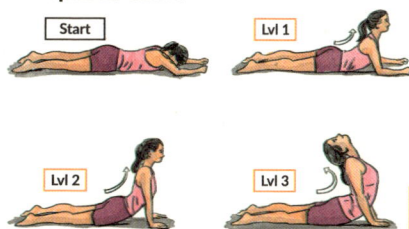

Start   Lvl 1   Lvl 2   Lvl 3   Level:

Duration: *(Goal: 30 sec)*
....

Day 55: Lower Body

1. Runner's Lunge

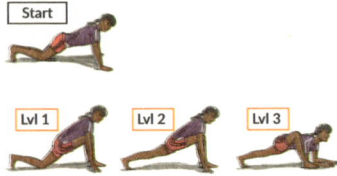

Start
Lvl 1   Lvl 2   Lvl 3

Duration:
....

(Goal: 30 sec each side)   Level:

2. Butterfly

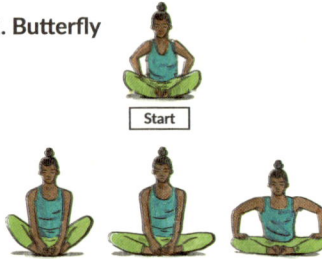

Start

Duration:
....

(Goal: 30 sec)   Level:

3. Scorpion Pose

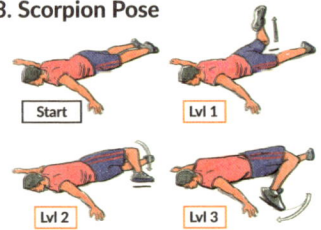

Start   Lvl 1
Lvl 2   Lvl 3

Duration:
....

(Goal: 30 sec each side)   Level:

4. Lying Hip Extension

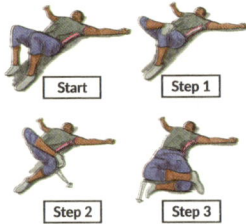

Start   Step 1
Step 2   Step 3

Duration:
....

(Goal: 30 sec each side)   Level:

5. Happy Baby Pose

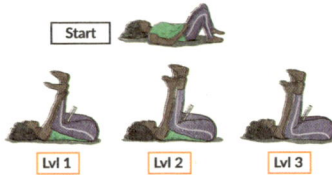

Start
Lvl 1   Lvl 2   Lvl 3

Duration:
....

(Goal: 30 sec)   Level:

6. Pigeon Stretch

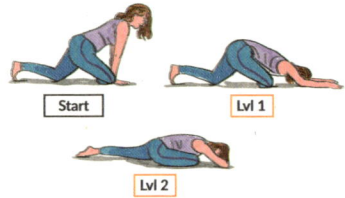

Start   Lvl 1
Lvl 2

Duration:
....

(Goal: 30 sec each side)   Level:

7. Figure 4

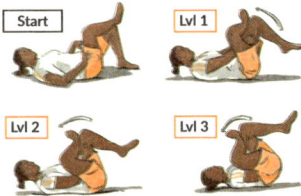

Start   Lvl 1
Lvl 2   Lvl 3

Duration:
....

(Goal: 30 sec each side)   Level:

8. Halfway Center Split

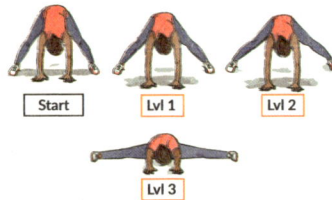

Start   Lvl 1   Lvl 2
Lvl 3

Duration:
....

(Goal: 30 sec)   Level:

9. Seated Single Leg Hamstring Stretch

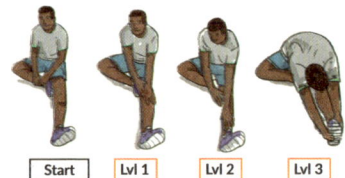

Start   Lvl 1   Lvl 2   Lvl 3

Duration:
....

(Goal: 30 sec each side)   Level:

10. Extended Triangle Pose

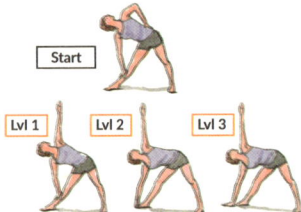

Start
Lvl 1   Lvl 2   Lvl 3

Duration:
....

(Goal: 30 sec each side)   Level:

11. Standing Quad Stretch

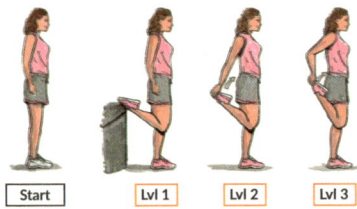

Start   Lvl 1   Lvl 2   Lvl 3

Duration:
....

(Goal: 30 sec each side)   Level:

12. Hanging Calf Stretch

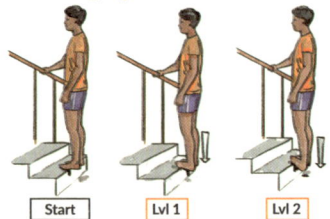

Start   Lvl 1   Lvl 2

Duration:
....

(Goal: 30 sec)   Level:

Daily Reflection

Benefits I'm Experiencing:

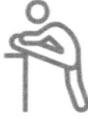

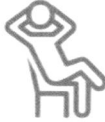

Feel Lighter	More Freedom of Movement	Improved Mental Clarity
Less Pain	Less Stressed	Improved Posture

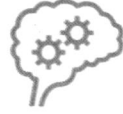

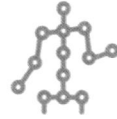

Notes On My Body:

Day 56: Dynamic Warm-Up

Full Session Exercise Guide:
habitnest.com/pages/stretching-day-56

1. World's Greatest Stretch

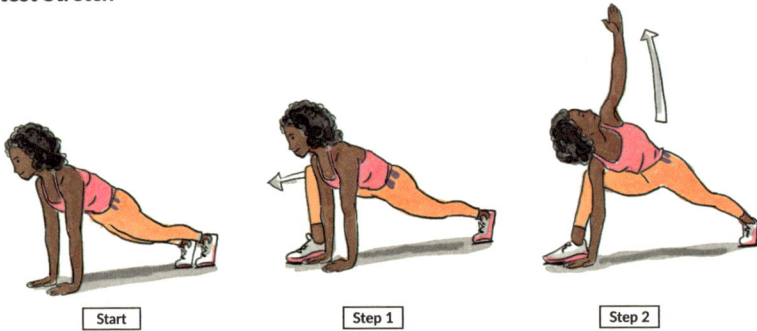

Start   Step 1   Step 2

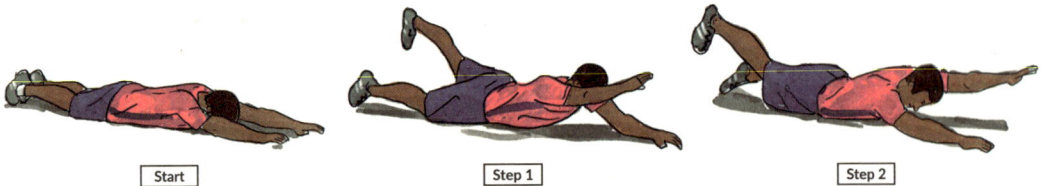

Reps: *(Goal: 10-20)*

2. Air Squat to Calf Raise

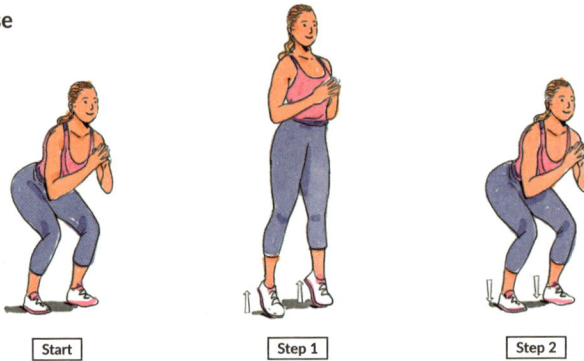

Start   Step 1   Step 2

Reps: *(Goal: 20-30)*

3. Aquaman

Start   Step 1   Step 2

Reps: *(Goal: 10-20)*

Day 56: Upper Body

1. Up & Down Neck Tilt

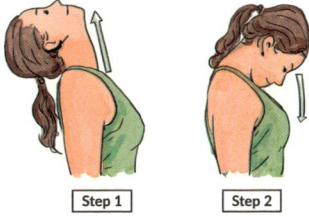

Step 1   Step 2

Duration:
....

(Goal: 30 sec, alternating)

2. Side Neck Tilt

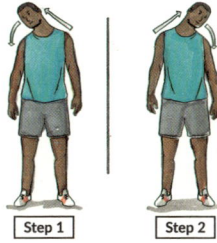

Step 1   Step 2

Duration:
....

(Goal: 15 sec each side)

3. Forward & Backward Neck Tilt

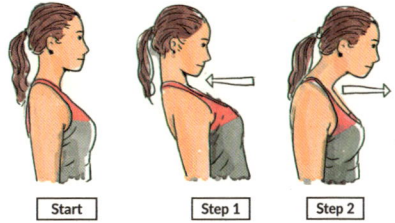

Start   Step 1   Step 2

Duration:
....

(Goal: 30 sec, alternating)

4. Child's Pose

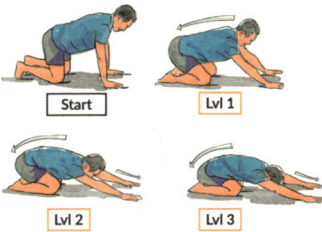

Start   Lvl 1   Lvl 2   Lvl 3

Duration:
....

(Goal: 60 sec)   Level:

5. Cat-Cow

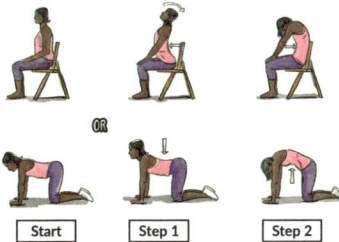

OR

Start   Step 1   Step 2

Duration:
....

(Goal: 30 sec, alternating)

6. Seated Spinal Twist

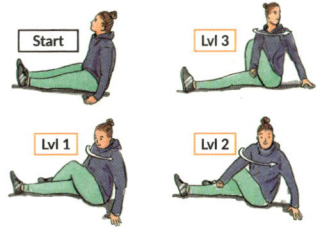

Start   Lvl 3   Lvl 1   Lvl 2

Duration:
....

(Goal: 15 sec each side)   Level:

7. Standing Oblique Stretch

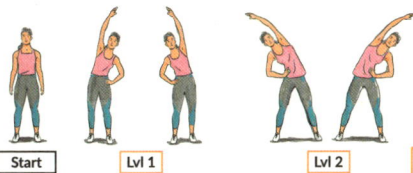

Start   Lvl 1   Lvl 2   Level:

Duration:
....

(Goal: 15 sec each side)

8. Open Book Chest Stretch

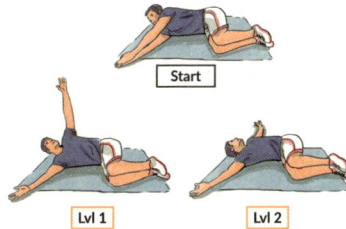

Start   Lvl 1   Lvl 2   Level:

Duration:
....

(Goal: 30 sec each side)

9. Cross Arm Shoulder Stretch

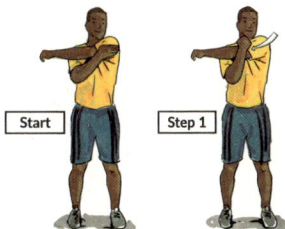

Start   Step 1

Duration:
....

(Goal: 15 sec each side)

10. Sphinx/Cobra

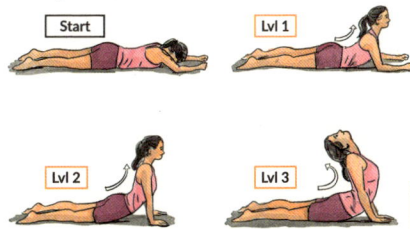

Start   Lvl 1   Lvl 2   Lvl 3   Level:

Duration:
....

(Goal: 30 sec)

Day 56: Lower Body

1. Runner's Lunge

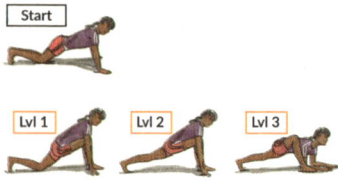

Start
Lvl 1   Lvl 2   Lvl 3

Duration:

(Goal: 30 sec each side)   Level:

2. Butterfly

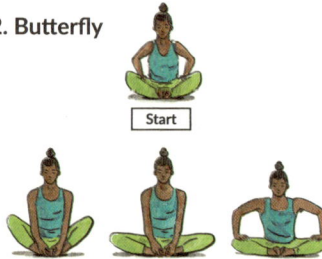

Start

Duration:

(Goal: 30 sec)   Level:

3. Scorpion Pose

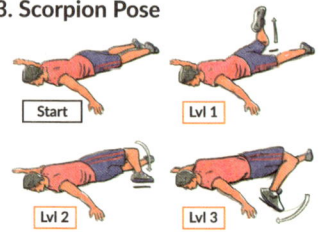

Start   Lvl 1
Lvl 2   Lvl 3

Duration:

(Goal: 30 sec each side)   Level:

4. Lying Hip Extension

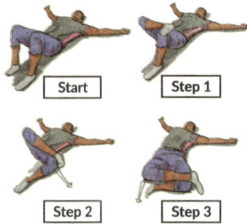

Start   Step 1
Step 2   Step 3

Duration:

(Goal: 30 sec each side)

5. Happy Baby Pose

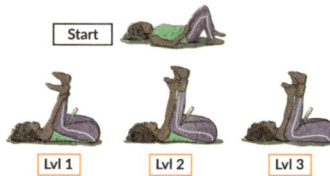

Start
Lvl 1   Lvl 2   Lvl 3

Duration:

(Goal: 30 sec)   Level:

6. Pigeon Stretch

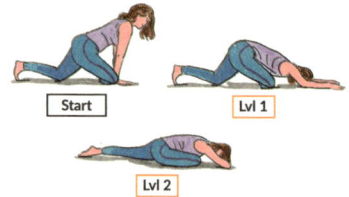

Start   Lvl 1
Lvl 2

Duration:

(Goal: 30 sec each side)   Level:

7. Figure 4

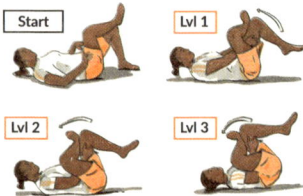

Start   Lvl 1
Lvl 2   Lvl 3

Duration:

(Goal: 30 sec each side)   Level:

8. Halfway Center Split

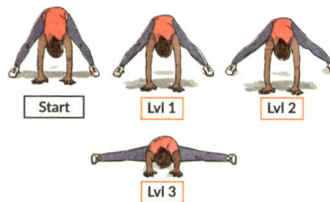

Start   Lvl 1   Lvl 2
Lvl 3

Duration:

(Goal: 30 sec)   Level:

9. Seated Single Leg Hamstring Stretch

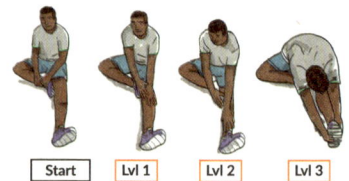

Start   Lvl 1   Lvl 2   Lvl 3

Duration:

(Goal: 30 sec each side)   Level:

10. Extended Triangle Pose

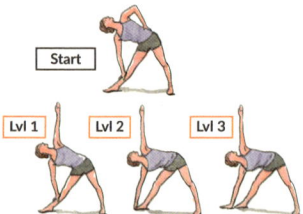

Start
Lvl 1   Lvl 2   Lvl 3

Duration:

(Goal: 30 sec each side)   Level:

11. Standing Quad Stretch

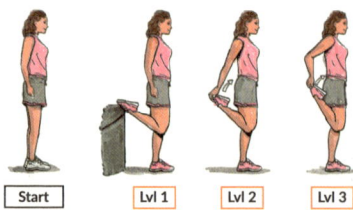

Start   Lvl 1   Lvl 2   Lvl 3

Duration:

(Goal: 30 sec each side)   Level:

12. Hanging Calf Stretch

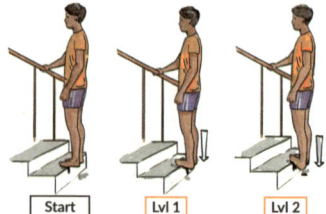

Start   Lvl 1   Lvl 2

Duration:

(Goal: 30 sec)   Level:

Daily Reflection

Benefits I'm Experiencing:

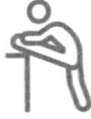

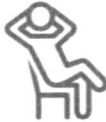

Feel Lighter	More Freedom of Movement	Improved Mental Clarity
Less Pain	Less Stressed	Improved Posture

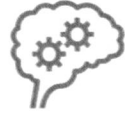

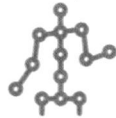

Notes On My Body:

....

....

....

....

....

....

....

....

Day 57: Dynamic Warm-Up

Full Session Exercise Guide:
habitnest.com/pages/stretching-day-57

1. Inch Worm Walk Out

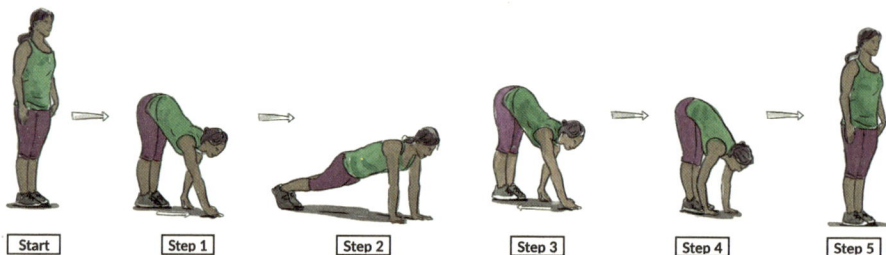

| Start | Step 1 | Step 2 | Step 3 | Step 4 | Step 5 |

Reps: .... *(Goal: 10-20)*

2. Standing Hip Circles

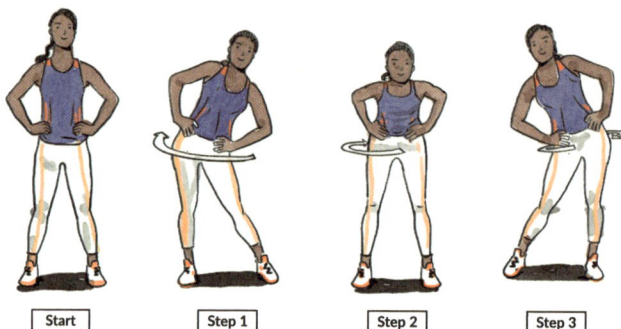

| Start | Step 1 | Step 2 | Step 3 |

Reps: .... *(Goal: 15-25 in each direction)*

3. Glute Bridge

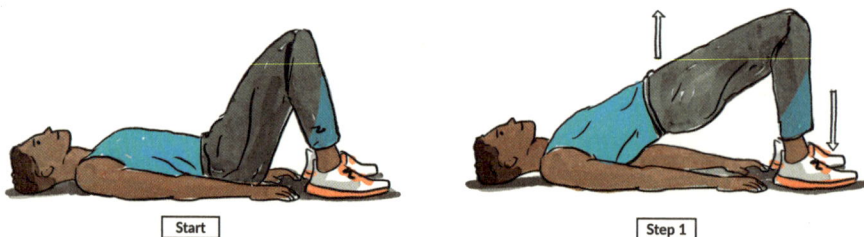

| Start | Step 1 |

Reps: .... *(Goal: 20-30)*

1. Lateral Side to Side Neck Rotation

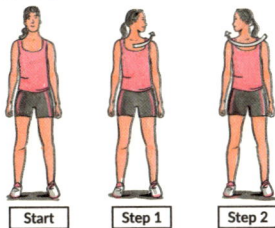

Start | Step 1 | Step 2

Duration:

(Goal: 30 sec, alternating)

2. Side Neck Stretch w/ Upside Down Palm on Wall

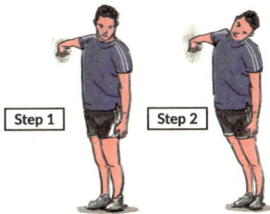

Step 1 | Step 2

Duration:

(Goal: 15 sec each side)

3. Levator Scap Neck Stretch

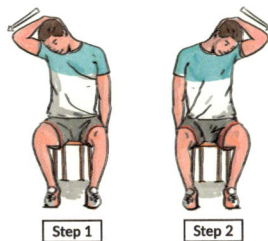

Step 1 | Step 2

Duration:

(Goal: 15 sec each side)

4. Sphinx/Cobra

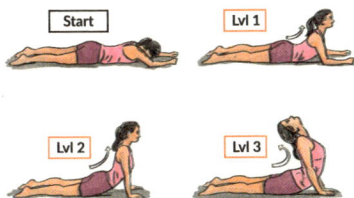

Start | Lvl 1 | Lvl 2 | Lvl 3

Duration:

(Goal: 30 sec)

Level:

5. Seated Forward Curl

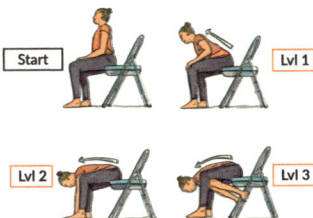

Start | Lvl 1 | Lvl 2 | Lvl 3

Duration:

(Goal: 30 sec)

Level:

6. Cross Arm Shoulder Stretch

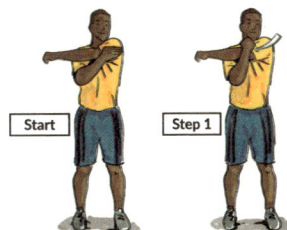

Start | Step 1

Duration:

(Goal: 15 sec each side)

7. Behind the Back Tricep Extension

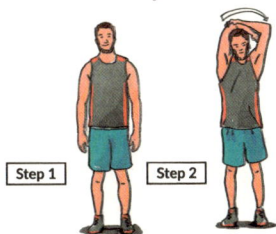

Step 1 | Step 2

Duration:

(Goal: 15 sec each side)

8. Leaning Long Arm Shoulder Stretch

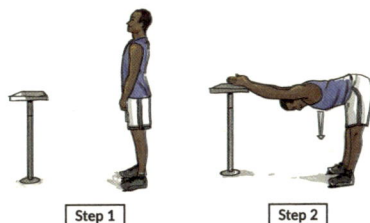

Step 1 | Step 2

Duration:

(Goal: 30 sec)

9. Corner Chest Stretch

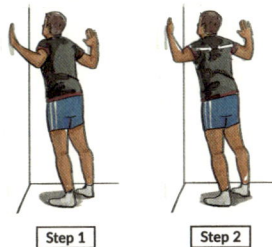

Step 1 | Step 2

Duration:

(Goal: 30 sec)

10. Locust Pose

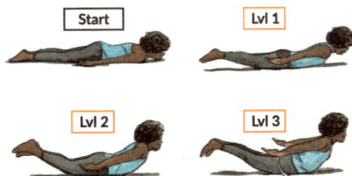

Start | Lvl 1 | Lvl 2 | Lvl 3

Level:

Duration:

(Goal: 30 sec)

Day 57: Lower Body

1. Frog Pose

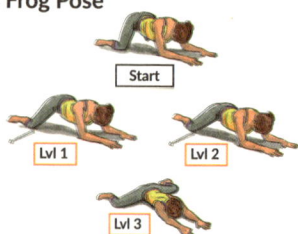

Duration:

(Goal: 60 sec)

Level:

2. Warrior II Pose

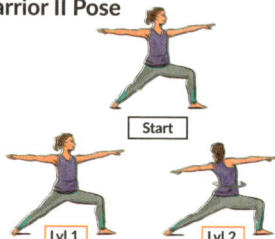

Duration:

(Goal: 30 sec each side)

Level:

3. Reclining Angle Bound Pose

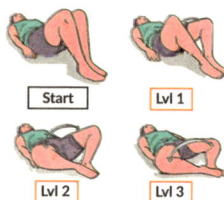

Duration:

(Goal: 30 sec)

Level:

4. Reverse Tabletop

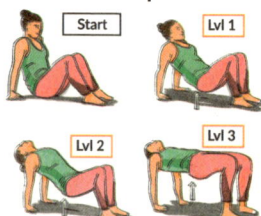

Duration:

(Goal: 30 sec)

Level:

5. Pry Squat

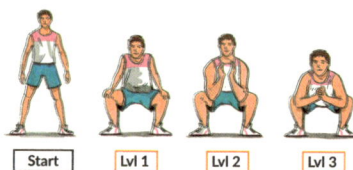

Duration:

(Goal: 30 sec)

Level:

6. Seated Forward Fold Hamstring Stretch

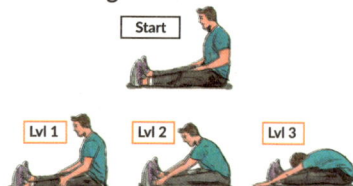

Duration:

(Goal: 30 sec)

Level:

7. Downward Dog

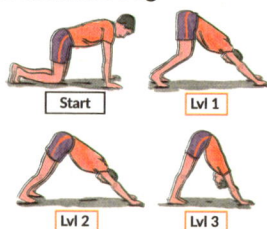

Duration:

(Goal: 30 sec)

Level:

8. Wig-Wag

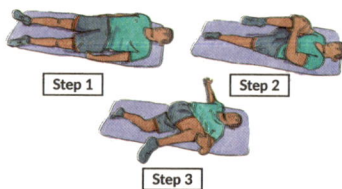

Duration:

(Goal: 30 sec each side)

9. Lateral Squat

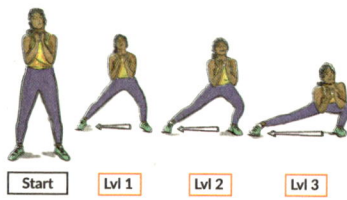

Duration:

(Goal: 30 sec each side)

Level:

10. Lateral Squat w/ Toe Raise

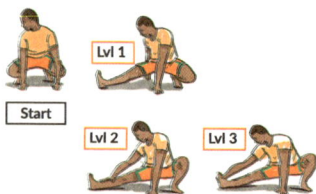

Duration:

(Goal: 30 sec each side)

Level:

11. Kneeling Quad Stretch

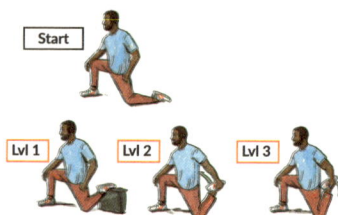

Duration:

(Goal: 30 sec each side)

Level:

12. Standing Wall Calf Stretch w/ Achilles Focus

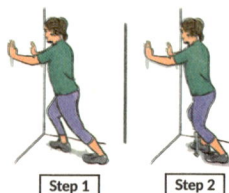

Duration:

(Goal: 15 sec each side)

Daily Reflection

Benefits I'm Experiencing:

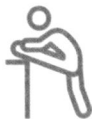

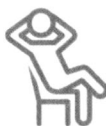

Feel Lighter	More Freedom of Movement	Improved Mental Clarity
Less Pain	Less Stressed	Improved Posture

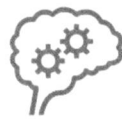

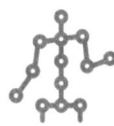

Notes On My Body:

....

....

....

....

....

....

....

....

Day 58: Dynamic Warm-Up

Full Session Exercise Guide:
habitnest.com/pages/stretching-day-58

1. Y Raise

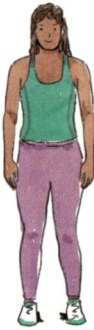
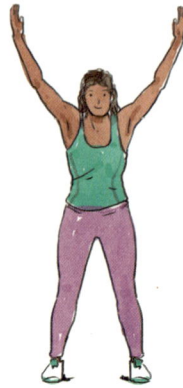

Step 1   Step 2

Reps: .... (Goal: 15-25)

2. Mountain Climber

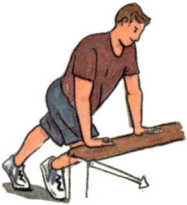
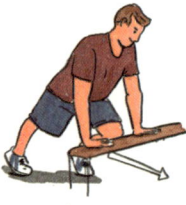
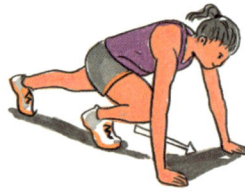

Lvl 1   Lvl 2

Level:

Reps: .... (Goal: 20-30 each side)

3. Standing Hamstring Scoop

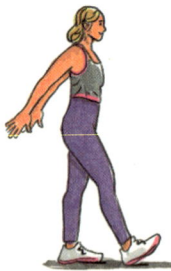
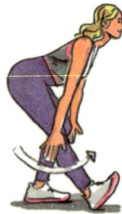
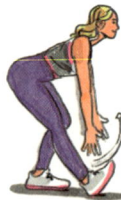
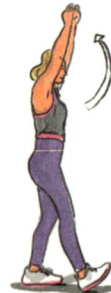

Start   Step 1   Step 2   Step 3

Reps: .... (Goal: 10-20 each side)

Day 58: Upper Body

1. Lateral Side to Side Neck Rotation

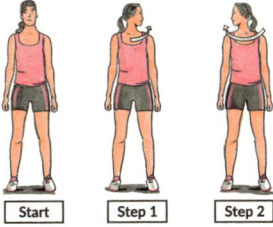

Start Step 1 Step 2

Duration:

(Goal: 30 sec, alternating)

2. Side Neck Stretch w/ Upside Down Palm on Wall

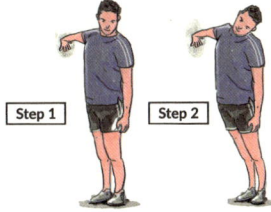

Step 1 Step 2

Duration:

(Goal: 15 sec each side)

3. Levator Scap Neck Stretch

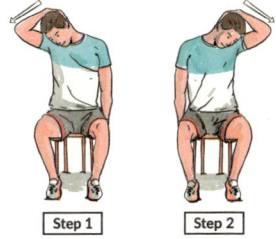

Step 1 Step 2

Duration:

(Goal: 15 sec each side)

4. Sphinx/Cobra

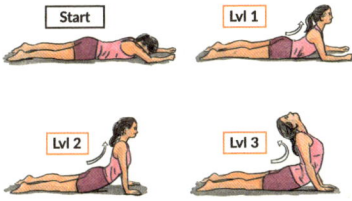

Start Lvl 1 Lvl 2 Lvl 3

Duration:

(Goal: 30 sec)

Level:

5. Seated Forward Curl

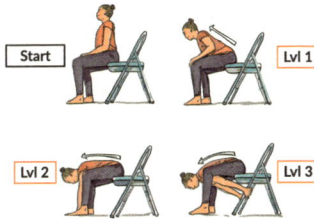

Start Lvl 1 Lvl 2 Lvl 3

Duration:

(Goal: 30 sec)

Level:

6. Cross Arm Shoulder Stretch

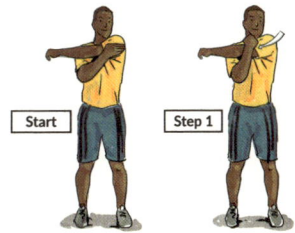

Start Step 1

Duration:

(Goal: 15 sec each side)

7. Behind the Back Tricep Extension

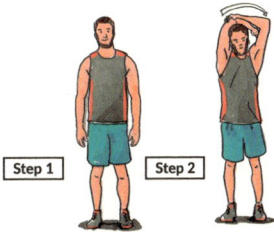

Step 1 Step 2

Duration:

(Goal: 15 sec each side)

8. Leaning Long Arm Shoulder Stretch

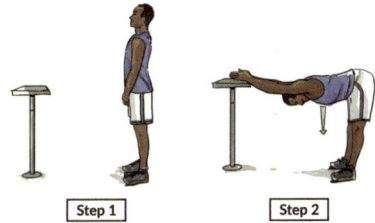

Step 1 Step 2

Duration:

(Goal: 30 sec)

9. Corner Chest Stretch

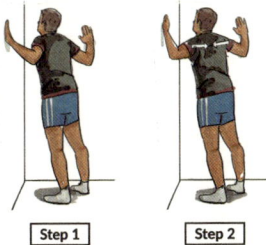

Step 1 Step 2

Duration:

(Goal: 30 sec)

10. Locust Pose

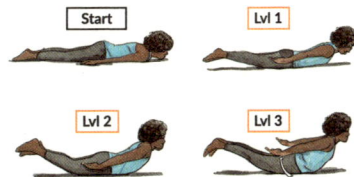

Start Lvl 1 Lvl 2 Lvl 3

Level:

Duration:

(Goal: 30 sec)

Day 58: Lower Body

1. Frog Pose

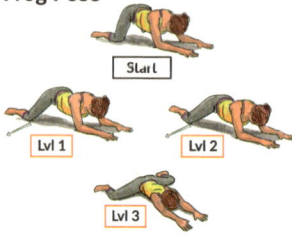

Duration:
....

(Goal: 60 sec)

Level:

2. Warrior II Pose

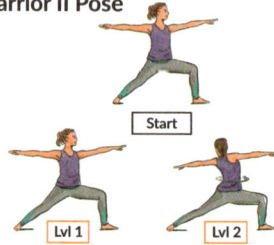

Duration:
....

(Goal: 30 sec each side)

Level:

3. Reclining Angle Bound Pose

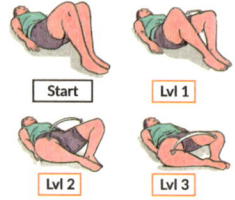

Duration:
....

(Goal: 30 sec)

Level:

4. Reverse Tabletop

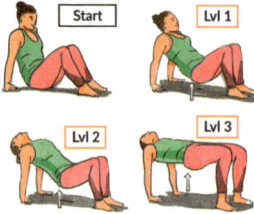

Duration:
....

(Goal: 30 sec)

Level:

5. Pry Squat

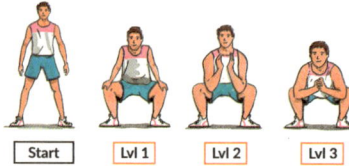

Duration:
....

(Goal: 30 sec)

Level:

6. Seated Forward Fold Hamstring Stretch

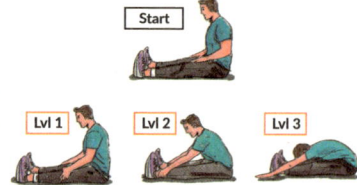

Duration:
....

(Goal: 30 sec)

Level:

7. Downward Dog

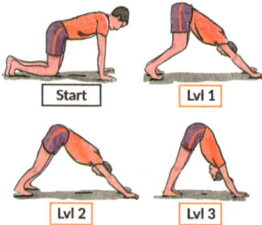

Duration:
....

(Goal: 30 sec)

Level:

8. Wig-Wag

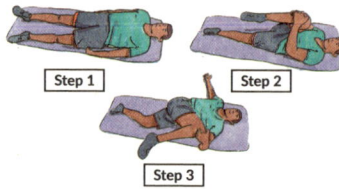

Duration:
....

(Goal: 30 sec each side)

9. Lateral Squat

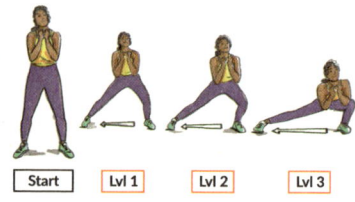

Duration:
....

(Goal: 30 sec each side)

Level:

10. Lateral Squat w/ Toe Raise

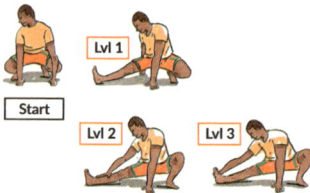

Duration:
....

(Goal: 30 sec each side)

Level:

11. Kneeling Quad Stretch

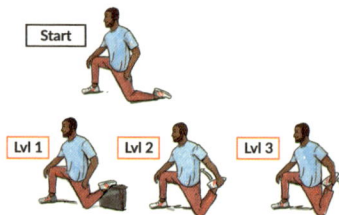

Duration:
....

(Goal: 30 sec each side)

Level:

12. Standing Wall Calf Stretch w/ Achilles Focus

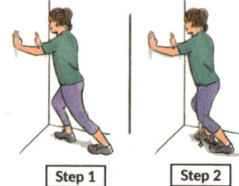

Duration:
....

(Goal: 15 sec each side)

Daily Reflection

Benefits I'm Experiencing:

Feel
Lighter

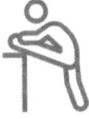

More Freedom
of Movement

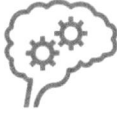

Improved
Mental Clarity

Less
Pain

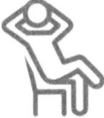

Less
Stressed

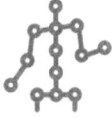

Improved
Posture

Notes On My Body:

Day 59: Dynamic Warm-Up

Full Session Exercise Guide:
habitnest.com/pages/stretching-day-59

1. Push-Up

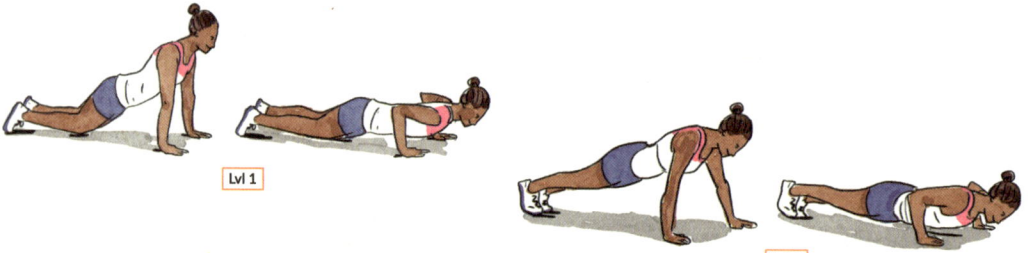

Lvl 1

Lvl 2

Level:

Reps: .... *(Goal: 15-25)*

2. Clam Opener w/ Side Plank

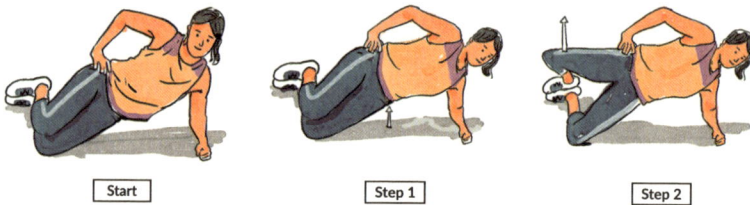

Start

Step 1

Step 2

Reps: .... *(Goal: 10-15 each side)*

3. Towel Snatch

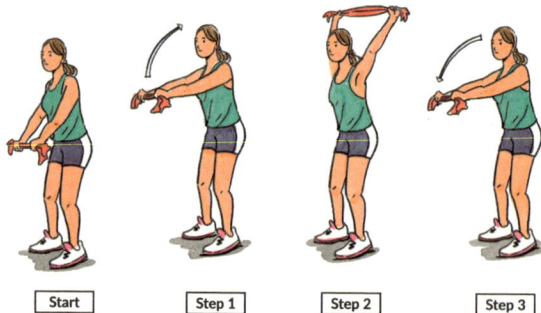

Start

Step 1

Step 2

Step 3

Reps: .... *(Goal: 10-20)*

Day 59: Upper Body

DATE

1. Lateral Side to Side Neck Rotation

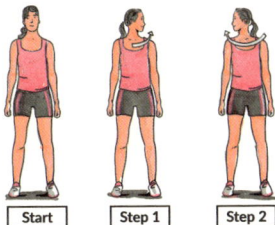

Start | Step 1 | Step 2

Duration:

(Goal: 30 sec, alternating)

2. Side Neck Stretch w/ Upside Down Palm on Wall

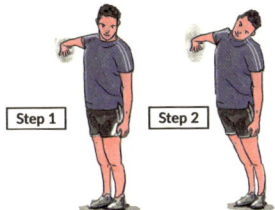

Step 1 | Step 2

Duration:

(Goal: 15 sec each side)

3. Levator Scap Neck Stretch

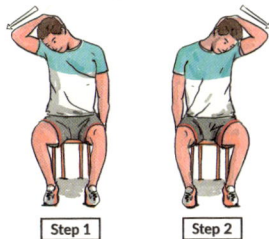

Step 1 | Step 2

Duration:

(Goal: 15 sec each side)

4. Sphinx/Cobra

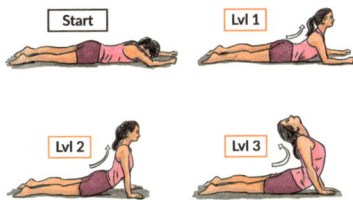

Start | Lvl 1 | Lvl 2 | Lvl 3

Duration:

(Goal: 30 sec)

Level:

5. Seated Forward Curl

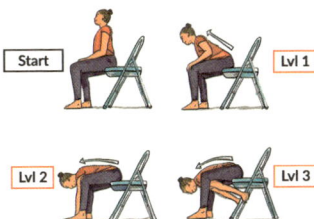

Start | Lvl 1 | Lvl 2 | Lvl 3

Duration:

(Goal: 30 sec)

Level:

6. Cross Arm Shoulder Stretch

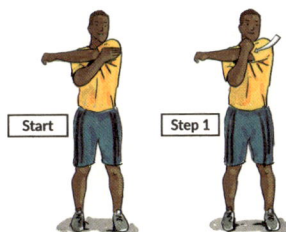

Start | Step 1

Duration:

(Goal: 15 sec each side)

7. Behind the Back Tricep Extension

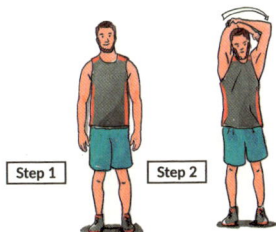

Step 1 | Step 2

Duration:

(Goal: 15 sec each side)

8. Leaning Long Arm Shoulder Stretch

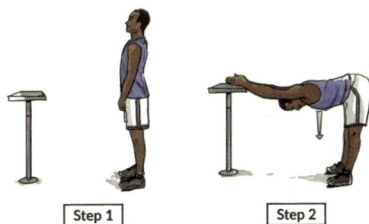

Step 1 | Step 2

Duration:

(Goal: 30 sec)

9. Corner Chest Stretch

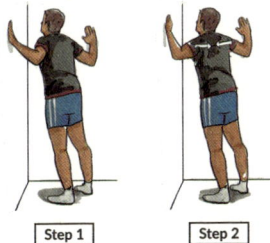

Step 1 | Step 2

Duration:

(Goal: 30 sec)

10. Locust Pose

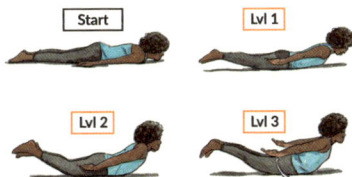

Start | Lvl 1 | Lvl 2 | Lvl 3

Level:

Duration:

(Goal: 30 sec)

283

Day 59: Lower Body

1. Frog Pose

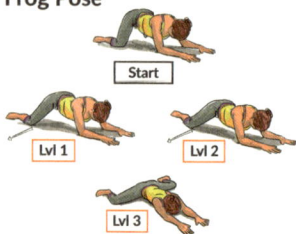

Start
Lvl 1
Lvl 2
Lvl 3

Duration:

(Goal: 60 sec)

Level:

2. Warrior II Pose

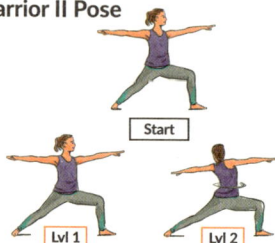

Start
Lvl 1
Lvl 2

Duration:

(Goal: 30 sec each side)

Level:

3. Reclining Angle Bound Pose

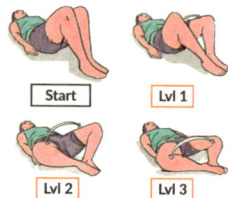

Start
Lvl 1
Lvl 2
Lvl 3

Duration:

(Goal: 30 sec)

Level:

4. Reverse Tabletop

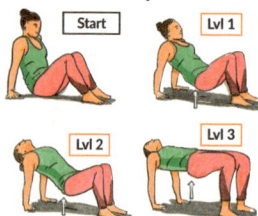

Start
Lvl 1
Lvl 2
Lvl 3

Duration:

(Goal: 30 sec)

Level:

5. Pry Squat

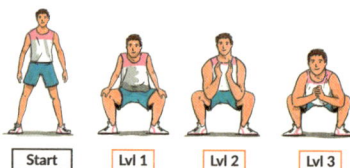

Start
Start
Lvl 1
Lvl 2
Lvl 3

Duration:

(Goal: 30 sec)

Level:

6. Seated Forward Fold Hamstring Stretch

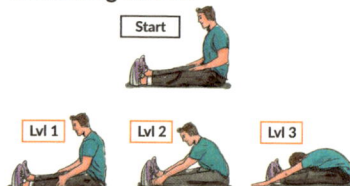

Start
Lvl 1
Lvl 2
Lvl 3

Duration:

(Goal: 30 sec)

Level:

7. Downward Dog

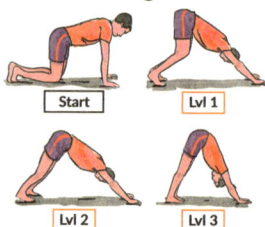

Start
Lvl 1
Lvl 2
Lvl 3

Duration:

(Goal: 30 sec)

Level:

8. Wig-Wag

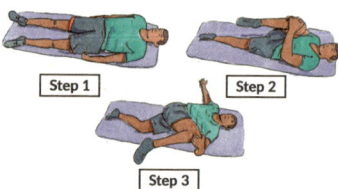

Step 1
Step 2
Step 3

Duration:

(Goal: 30 sec each side)

9. Lateral Squat

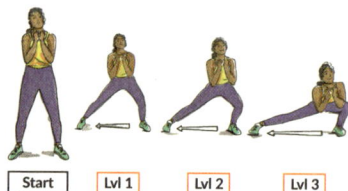

Start
Lvl 1
Lvl 2
Lvl 3

Duration:

(Goal: 30 sec each side)

Level:

10. Lateral Squat w/ Toe Raise

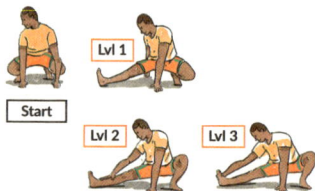

Lvl 1
Start
Lvl 2
Lvl 3

Duration:

(Goal: 30 sec each side)

Level:

11. Kneeling Quad Stretch

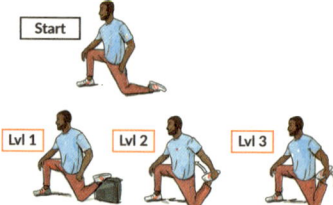

Start
Lvl 1
Lvl 2
Lvl 3

Duration:

(Goal: 30 sec each side)

Level:

12. Standing Wall Calf Stretch w/ Achilles Focus

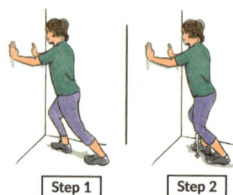

Step 1
Step 2

Duration:

(Goal: 15 sec each side)

Daily Reflection

Benefits I'm Experiencing:

Feel
Lighter

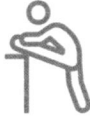

More Freedom
of Movement

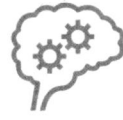

Improved
Mental Clarity

Less
Pain

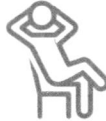

Less
Stressed

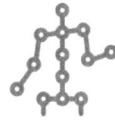

Improved
Posture

Notes On My Body:

1. World's Greatest Stretch

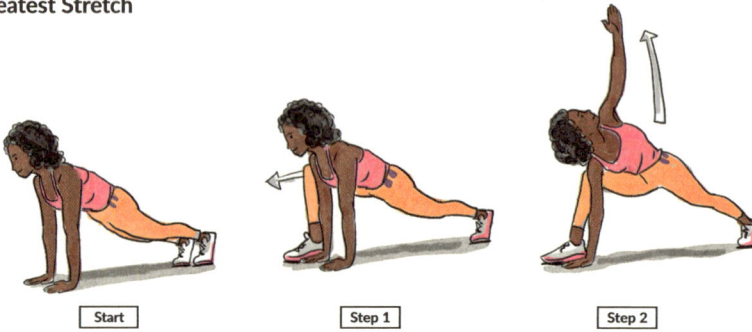

Start   Step 1   Step 2

Reps: *(Goal: 10-20)*

2. Good Morning

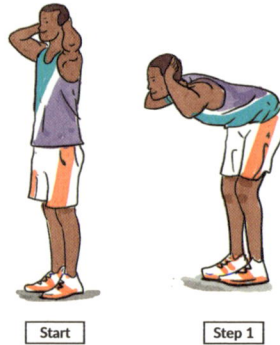

Start   Step 1

Reps: *(Goal: 15-20)*

3. Bird-Dog

Start   Step 1   Step 2   Step 3

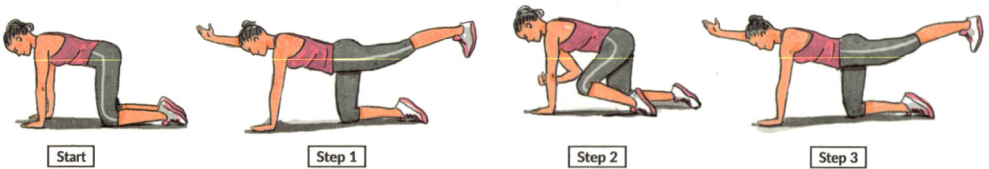

Reps: *(Goal: 10-15 each side)*

Day 60: Upper Body

DATE

1. Lateral Side to Side Neck Rotation

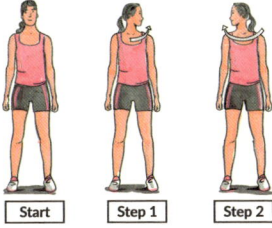

Start Step 1 Step 2

Duration: ....

(Goal: 30 sec, alternating)

2. Side Neck Stretch w/ Upside Down Palm on Wall

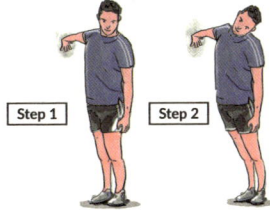

Step 1 Step 2

Duration: ....

(Goal: 15 sec each side)

3. Levator Scap Neck Stretch

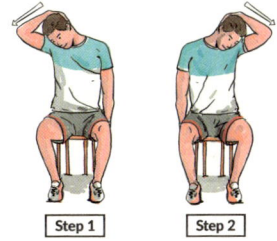

Step 1 Step 2

Duration: ....

(Goal: 15 sec each side)

4. Sphinx/Cobra

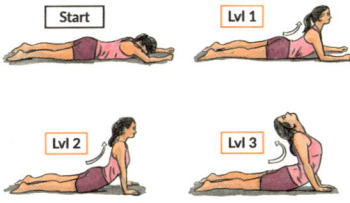

Start Lvl 1 Lvl 2 Lvl 3

Duration: ....

(Goal: 30 sec)

Level: ____

5. Seated Forward Curl

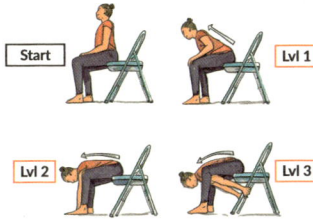

Start Lvl 1 Lvl 2 Lvl 3

Duration: ....

(Goal: 30 sec)

Level: ____

6. Cross Arm Shoulder Stretch

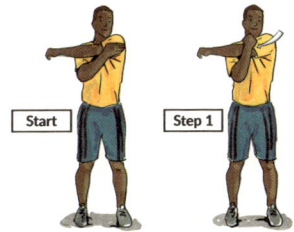

Start Step 1

Duration: ....

(Goal: 15 sec each side)

7. Behind the Back Tricep Extension

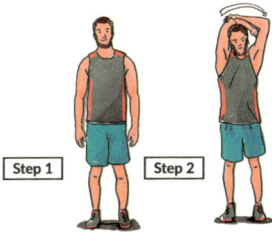

Step 1 Step 2

Duration: ....

(Goal: 15 sec each side)

8. Leaning Long Arm Shoulder Stretch

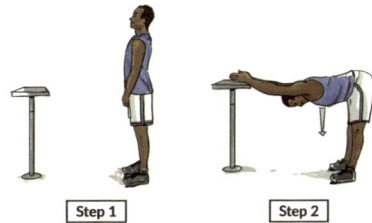

Step 1 Step 2

Duration: ....

(Goal: 30 sec)

9. Corner Chest Stretch

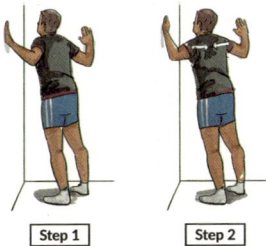

Step 1 Step 2

Duration: ....

(Goal: 30 sec)

10. Locust Pose

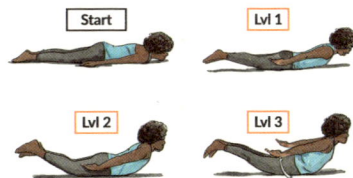

Start Lvl 1 Lvl 2 Lvl 3

Level: ____

Duration: ....

(Goal: 30 sec)

Day 60: Lower Body

1. Frog Pose

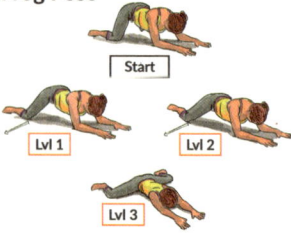

Start
Lvl 1
Lvl 2
Lvl 3

Duration: ....

(Goal: 60 sec)

Level:

2. Warrior II Pose

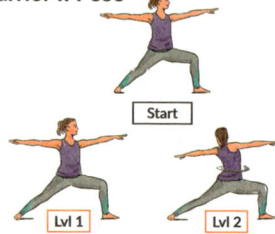

Start
Lvl 1
Lvl 2

Duration: ....

(Goal: 30 sec each side)

Level:

3. Reclining Angle Bound Pose

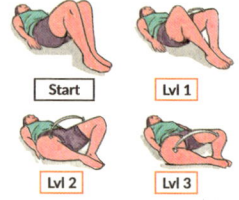

Start
Lvl 1
Lvl 2
Lvl 3

Duration: ....

(Goal: 30 sec)

Level:

4. Reverse Tabletop

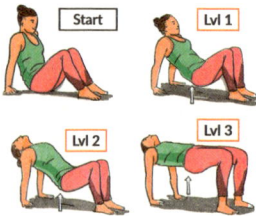

Start
Lvl 1
Lvl 2
Lvl 3

Duration: ....

(Goal: 30 sec)

Level:

5. Pry Squat

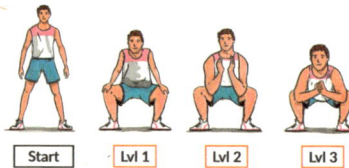

Start
Lvl 1
Lvl 2
Lvl 3

Duration: ....

(Goal: 30 sec)

Level:

6. Seated Forward Fold Hamstring Stretch

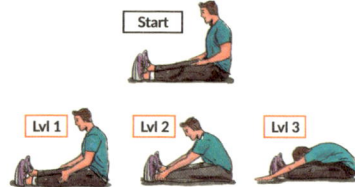

Start
Lvl 1
Lvl 2
Lvl 3

Duration: ....

(Goal: 30 sec)

Level:

7. Downward Dog

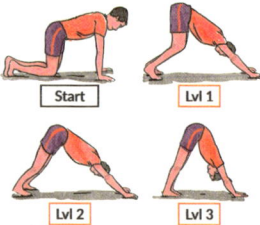

Start
Lvl 1
Lvl 2
Lvl 3

Duration: ....

(Goal: 30 sec)

Level:

8. Wig-Wag

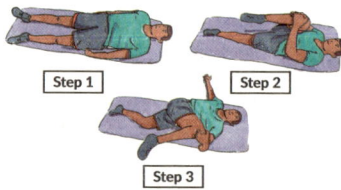

Step 1
Step 2
Step 3

Duration: ....

(Goal: 30 sec each side)

9. Lateral Squat

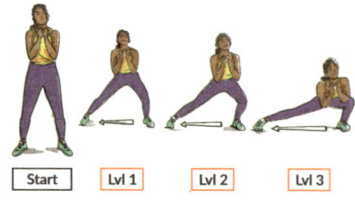

Start
Lvl 1
Lvl 2
Lvl 3

Duration: ....

(Goal: 30 sec each side)

Level:

10. Lateral Squat w/ Toe Raise

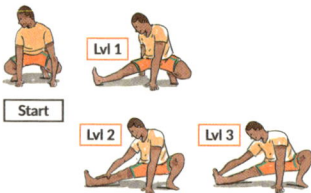

Lvl 1
Start
Lvl 2
Lvl 3

Duration: ....

(Goal: 30 sec each side)

Level:

11. Kneeling Quad Stretch

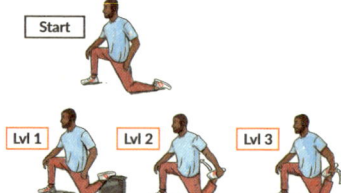

Start
Lvl 1
Lvl 2
Lvl 3

Duration: ....

(Goal: 30 sec each side)

Level:

12. Standing Wall Calf Stretch w/ Achilles Focus

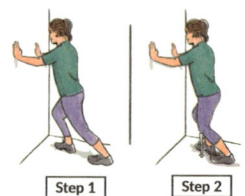

Step 1
Step 2

Duration: ....

(Goal: 15 sec each side)

Daily Reflection

Benefits I'm Experiencing:

Feel
Lighter

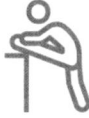

More Freedom
of Movement

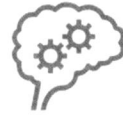

Improved
Mental Clarity

Less
Pain

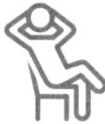

Less
Stressed

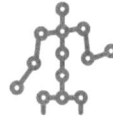

Improved
Posture

Notes On My Body:

Day 61: Dynamic Warm-Up

Full Session Exercise Guide:
habitnest.com/pages/stretching-day-61

1. Pike Push-Up

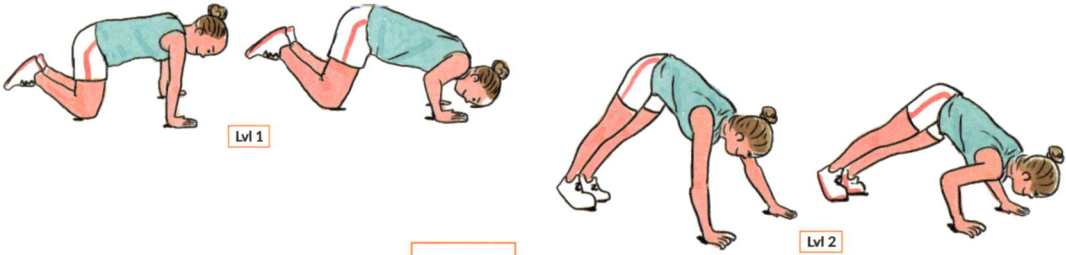

Lvl 1

Lvl 2

Level:

Reps: .... *(Goal: 15-25)*

2. Side Plank w/ Twist

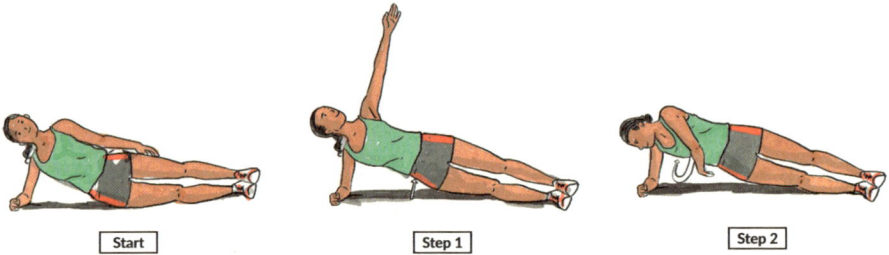

Start

Step 1

Step 2

Reps: .... *(Goal: 10-15 each side)*

3. Good Morning

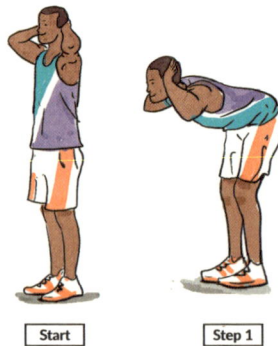

Start

Step 1

Reps: .... *(Goal: 15-20)*

Day 61: Upper Body

1. Lateral Side to Side Neck Rotation

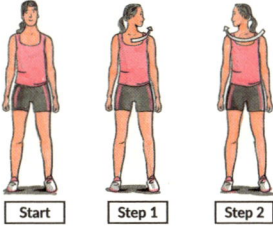

Start | Step 1 | Step 2

Duration:

(Goal: 30 sec, alternating)

2. Side Neck Stretch w/ Upside Down Palm on Wall

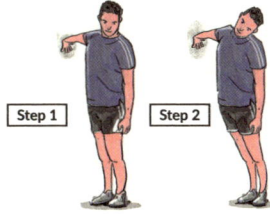

Step 1 | Step 2

Duration:

(Goal: 15 sec each side)

3. Levator Scap Neck Stretch

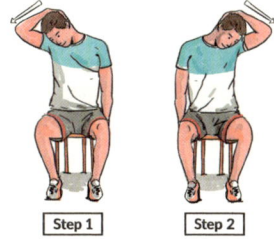

Step 1 | Step 2

Duration:

(Goal: 15 sec each side)

4. Sphinx/Cobra

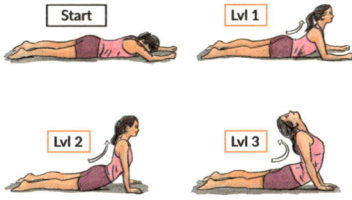

Start | Lvl 1 | Lvl 2 | Lvl 3

Duration:

(Goal: 30 sec)

Level:

5. Seated Forward Curl

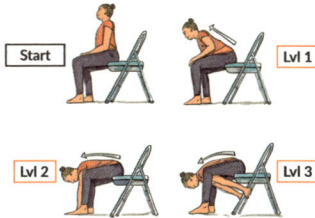

Start | Lvl 1 | Lvl 2 | Lvl 3

Duration:

(Goal: 30 sec)

Level:

6. Cross Arm Shoulder Stretch

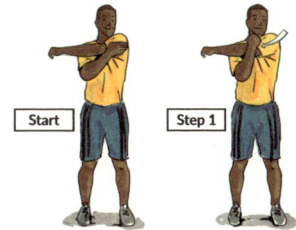

Start | Step 1

Duration:

(Goal: 15 sec each side)

7. Behind the Back Tricep Extension

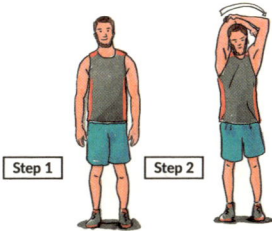

Step 1 | Step 2

Duration:

(Goal: 15 sec each side)

8. Leaning Long Arm Shoulder Stretch

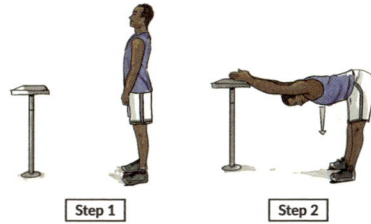

Step 1 | Step 2

Duration:

(Goal: 30 sec)

9. Corner Chest Stretch

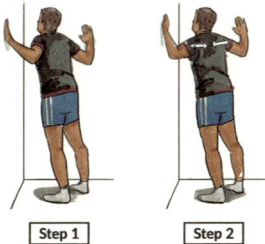

Step 1 | Step 2

Duration:

(Goal: 30 sec)

10. Locust Pose

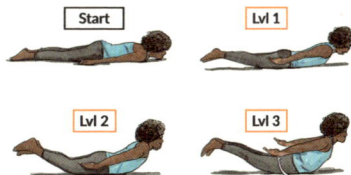

Start | Lvl 1 | Lvl 2 | Lvl 3

Level:

Duration:

(Goal: 30 sec)

Day 61: Lower Body

1. Frog Pose

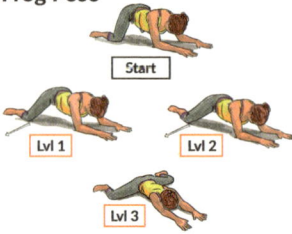
Start
Lvl 1
Lvl 2
Lvl 3

Duration:
....

(Goal: 60 sec)

Level:

2. Warrior II Pose

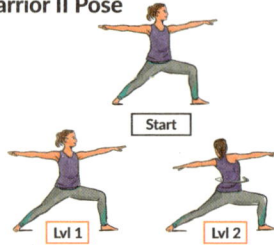
Start
Lvl 1
Lvl 2

Duration:
....

(Goal: 30 sec each side)

Level:

3. Reclining Angle Bound Pose

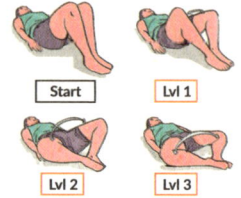
Start
Lvl 1
Lvl 2
Lvl 3

Duration:
....

(Goal: 30 sec)

Level:

4. Reverse Tabletop

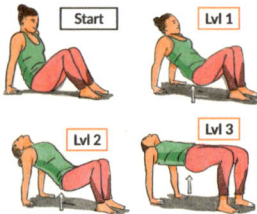
Start
Lvl 1
Lvl 2
Lvl 3

Duration:
....

(Goal: 30 sec)

Level:

5. Pry Squat

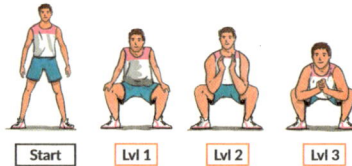
Start
Start
Lvl 1
Lvl 2
Lvl 3

Duration:
....

(Goal: 30 sec)

Level:

6. Seated Forward Fold Hamstring Stretch

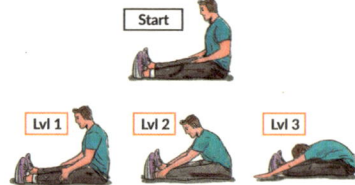
Start
Lvl 1
Lvl 2
Lvl 3

Duration:
....

(Goal: 30 sec)

Level:

7. Downward Dog

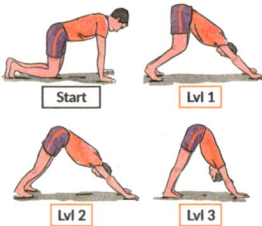
Start
Lvl 1
Lvl 2
Lvl 3

Duration:
....

(Goal: 30 sec)

Level:

8. Wig-Wag

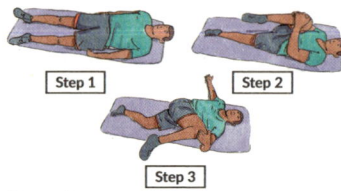
Step 1
Step 2
Step 3

Duration:
....

(Goal: 30 sec each side)

9. Lateral Squat

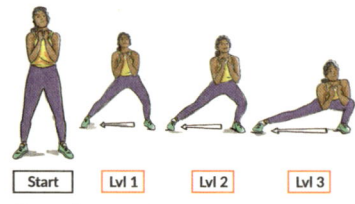
Start
Lvl 1
Lvl 2
Lvl 3

Duration:
....

(Goal: 30 sec each side)

Level:

10. Lateral Squat w/ Toe Raise

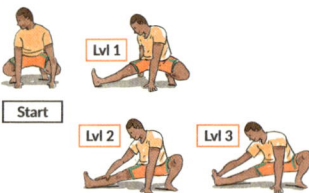
Lvl 1
Start
Lvl 2
Lvl 3

Duration:
....

(Goal: 30 sec each side)

Level:

11. Kneeling Quad Stretch

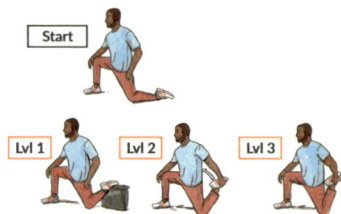
Start
Lvl 1
Lvl 2
Lvl 3

Duration:
....

(Goal: 30 sec each side)

Level:

12. Standing Wall Calf Stretch w/ Achilles Focus

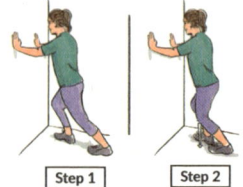
Step 1
Step 2

Duration:
....

(Goal: 15 sec each side)

Daily Reflection

Benefits I'm Experiencing:

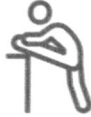

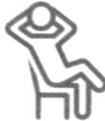

Feel Lighter	More Freedom of Movement	Improved Mental Clarity
Less Pain	Less Stressed	Improved Posture

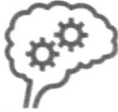

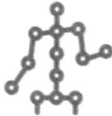

Notes On My Body:

1. Roundhouse Kick to Squat

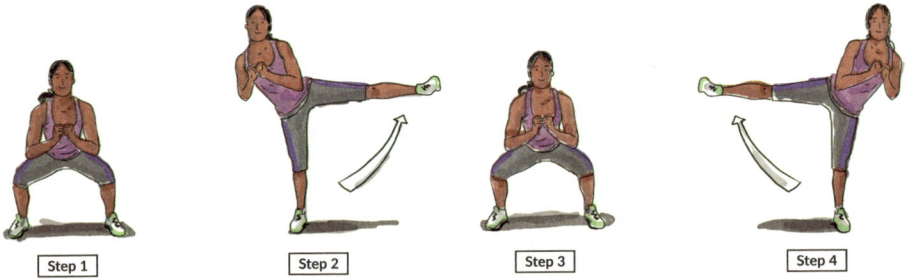

Step 1

Step 2

Step 3

Step 4

Reps: .... *(Goal: 10-15 each side)*

2. Aquaman

Start

Step 1

Step 2

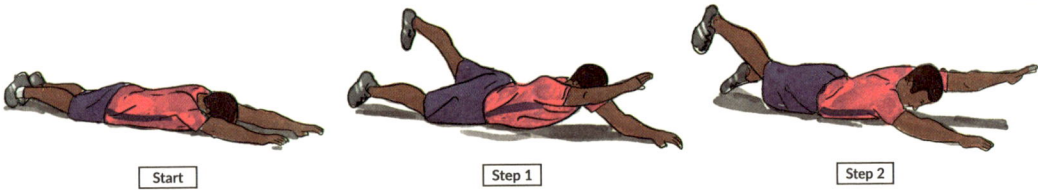

Reps: .... *(Goal: 10-20)*

3. Glute Bridge

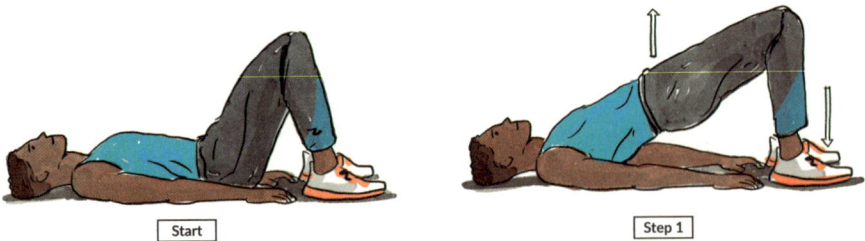

Start

Step 1

Reps: .... *(Goal: 20-30)*

Day 62: Upper Body

DATE

1. Lateral Side to Side Neck Rotation

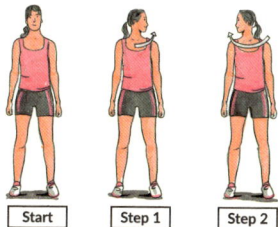

Start | Step 1 | Step 2

Duration:

(Goal: 30 sec, alternating)

2. Side Neck Stretch w/ Upside Down Palm on Wall

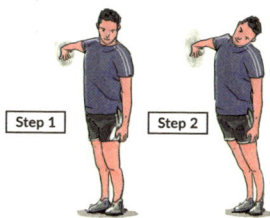

Step 1 | Step 2

Duration:

(Goal: 15 sec each side)

3. Levator Scap Neck Stretch

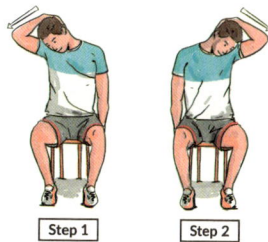

Step 1 | Step 2

Duration:

(Goal: 15 sec each side)

4. Sphinx/Cobra

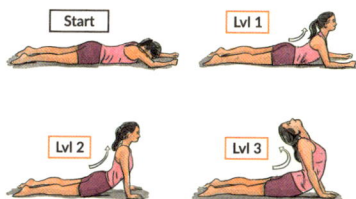

Start | Lvl 1 | Lvl 2 | Lvl 3

Duration:

(Goal: 30 sec)

Level:

5. Seated Forward Curl

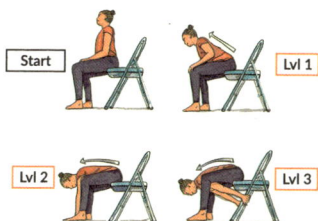

Start | Lvl 1 | Lvl 2 | Lvl 3

Duration:

(Goal: 30 sec)

Level:

6. Cross Arm Shoulder Stretch

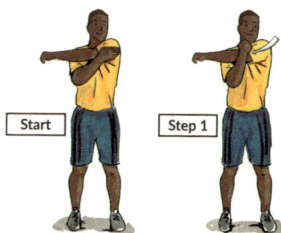

Start | Step 1

Duration:

(Goal: 15 sec each side)

7. Behind the Back Tricep Extension

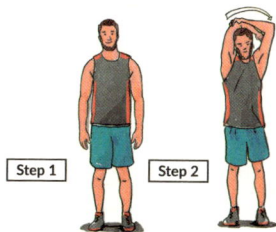

Step 1 | Step 2

Duration:

(Goal: 15 sec each side)

8. Leaning Long Arm Shoulder Stretch

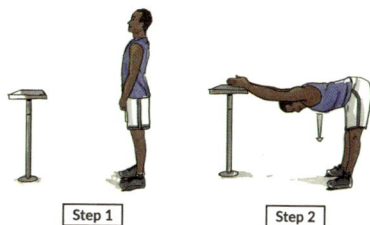

Step 1 | Step 2

Duration:

(Goal: 30 sec)

9. Corner Chest Stretch

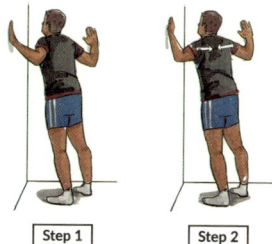

Step 1 | Step 2

Duration:

(Goal: 30 sec)

10. Locust Pose

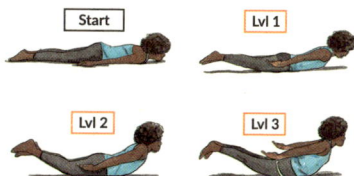

Start | Lvl 1 | Lvl 2 | Lvl 3

Level:

Duration:

(Goal: 30 sec)

295

Day 62: Lower Body

1. Frog Pose

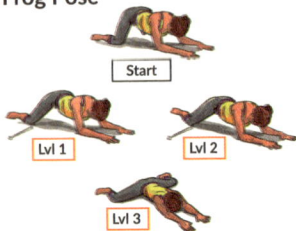

Start
Lvl 1
Lvl 2
Lvl 3

Duration:

(Goal: 60 sec)

Level:

2. Warrior II Pose

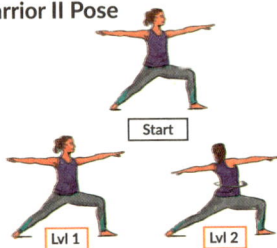

Start
Lvl 1
Lvl 2

Duration:

(Goal: 30 sec each side)

Level:

3. Reclining Angle Bound Pose

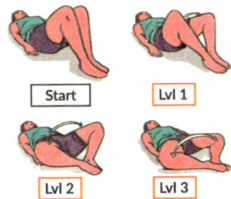

Start
Lvl 1
Lvl 2
Lvl 3

Duration:

(Goal: 30 sec)

Level:

4. Reverse Tabletop

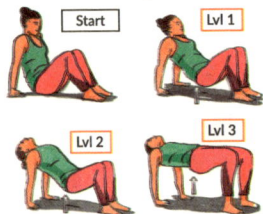

Start
Lvl 1
Lvl 2
Lvl 3

Duration:

(Goal: 30 sec)

Level:

5. Pry Squat

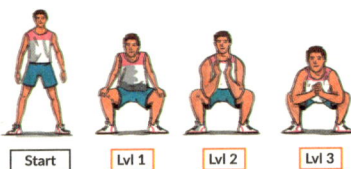

Start
Lvl 1
Lvl 2
Lvl 3

Duration:

(Goal: 30 sec)

Level:

6. Seated Forward Fold Hamstring Stretch

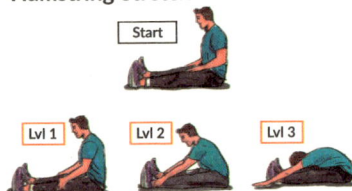

Start
Lvl 1
Lvl 2
Lvl 3

Duration:

(Goal: 30 sec)

Level:

7. Downward Dog

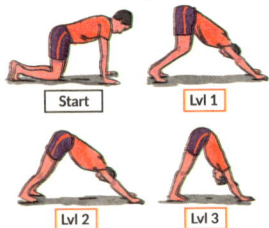

Start
Lvl 1
Lvl 2
Lvl 3

Duration:

(Goal: 30 sec)

Level:

8. Wig-Wag

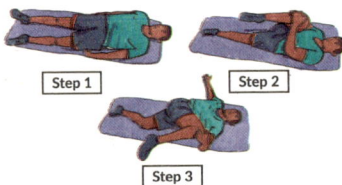

Step 1
Step 2
Step 3

Duration:

(Goal: 30 sec each side)

9. Lateral Squat

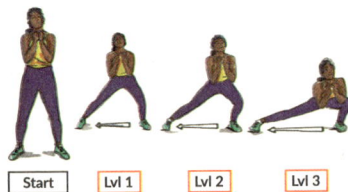

Start
Lvl 1
Lvl 2
Lvl 3

Duration:

(Goal: 30 sec each side)

Level:

10. Lateral Squat w/ Toe Raise

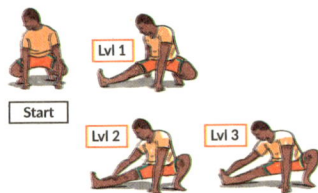

Lvl 1
Start
Lvl 2
Lvl 3

Duration:

(Goal: 30 sec each side)

Level:

11. Kneeling Quad Stretch

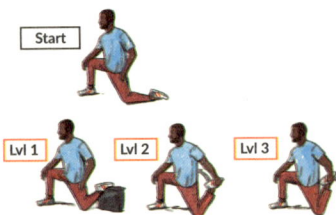

Start
Lvl 1
Lvl 2
Lvl 3

Duration:

(Goal: 30 sec each side)

Level:

12. Standing Wall Calf Stretch w/ Achilles Focus

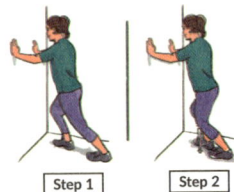

Step 1
Step 2

Duration:

(Goal: 15 sec each side)

Daily Reflection

Benefits I'm Experiencing:

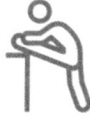

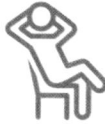

Feel Lighter	More Freedom of Movement	Improved Mental Clarity
Less Pain	Less Stressed	Improved Posture

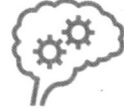

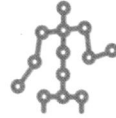

Notes On My Body:

....

....

....

....

....

....

....

....

Day 63: Dynamic Warm-Up

Full Session Exercise Guide:
habitnest.com/pages/stretching-day-63

1. Inch Worm Walk Out

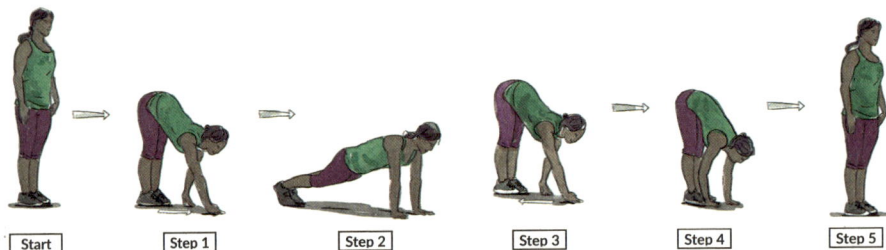

| Start | Step 1 | Step 2 | Step 3 | Step 4 | Step 5 |

Reps: .... *(Goal: 10-20)*

2. Y Raise

| Step 1 | Step 2 |

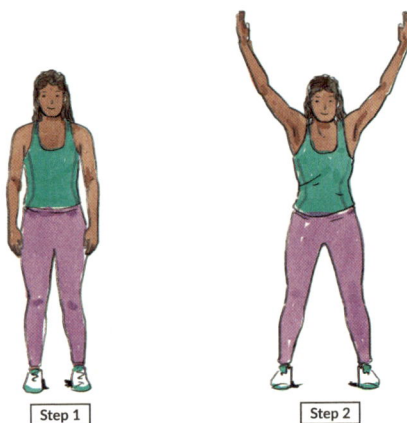

Reps: .... *(Goal: 15-25)*

3. Standing Hip Circles

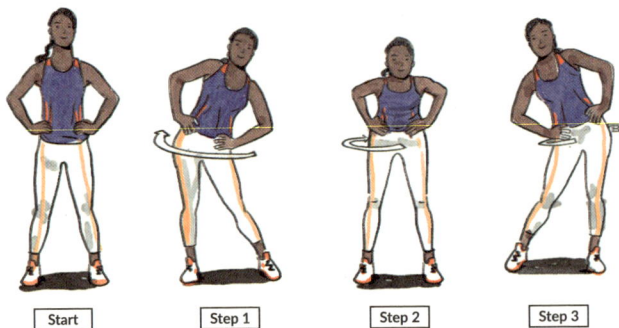

| Start | Step 1 | Step 2 | Step 3 |

Reps: .... *(Goal: 15-20 in each direction)*

1. Lateral Side to Side Neck Rotation

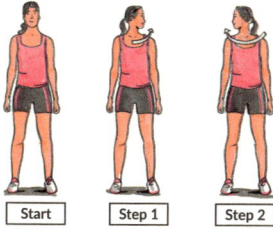

Start | Step 1 | Step 2

Duration:

(Goal: 30 sec, alternating)

2. Side Neck Stretch w/ Upside Down Palm on Wall

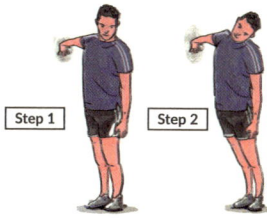

Step 1 | Step 2

Duration:

(Goal: 15 sec each side)

3. Levator Scap Neck Stretch

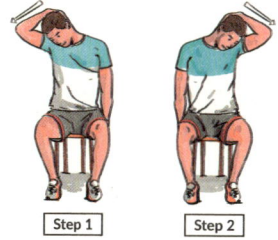

Step 1 | Step 2

Duration:

(Goal: 15 sec each side)

4. Sphinx/Cobra

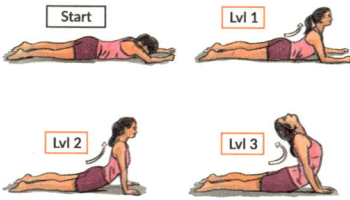

Start | Lvl 1 | Lvl 2 | Lvl 3

Duration:

(Goal: 30 sec)

Level:

5. Seated Forward Curl

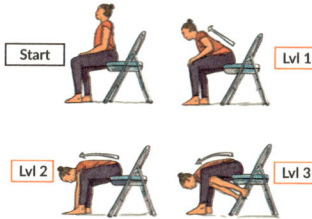

Start | Lvl 1 | Lvl 2 | Lvl 3

Duration:

(Goal: 30 sec)

Level:

6. Cross Arm Shoulder Stretch

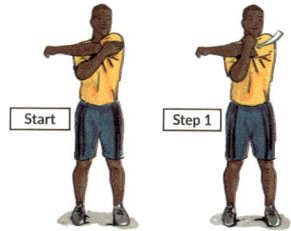

Start | Step 1

Duration:

(Goal: 15 sec each side)

7. Behind the Back Tricep Extension

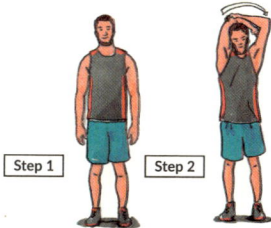

Step 1 | Step 2

Duration:

(Goal: 15 sec each side)

8. Leaning Long Arm Shoulder Stretch

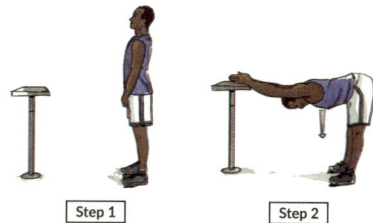

Step 1 | Step 2

Duration:

(Goal: 30 sec)

9. Corner Chest Stretch

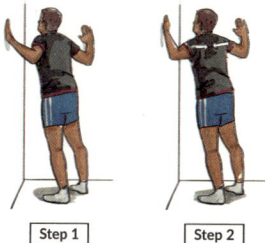

Step 1 | Step 2

Duration:

(Goal: 30 sec)

10. Locust Pose

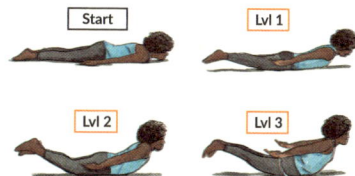

Start | Lvl 1 | Lvl 2 | Lvl 3

Level:

Duration:

(Goal: 30 sec)

Day 63: Lower Body

1. Frog Pose

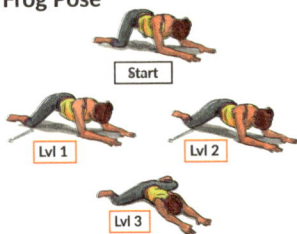

Start
Lvl 1   Lvl 2
Lvl 3

Duration:

(Goal: 60 sec)

Level:

2. Warrior II Pose

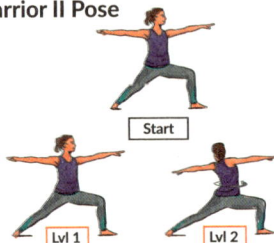

Start
Lvl 1   Lvl 2

Duration:

(Goal: 30 sec each side)

Level:

3. Reclining Angle Bound Pose

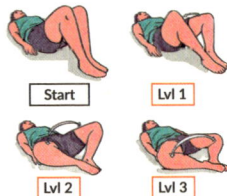

Start   Lvl 1
Lvl 2   Lvl 3

Duration:

(Goal: 30 sec)

Level:

4. Reverse Tabletop

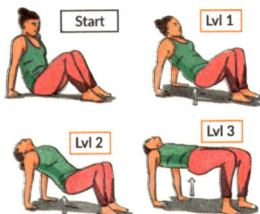

Start   Lvl 1
Lvl 2   Lvl 3

Duration:

(Goal: 30 sec)

Level:

5. Pry Squat

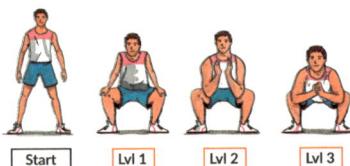

Start   Lvl 1   Lvl 2   Lvl 3

Duration:

(Goal: 30 sec)

Level:

6. Seated Forward Fold Hamstring Stretch

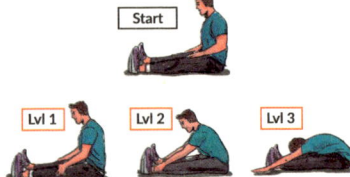

Start
Lvl 1   Lvl 2   Lvl 3

Duration:

(Goal: 30 sec)

Level:

7. Downward Dog

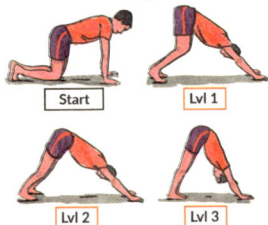

Start   Lvl 1
Lvl 2   Lvl 3

Duration:

(Goal: 30 sec)

Level:

8. Wig-Wag

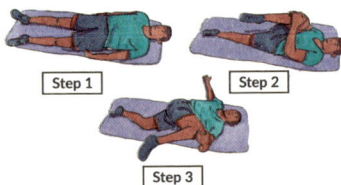

Step 1   Step 2
Step 3

Duration:

(Goal: 30 sec each side)

9. Lateral Squat

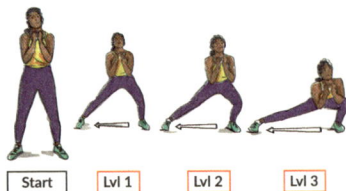

Start   Lvl 1   Lvl 2   Lvl 3

Duration:

(Goal: 30 sec each side)

Level:

10. Lateral Squat w/ Toe Raise

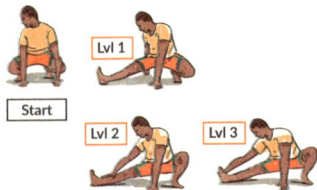

Lvl 1
Start
Lvl 2   Lvl 3

Duration:

(Goal: 30 sec each side)

Level:

11. Kneeling Quad Stretch

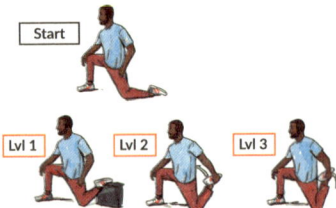

Start
Lvl 1   Lvl 2   Lvl 3

Duration:

(Goal: 30 sec each side)

Level:

12. Standing Wall Calf Stretch w/ Achilles Focus

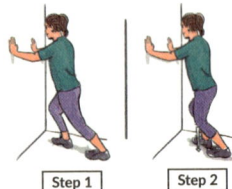

Step 1   Step 2

Duration:

(Goal: 15 sec each side)

Daily Reflection

Benefits I'm Experiencing:

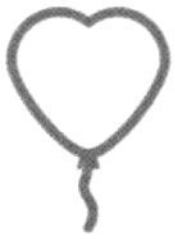

Feel
Lighter

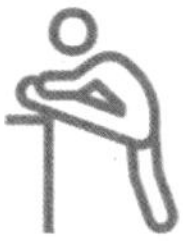

More Freedom
of Movement

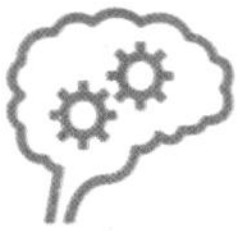

Improved
Mental Clarity

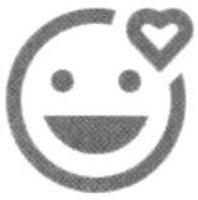

Less
Pain

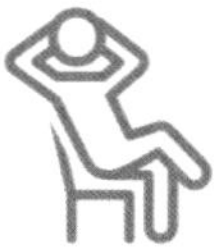

Less
Stressed

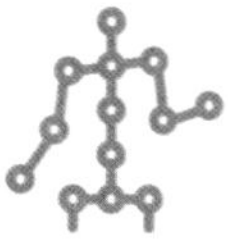

Improved
Posture

Notes On My Body:

Day 64: Dynamic Warm-Up

Full Session Exercise Guide:
habitnest.com/pages/stretching-day-64

1. Pike Push-Up

Lvl 1

Lvl 2

Level:

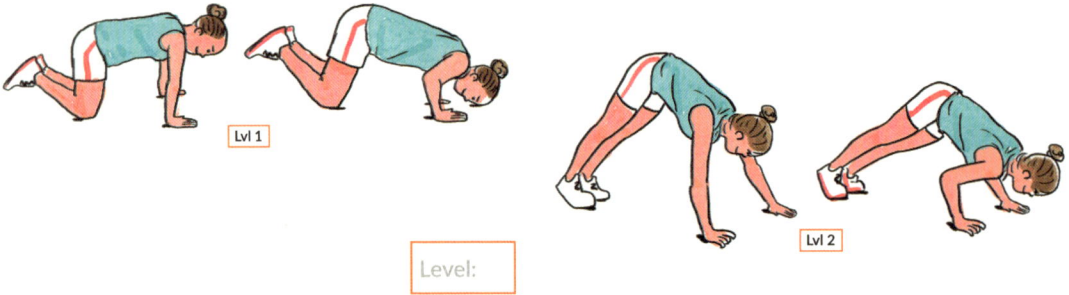

Reps: *(Goal: 15-25)*

2. Y Raise

Step 1

Step 2

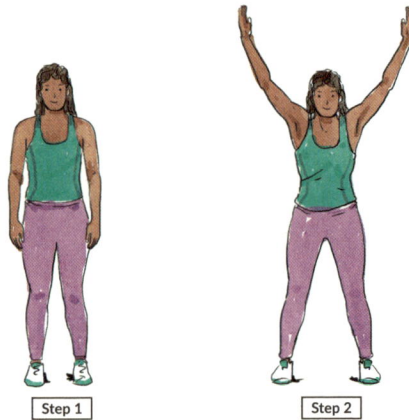

Reps: *(Goal: 20-30)*

3. Air Squat to Calf Raise

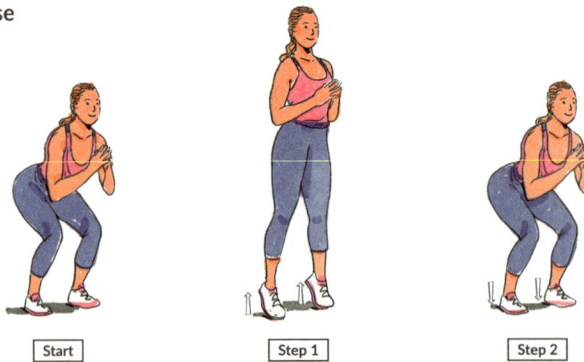

Start

Step 1

Step 2

Reps: *(Goal: 20-30)*

Day 64: Upper Body

1. Up & Down Neck Tilt

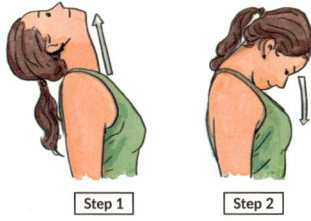

Step 1 Step 2

Duration:

(Goal: 30 sec, alternating)

2. Side Neck Tilt

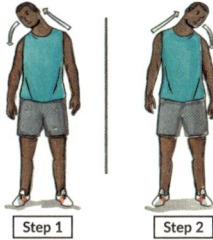

Step 1 Step 2

Duration:

(Goal: 15 sec each side)

3. Forward & Backward Neck Tilt

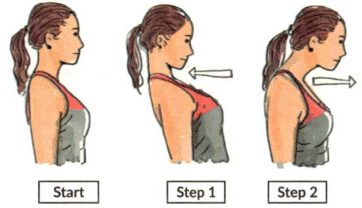

Start Step 1 Step 2

Duration:

(Goal: 30 sec, alternating)

4. Child's Pose

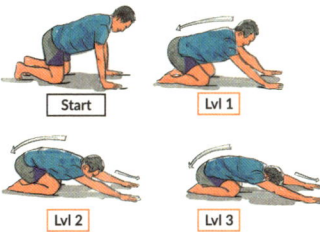

Start Lvl 1 Lvl 2 Lvl 3

Duration:

(Goal: 60 sec)

Level:

5. Cat-Cow

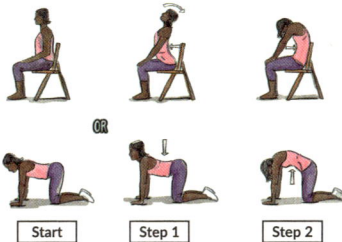

OR

Start Step 1 Step 2

Duration:

(Goal: 30 sec, alternating)

6. Sphinx/Cobra

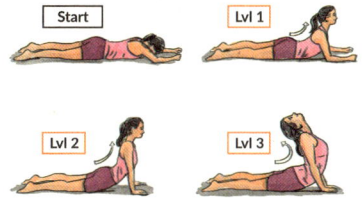

Start Lvl 1 Lvl 2 Lvl 3

Duration:

(Goal: 30 sec)

Level:

7. Standing Oblique Stretch

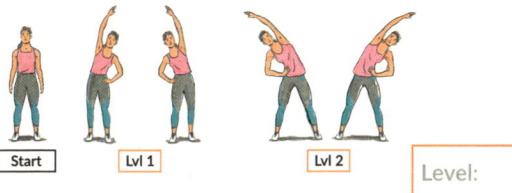

Start Lvl 1 Lvl 2

Level:

Duration:

(Goal: 15 sec each side)

8. Doorway Pectoral Stretch

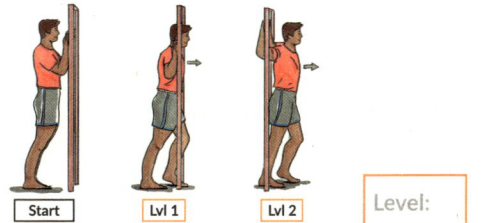

Start Lvl 1 Lvl 2

Level:

Duration:

(Goal: 30 sec)

9. Floor Angel

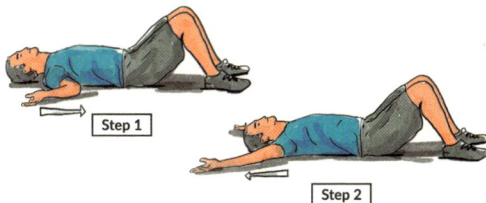

Step 1 Step 2

Duration:

(Goal: 30 sec, alternating)

10. Reverse Prayer

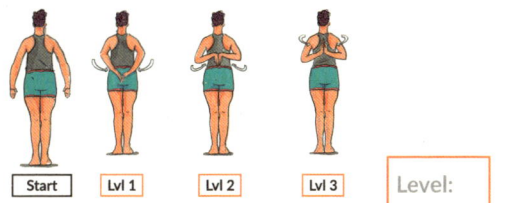

Start Lvl 1 Lvl 2 Lvl 3

Level:

Duration:

(Goal: 30 sec)

Day 64: Lower Body

1. Frog Pose

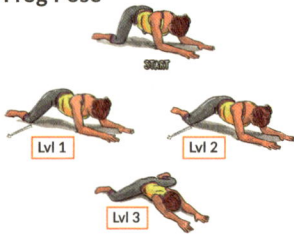

Duration: ....

(Goal: 60 sec)

Level:

2. Runner's Lunge

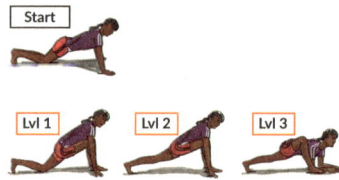

Duration: ....

(Goal: 30 sec each side)

Level:

3. Lying Hip Extension

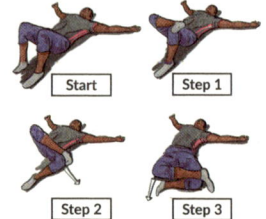

Duration: ....

(Goal: 30 sec each side)

Level:

4. Butterfly

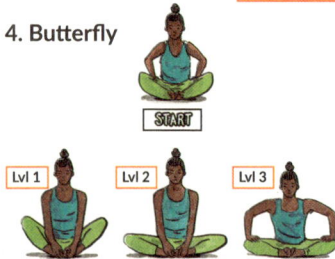

Duration: ....

(Goal: 30 sec)

Level:

5. Scorpion Pose

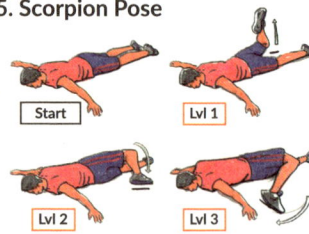

Duration: ....

(Goal: 30 sec each side)

Level:

6. Pigeon Stretch

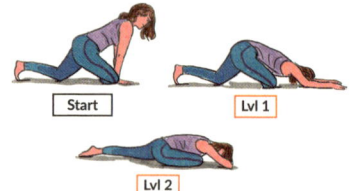

Duration: ....

(Goal: 30 sec each side)

Level:

7. Figure 4

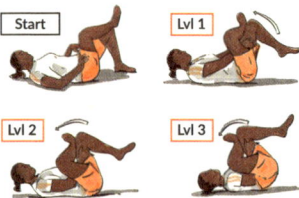

Duration: ....

(Goal: 30 sec each side)

Level:

8. Lateral Squat

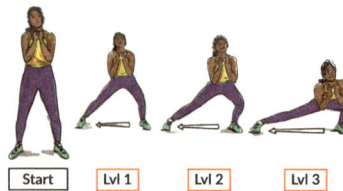

Duration: ....

(Goal: 30 sec each side)

Level:

9. Lateral Squat w/ Toe Raise

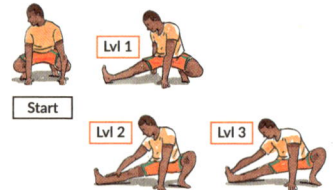

Duration: ....

(Goal: 30 sec each side)

Level:

10. Downward Dog

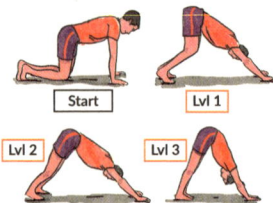

Duration: ....

(Goal: 30 sec)

Level:

11. Lying Quad Stretch

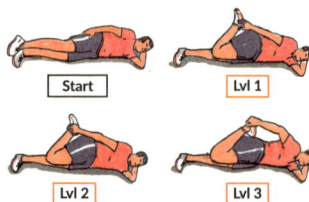

Duration: ....

(Goal: 30 sec each side)

Level:

12. Standing Wall Calf Stretch

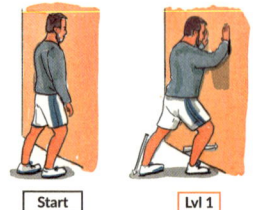

Duration: ....

(Goal: 15 sec each side)

Daily Reflection

Benefits I'm Experiencing:

Feel
Lighter

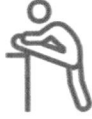

More Freedom
of Movement

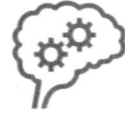

Improved
Mental Clarity

Less
Pain

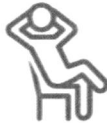

Less
Stressed

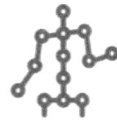

Improved
Posture

Notes On My Body:

....

....

....

....

....

....

....

....

Day 65: Dynamic Warm-Up

Full Session Exercise Guide:
habitnest.com/pages/stretching-day-65

1. World's Greatest Stretch

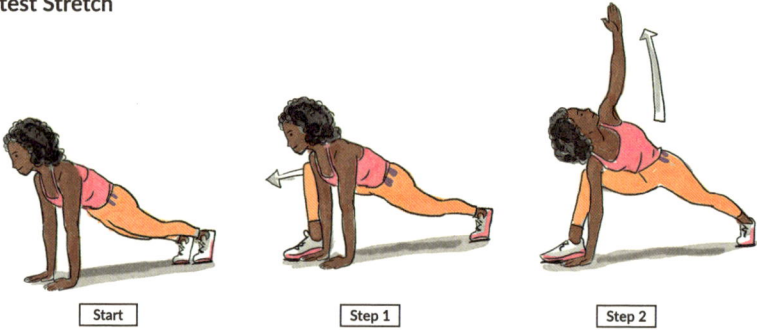

Start

Step 1

Step 2

Reps: .... *(Goal: 10-20)*

2. Bird-Dog

Start

Step 1

Step 2

Step 3

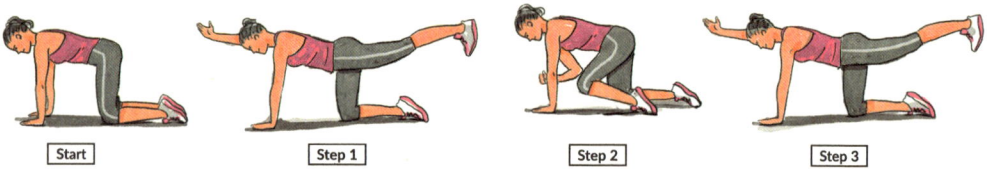

Reps: .... *(Goal: 10-15 each side)*

3. Glute Bridge

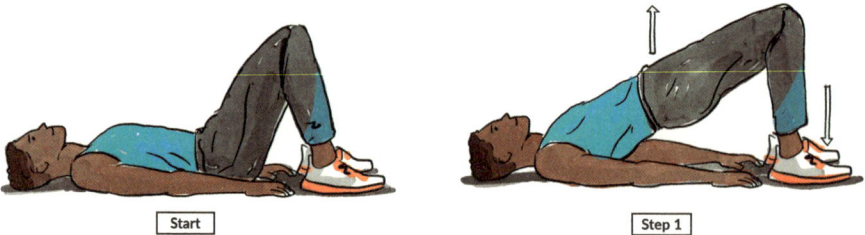

Start

Step 1

Reps: .... *(Goal: 20-30)*

Day 65: Upper Body

1. Up & Down Neck Tilt

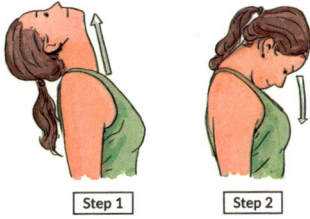

Step 1 Step 2

Duration:
....
(Goal: 30 sec, alternating)

2. Side Neck Tilt

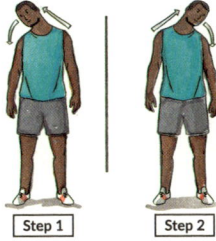

Step 1 Step 2

Duration:
....
(Goal: 15 sec each side)

3. Forward & Backward Neck Tilt

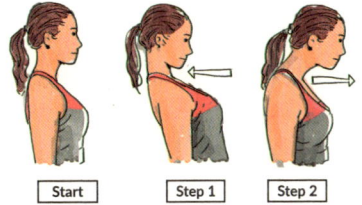

Start Step 1 Step 2

Duration:
....
(Goal: 30 sec, alternating)

4. Child's Pose

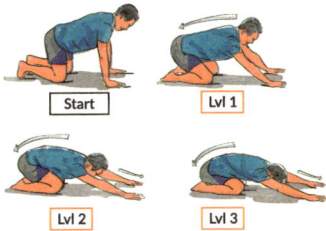

Start Lvl 1
Lvl 2 Lvl 3

Duration:
....
(Goal: 60 sec)   Level:

5. Cat-Cow

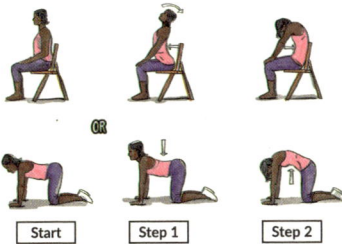

OR

Start Step 1 Step 2

Duration:
....
(Goal: 30 sec, alternating)

6. Sphinx/Cobra

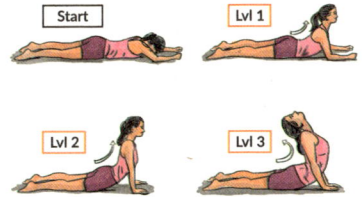

Start Lvl 1
Lvl 2 Lvl 3

Duration:
....
(Goal: 30 sec)   Level:

7. Standing Oblique Stretch

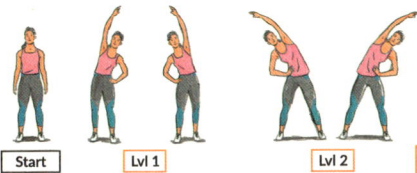

Start Lvl 1 Lvl 2 Level:

Duration: *(Goal: 15 sec each side)*
....

8. Doorway Pectoral Stretch

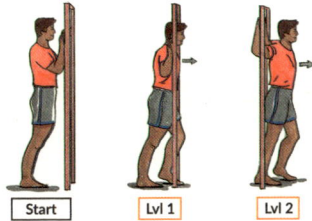

Start Lvl 1 Lvl 2 Level:

Duration: *(Goal: 30 sec)*
....

9. Floor Angel

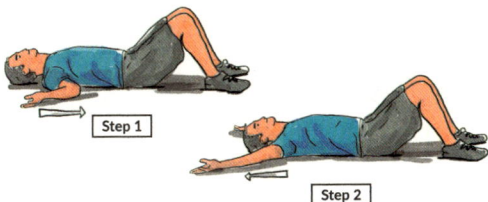

Step 1
Step 2

Duration: *(Goal: 30 sec, alternating)*
....

10. Reverse Prayer

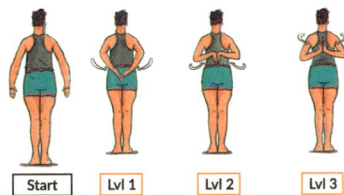

Start Lvl 1 Lvl 2 Lvl 3 Level:

Duration: *(Goal: 30 sec)*
....

Day 65: Lower Body

1. Frog Pose

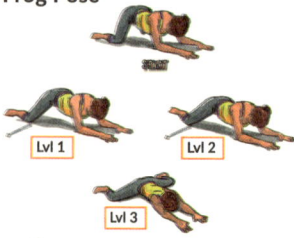

Lvl 1   Lvl 2

Lvl 3

Duration:
....

(Goal: 60 sec)

Level:

2. Runner's Lunge

Start

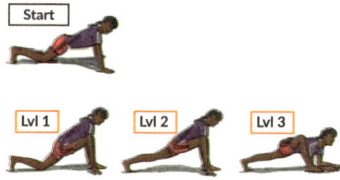

Lvl 1   Lvl 2   Lvl 3

Duration:
....

(Goal: 30 sec each side)

Level:

3. Lying Hip Extension

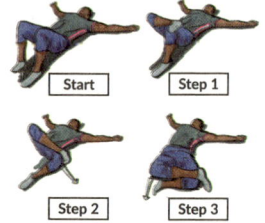

Start   Step 1

Step 2   Step 3

Duration:
....

(Goal: 30 sec each side)

4. Butterfly

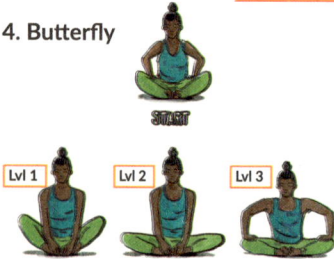

Lvl 1   Lvl 2   Lvl 3

Duration:
....

(Goal: 30 sec)

Level:

5. Scorpion Pose

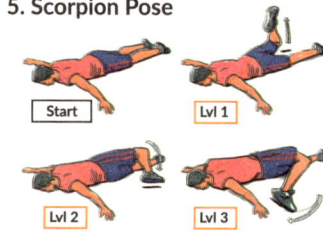

Start   Lvl 1

Lvl 2   Lvl 3

Duration:
....

(Goal: 30 sec each side)

Level:

6. Pigeon Stretch

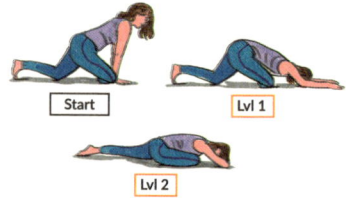

Start   Lvl 1

Lvl 2

Duration:
....

(Goal: 30 sec each side)

Level:

7. Figure 4

Start   Lvl 1

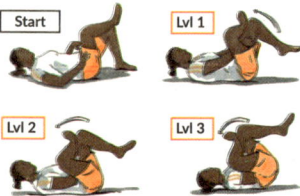

Lvl 2   Lvl 3

Duration:
....

(Goal: 30 sec each side)

Level:

8. Lateral Squat

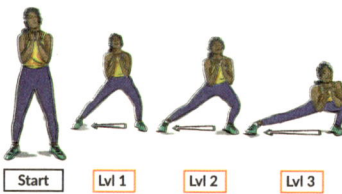

Start   Lvl 1   Lvl 2   Lvl 3

Duration:
....

(Goal: 30 sec each side)

Level:

9. Lateral Squat w/ Toe Raise

Lvl 1

Start

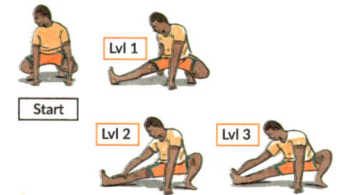

Lvl 2   Lvl 3

Duration:
....

(Goal: 30 sec each side)

Level:

10. Downward Dog

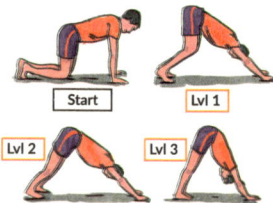

Start   Lvl 1

Lvl 2   Lvl 3

Duration:
....

(Goal: 30 sec)

Level:

11. Lying Quad Stretch

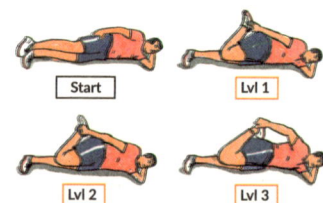

Start   Lvl 1

Lvl 2   Lvl 3

Duration:
....

(Goal: 30 sec each side)

Level:

12. Standing Wall Calf Stretch

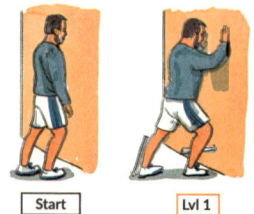

Start   Lvl 1

Duration:
....

(Goal: 15 sec each side)

Daily Reflection

Benefits I'm Experiencing:

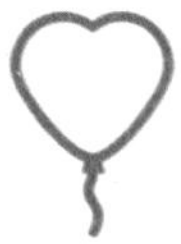

Feel
Lighter

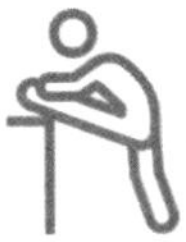

More Freedom
of Movement

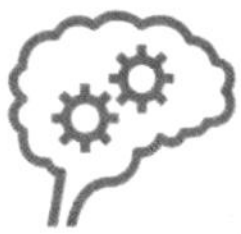

Improved
Mental Clarity

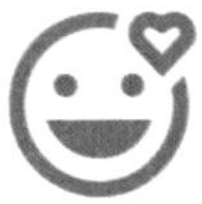

Less
Pain

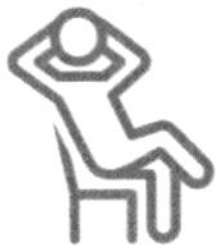

Less
Stressed

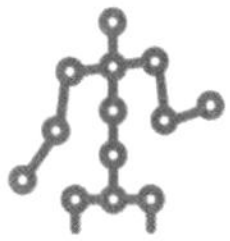

Improved
Posture

Notes On My Body:

Day 66: Dynamic Warm-Up

Full Session Exercise Guide:
habitnest.com/pages/stretching–day–66

1. Inch Worm Walk Out

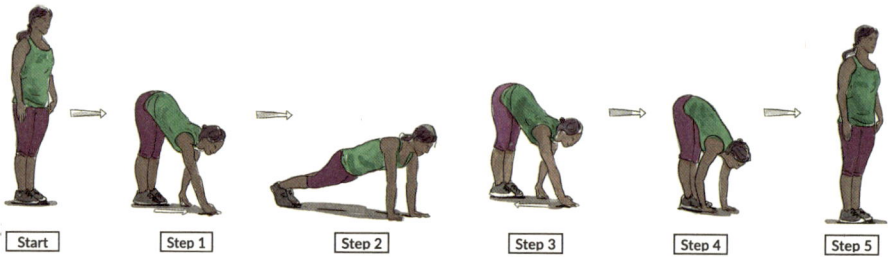

Start → Step 1 → Step 2 → Step 3 → Step 4 → Step 5

Reps: .... (Goal: 10-15)

2. Push-Up

Lvl 1

Lvl 2

Level:

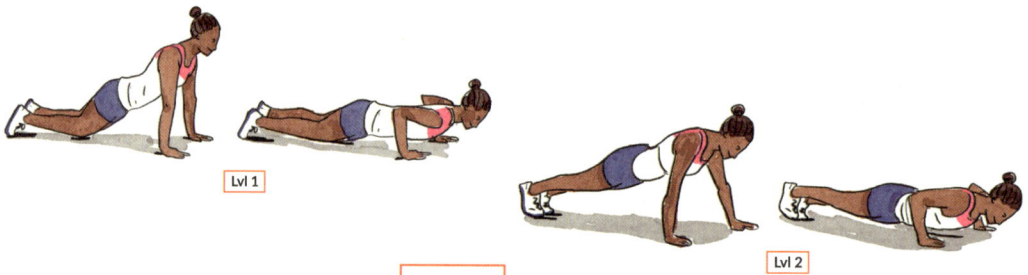

Reps: .... (Goal: 15-25)

3. Clam Opener w/ Side Plank

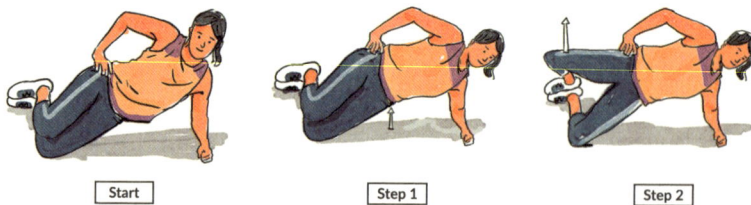

Start

Step 1

Step 2

Reps: .... (Goal: 10-15 each side)

Day 66: Upper Body

1. Up & Down Neck Tilt

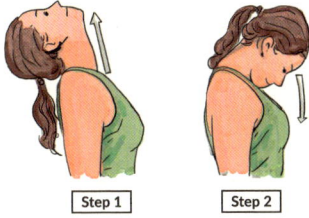

Step 1 Step 2

Duration:

(Goal: 30 sec, alternating)

2. Side Neck Tilt

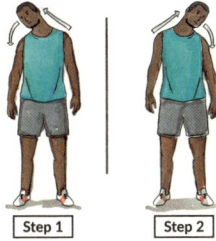

Step 1 Step 2

Duration:

(Goal: 15 sec each side)

3. Forward & Backward Neck Tilt

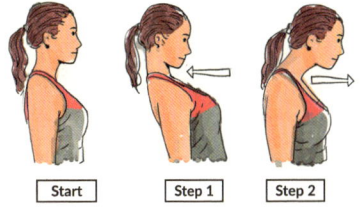

Start Step 1 Step 2

Duration:

(Goal: 30 sec, alternating)

4. Child's Pose

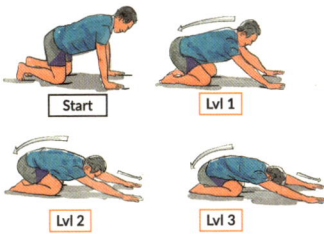

Start Lvl 1 Lvl 2 Lvl 3

Duration:

(Goal: 60 sec)

Level:

5. Cat-Cow

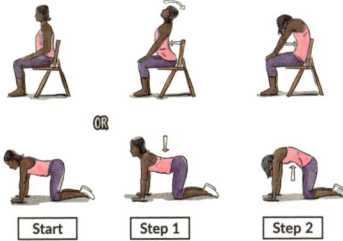

OR

Start Step 1 Step 2

Duration:

(Goal: 30 sec, alternating)

6. Sphinx/Cobra

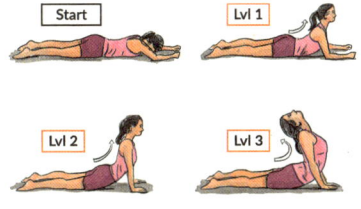

Start Lvl 1 Lvl 2 Lvl 3

Duration:

(Goal: 30 sec)

Level:

7. Standing Oblique Stretch

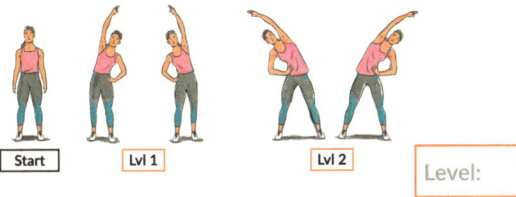

Start Lvl 1 Lvl 2

Level:

Duration:

(Goal: 15 sec each side)

8. Doorway Pectoral Stretch

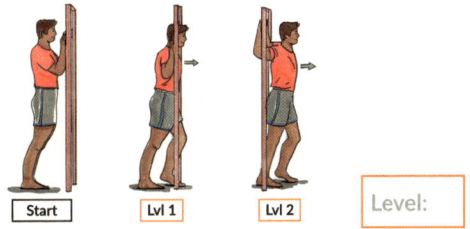

Start Lvl 1 Lvl 2

Level:

Duration:

(Goal: 30 sec)

9. Floor Angel

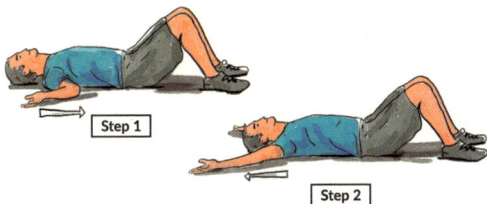

Step 1 Step 2

Duration:

(Goal: 30 sec, alternating)

10. Reverse Prayer

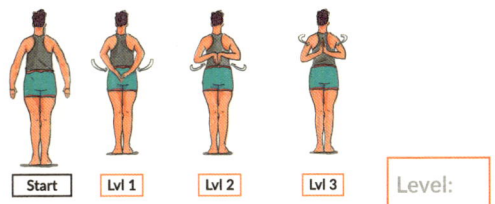

Start Lvl 1 Lvl 2 Lvl 3

Level:

Duration:

(Goal: 30 sec)

Day 66: Lower Body

1. Frog Pose

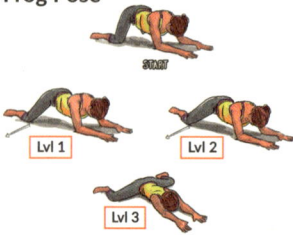

START

Lvl 1   Lvl 2

Lvl 3

Duration:

(Goal: 60 sec)

Level:

2. Runner's Lunge

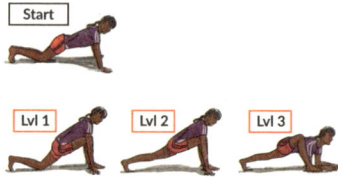

Start

Lvl 1   Lvl 2   Lvl 3

Duration:

(Goal: 30 sec each side)

Level:

3. Lying Hip Extension

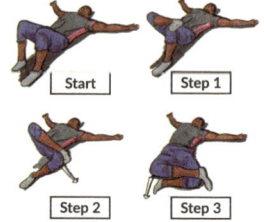

Start   Step 1

Step 2   Step 3

Duration:

(Goal: 30 sec each side)

4. Butterfly

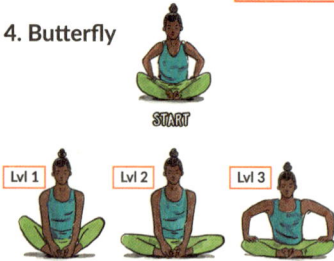

START

Lvl 1   Lvl 2   Lvl 3

Duration:

(Goal: 30 sec)

Level:

5. Scorpion Pose

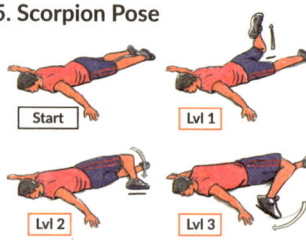

Start   Lvl 1

Lvl 2   Lvl 3

Duration:

(Goal: 30 sec each side)

Level:

6. Pigeon Stretch

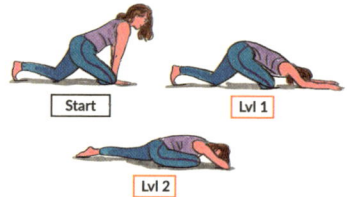

Start   Lvl 1

Lvl 2

Duration:

(Goal: 30 sec each side)

Level:

7. Figure 4

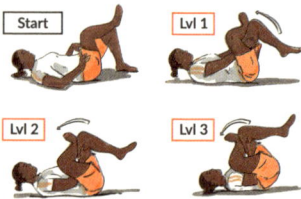

Start   Lvl 1

Lvl 2   Lvl 3

Duration:

(Goal: 30 sec each side)

Level:

8. Lateral Squat

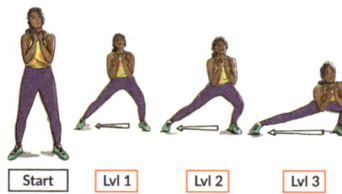

Start   Lvl 1   Lvl 2   Lvl 3

Duration:

(Goal: 30 sec each side)

Level:

9. Lateral Squat w/ Toe Raise

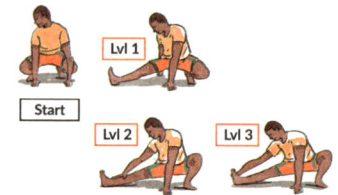

Lvl 1

Start

Lvl 2   Lvl 3

Duration:

(Goal: 30 sec each side)

Level:

10. Downward Dog

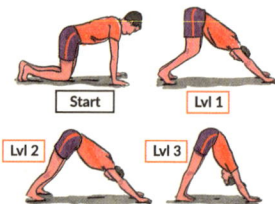

Start   Lvl 1

Lvl 2   Lvl 3

Duration:

(Goal: 30 sec)

Level:

11. Lying Quad Stretch

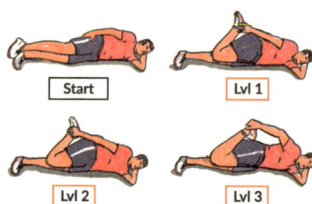

Start   Lvl 1

Lvl 2   Lvl 3

Duration:

(Goal: 30 sec each side)

Level:

12. Standing Wall Calf Stretch

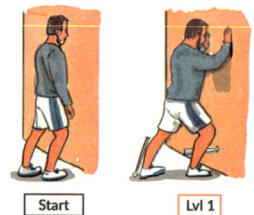

Start   Lvl 1

Duration:

(Goal: 15 sec each side)

Daily Reflection

Benefits I'm Experiencing:

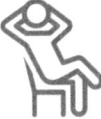

Feel Lighter	More Freedom of Movement	Improved Mental Clarity
Less Pain	Less Stressed	Improved Posture

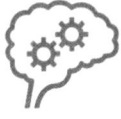

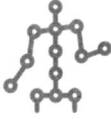

Notes On My Body:

Congratulations!!!

You've made it to the end of the journal, and you are amazing.

You absolute monster!! You just gave yourself such a beautiful gift - 66 days of stretching.

Sixty-six days in which you chose time and time again to make your body happy.

We hope this journey has been a special experience for you, and we wish for you to continue your stretching journey for the rest of your life.

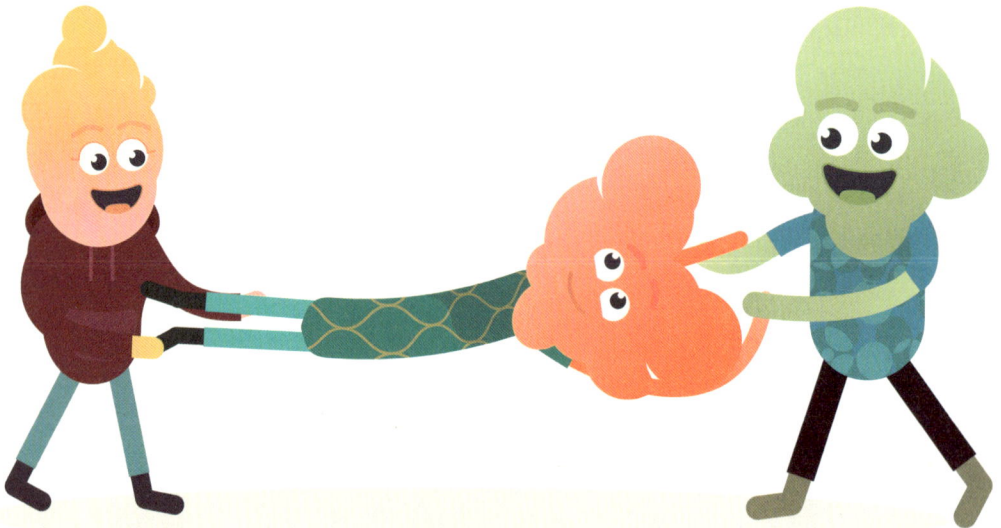

Note: We LOVE sharing stories of our users and what their lives looked like BEFORE using the journal compared to where they are NOW!

If you want to share your story with us, you can do so here:

habitnest.com/stretchingtestimonial

Recap Questions

1. How does my flexibility, range of motion, and comfort in mobility compare to when I started this journey?

2. In what other ways has stretching regularly impacted my quality of life?

3. What stretches do I know I want to perform for the rest of my life?

4. What steps can I take to ensure I will continue to stretch consistently?

Congratulations!

You've mastered the Stretching Routine Journal!

Phase 3 Done.

- Fin -

So... What Now?

Although you should feel very accomplished for getting through this entire journal... know that you built this habit to continually improve your life. Don't stop now. This is only the beginning.

One huge factor to sticking with any habit is tracking your progress.

Once you stop tracking, it makes it exponentially easier for you to forget about a consistent stretching routine (due to a lack of accountability with yourself).

Remember: **Every single day of your life that you take the time to stretch will be a better day.**

Now that you're done with the initial stretching journey, you have two tasks:

1. Keep stretching every day. You know more than enough to build your own routines.

2. Choose a new habit you will work on building. A morning routine or meditation practice work really well with stretching.

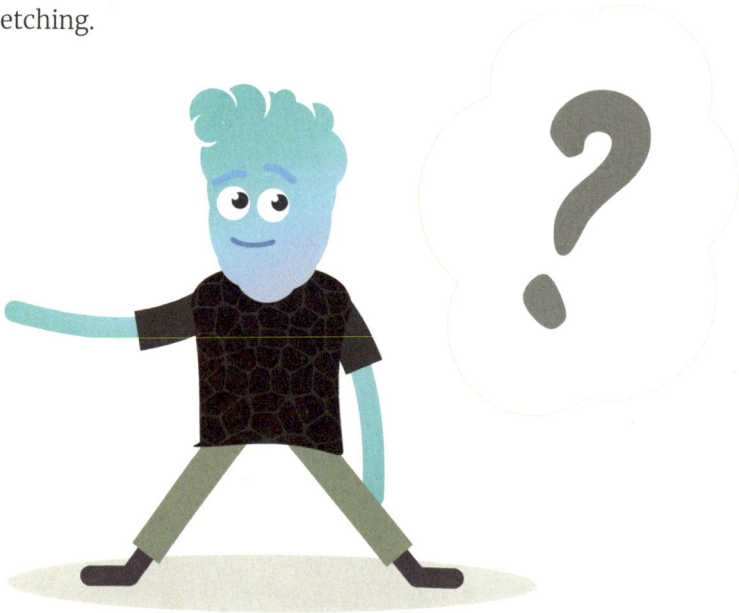

Shop Habit Nest Products

Lifestyle Products

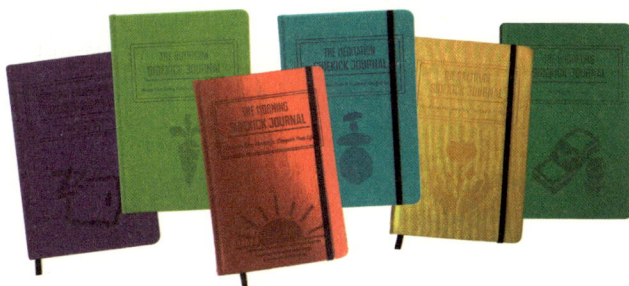

All of our lifestyle journals come with **daily content** (including Pro-Tips, Daily Challenges, Practical Resources, & more) to inspire you and give you bite-sized information to use along your journey. They also contain **daily questions aimed at holding you accountable** to ingraining that habit into your life.

The Morning Sidekick Journal Series

A set of guided morning planners that help you conquer your mornings and conquer your life. This complete 4-volume series covers one year of morning routines.

The Evening Routine & Sleep Sidekick Journal

Helps you to wind down your days peacefully, prepare for each next day, and get the most rejuvenating sleep of your life.

The Gratitude Sidekick Journal Series

A set of research-based journals that will help make an attitude of appreciation a core part of who you are. There are 3 Volumes in total.

The Meditation Sidekick Journal

Built to give you all the tools you need to stay consistent with a meditation practice.

The Nutrition Sidekick Journal

Your nutrition tracker, informational guide, and coach, all in one.

The Budgeting Sidekick Journal Series

The most simple-yet-effective budgeting guide in the world, helping you find full clarity on your budgeting goals and to achieve financial freedom. Set spending goals, track your daily spending, and reconcile along the way. Contains 2 volumes which cover well over a year of budgeting.

Fitness Products

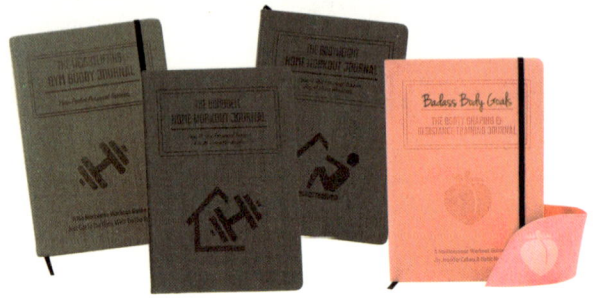

Our no-nonsense fitness books have fully guided fitness routines. No thinking required; just open the books and follow along.

The Weightlifting Gym Buddy Journal Series

A set of guided personal training programs aimed at helping you have the best workouts of your life. This complete 4-volume series covers one year of weightlifting workouts.

The Bodyweight / Dumbbell Home Workout Journals

Specifically focus on HOME workout programs that require minimal-to-no equipment to complete.

The Badass Body Goals Journal

An at-home-friendly fitness journal that focuses on HIIT and circuit workouts. This journal comes with a full video guide you can play and follow along.

Other Products

The Habit Nest Daily Planner

Plan your day including your top priorities, smaller 5-minute tasks, and all your to-dos. Get optional suggestions for ways to start your mornings and end your evenings with as well.

George The Short-Necked Giraffe (Children's Book)

Follow along George's journey as he learns the hard way that fully accepting himself, exactly the way he is, is the only path to living his happiest life.

Shop all products here: **habitnest.com/store**

The Habit Nest Mobile App

The Habit Nest app offers a **digital representation of our journals**, with the benefit of improved tracking, varying ways to showcase content, and gamification, and more.

When Habit Nest was initially founded, it was supposed to be in mobile app form from the start.

As a team of three young founders with no outside funding to get a mobile app built, we started with paper journals that worked using the same concept, which you're currently holding.

5 years and hundreds of thousands of journals sold later, we were finally able to create our mobile app and released it at the end of 2021.

We will always continue to print physical journals for every habit we release, only now, they'll also be put into the app so that everyone can experience our habit journeys in the way that suits them best.

If you're interested in seeing seeing whether the app is right for you, feel free to see more at **habitnest.com/app**

With a lot of love,

Mikey Ahdoot, Ari Banayan, & Amir Atighehchi
Co-Founders of Habit Nest

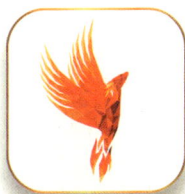

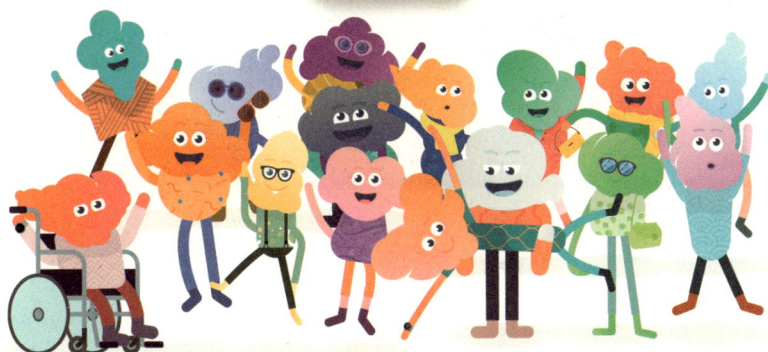

The Phoenixes Access Pass

We released *The Phoenixes* – Habit Nest's Special Access Pass – in 2022.

Anyone who purchases a Phoenix gets:

1. **Lifetime access** to the Habit Nest app.

2. Access to a **Learn2Earn system** we're building within the app, in which you will have chances to earn prizes/rewards for using our app to build better habits.

3. **First dibs** on new journal releases & our best discounts.

If you're interested in purchasing a Phoenix, visit:
https://habitnest.com/vip

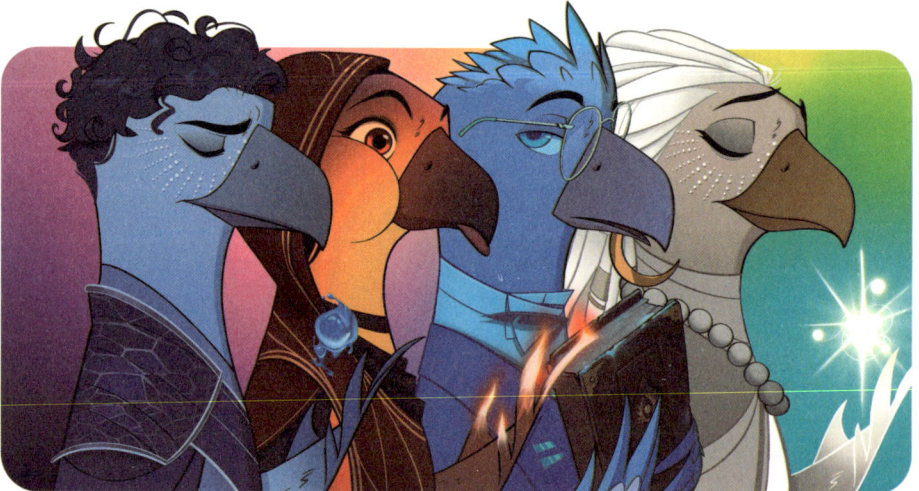

For more information, follow The Phoenixes on Twitter: **@thephoenixesnft**

Stretching Index

Dynamic Warm-Ups

Air Squat to Calf Raise

1. Stand upright, with your feet a little wider than hip-width apart, and your toes turned slightly out. If you can, engage your abdominal muscles and broaden your chest by gently pulling your shoulder blades in toward each other.

2. Bend your knees slowly, pushing your glutes and hips out and down behind you, as if you're sitting down on a chair. Keep your head and shoulders aligned with your knees and your knees aligned with your ankles.

3. Lower your body until your thighs are parallel to the ground. Keep your knees alined with your toes (without surpassing them) as you lower yourself as straight down as possible. Straighten your legs to come up and squeeze your glutes as you approach the starting position.

4. Don't stop at the starting position. Rather, when your legs are straight, lift up onto your tippy toes while also lifting your arms straight up above your head, reaching for the ceiling.

5. Come down onto your feet, and relax your arms before beginning again with the squat.

6. Repeat the entire sequence for the stated amount of repetitions.

Aquaman

1. Lie face down on the ground, toes pointed, ankles touching the ground. Extend your arms forward like Superman in flight, palms down, touching the ground.

2. Pull one arm and the opposite leg off the ground by engaging your glutes, shoulders, core, and back. They should raise up 2-3 inches.

3. Ensure that your arms are also fully contracted.

4. Hold this position for 1-2 seconds.

5. Slowly lower your arm and leg back to the starting position. Repeat, using the other arm and opposite leg.

6. Perform 10-15 repetitions on each side for a total of 20-30 repetitions.

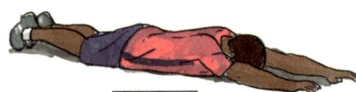

Start

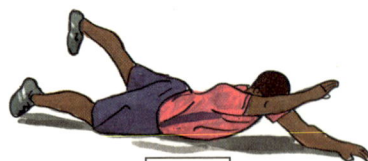

Step 1

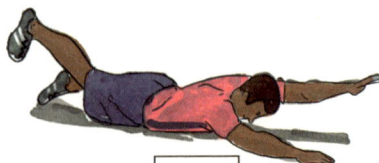

Step 2

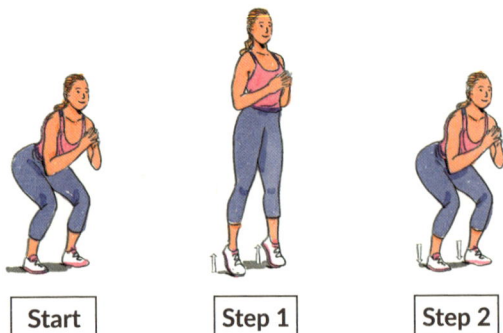

Start   **Step 1**   **Step 2**

Dynamic Warm-Ups

Bird-Dog

1. Begin on all fours in a table-top position, with your knees directly under your hips and your hands under your shoulders.

2. Maintain a neutral spine by engaging your abdominal muscles and slightly draw your shoulder blades together.

3. At the same time, slowly, and in a controlled manner, raise your right arm and your left leg as high as you can while keeping your shoulders and hips parallel to the floor.

4. Hold the position for a few moments, and then return to the original table-top position.

5. Then, raise your left arm and your right leg as high as you can while keeping your shoulders and hips parallel to the floor.

6. Perform the exercise on each side 10-15 times for a total of 20-30 repetitions.

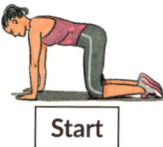

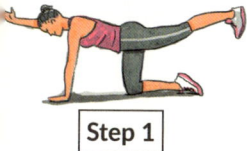

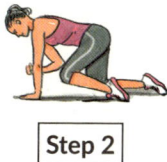

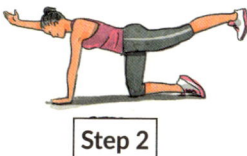

Clam Opener w/ Side Plank

1. Lie on your right side on the floor, using your right forearm to hold your upper body up and with your legs on top of each and your knees bent up to about hip level.

2. In one motion, while squeezing your glutes and keeping your core nice and tight, open your knees as widely as you can, and lift the right side of your body off the floor by pushing off the floor with your right knee and forearm.

3. Hold for 1-2 seconds, and then return to the starting position.

4. Repeat this 10-15 times on the right side, and then 10-15 times on the left side, for a total of 20-30 repetitions.

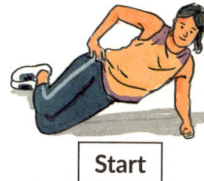

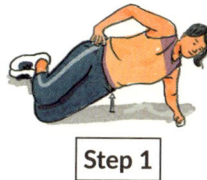

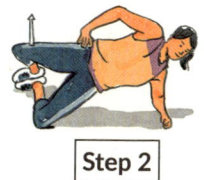

Start

Step 1

Step 2

Start

Step 1

Step 2

Dynamic Warm-Ups

Glute Bridge

1. Position yourself with your back on the ground, knees bent and feet on the floor, hip-width apart, shins perpendicular to the floor.

2. Engage your core by first flattening your back onto the ground. Imagine a string pulling your belly button into your spine.

3. Brace your core and drive your hips and chest upward at the same time until your torso, hips, and thighs form a 45° angle to the floor.

4. Contract your glute muscles and hold for a count of 2.

5. In a controlled movement, return to starting position.

6. Repeat 20-30 times.

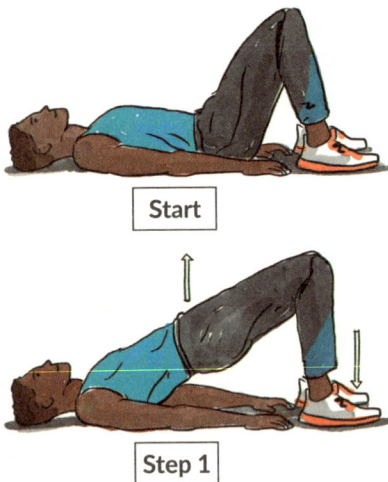

Good Morning

1. With feet hip-width apart, stand upright, knees slightly bent, and place your hands at the back of your head, elbows opened wide.

2. Engage your abdominal muscles by pulling them into your spine.

3. Keeping your spine neutral and pressing your rear backward, bend forward at the hips and continue doing so until your back is nearly parallel to the floor.

4. Slowly return to standing, engaging your core and squeezing your glutes at the top of the movement.

5. Perform the movement 15-20 times.

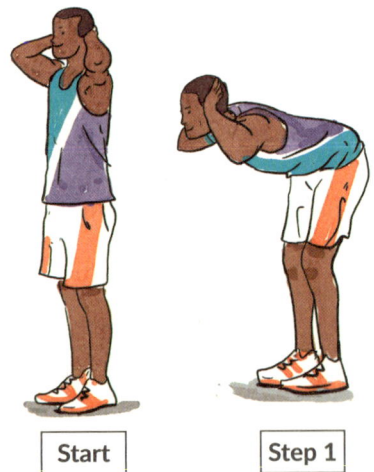

Dynamic Warm-Ups

High Knees

1. Stand with your feet about shoulder-width apart.

2. Lift one leg as you drive your knee up toward your chest and raise your opposite arm. Slightly arch or round your lower back to keep your pelvis stationary and reduce strain on your back.

3. With maximum control and stability, quickly place your foot back on the ground.

4. Bring your opposite leg upward in the same motion, driving your knee to your chest, while raising your opposite arm. (This movement is essentially running in place to increase your heart rate.)

5. Alternate sides for 20-30 total repetitions (10-15 on each leg).

Inch Worm Walk Out

1. Stand straight up with feet hip-width apart. Keep knees slightly bent.

2. Bend at the waist and fold over in a slow and controlled manner to reach your hands to the ground. Bend your knees as much as necessary to actually have your hands firmly planted on the ground.

3. Walk your hands forward until you find yourself in a push-up position.

4. Hold the push-up position for 1-2 seconds, squeezing your core, butt, and hamstring muscles.

5. Walk your hands back to your feet until you're comfortable enough to stand up again.

6. Repeat for 10-15 repetitions total.

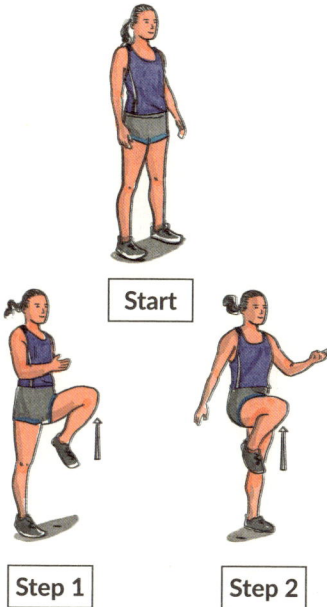

Start

Step 1

Step 2

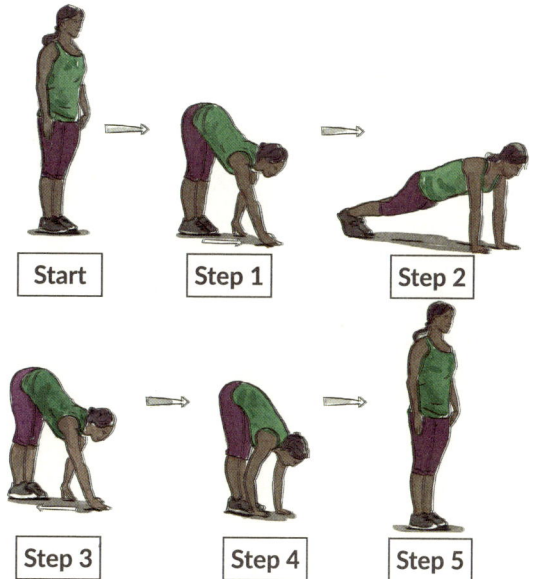

Start

Step 1

Step 2

Step 3

Step 4

Step 5

Dynamic Warm-Ups

Knee Hug

1. Stand with your feet shoulder-width apart.

2. Keep your core tight and your spine straight throughout the following movements.

3. Lift your right knee up to your chest as high as possible, then grab it with both hands and pull it towards your chest until you feel a stretch in the top of your butt.

4. Hold for a few moments, and then return to a simple standing position.

5. Repeat the motion with the left leg.

6. Perform the movement on each leg 10-15 times for a total of 20-30 repetitions.

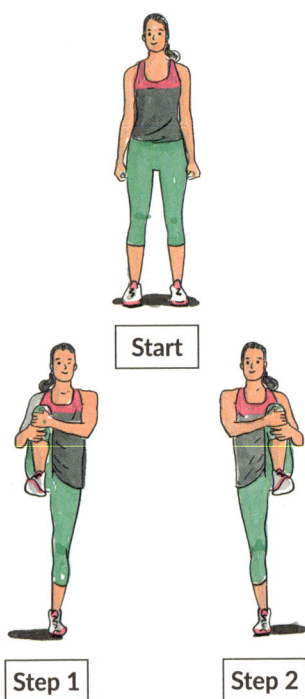

Low Lunge w/ Elbow Twist

1. Stand tall with feet hip-width apart.

2. Step forward with your right foot.

3. Bend your knee to get into a low lunge position. Make sure not to bend your knee past your toes. There should be a straight line from your knee down to your ankle.

4. Tilt your torso forward and down by bending at the hip.

5. Put your left hand on the floor for stabilization, and twist your spine to the extent it's comfortable and try to get as close as you can to touching your right elbow to your right foot (or the floor next to your foot).

6. Return to the starting position (standing up).

7. Step with the left foot, and perform the same movement with the other side.

8. Alternate each time, and perform a total of 20-30 repetitions.

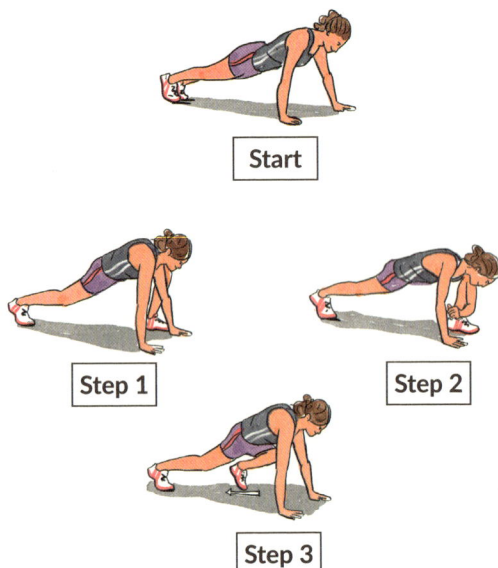

Start

Step 1

Step 2

Start

Step 1

Step 2

Step 3

Dynamic Warm-Ups

Mountain Climber

1. Get in a push-up or plank position. Keep your abdominal muscles tight and your body straight while holding yourself off the floor.

2. Pull your right knee into your chest. Make sure that your body doesn't come out of its push-up or plank position. Keep your spine in a straight line and don't let your head slump. Having core body stability is very crucial for this movement.

3. Quickly place your right leg back down while simultaneously switching legs and pulling your left knee into your chest. Make sure that at the same time you push your right leg back, you pull your left knee into your chest using the same form. (This movement is essentially running in place while maintaining a straight and aligned body.)

4. Alternate sides for 20-30 repetitions.

Pike Push-Up

1. Position your body as though you were going to perform a plank, with your body forming a straight line from head to hips to heels.

2. Engage your core and begin to lift your hips toward the ceiling. At the same time, walk your hands towards your feet.

3. Once your torso is nearly perpendicular to the ground, position your hands wider than your shoulders. Shift your weight to your hands and move your feet so you are on your toes.

4. Gaze toward your toes to keep your head neutral and begin to bend your elbows, lowering your head toward the floor.

5. Once you've lowered as far as you can, push yourself back up to complete one rep.

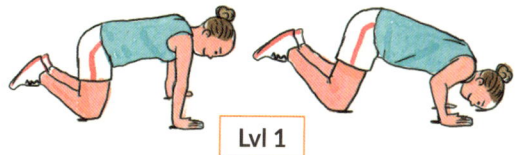

Lvl 1

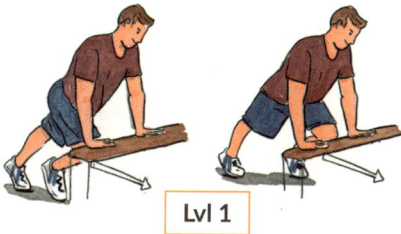

Lvl 1

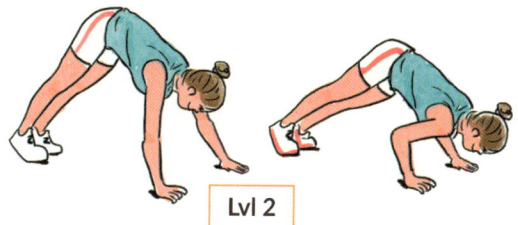

Lvl 2

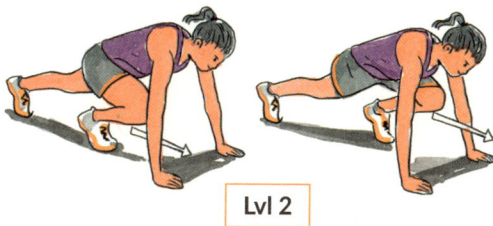

Lvl 2

Dynamic Warm-Ups

Plank

1. Place your forearms on the ground, with your elbows aligned beneath your shoulders. Keep your arms parallel to your body at about shoulder-width distance. (You should be in a push-up position, only on your forearms rather than your hands).

2. Ground your toes on the floor and squeeze your glutes to stabilize your body. Be careful not to lock or hyperextend your knees.

3. Neutralize your neck and spine by looking at a spot on the floor about a foot in front of your hands. Your head should be in line with your back.

4. Contract your abdominals to keep yourself up and prevent your booty from sticking up towards the ceiling.

5. Keep your back flat and hold the position for 30-60 seconds.

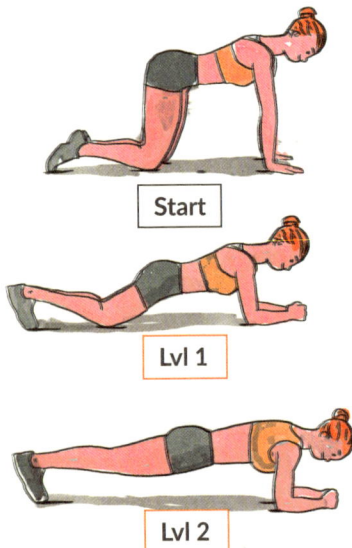

Plank w/ Shoulder Tap

1. Start in a straight-arm plank (push-up position), with your wrists under your shoulders and your feet hip-width apart.

2. Tighten your core, ground your toes on the floor, and squeeze your glute muscles to stabilize your body and keep it in one straight line from the top of your head down to your heels.

3. Slowly and in a controlled manner, lift your right hand, tap your left shoulder, and then return to the plank position.

4. Then, tap your right shoulder with your left hand and continue alternating sides.

5. Tap each shoulder 10-15 times for a total of 20-30 repetitions.

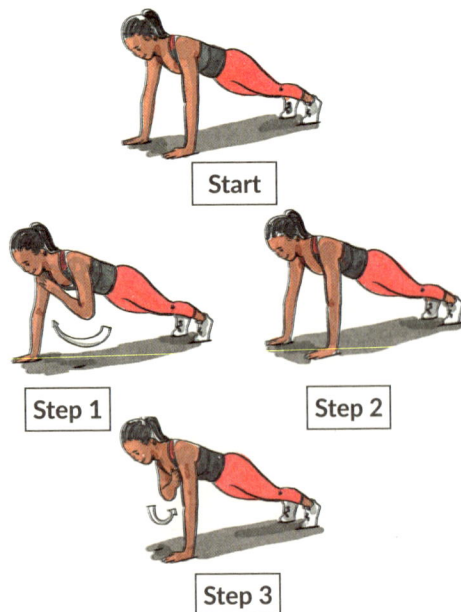

Start

Start

Lvl 1

Step 1

Step 2

Lvl 2

Step 3

Dynamic Warm-Ups

Push-Up

1. Lie on the ground face down and place your hands shoulder-width apart. Push your body off the ground through your hands while keeping your back as straight as possible.

2. Lower yourself back down until your chest nearly touches the ground as you inhale.

3. Exhale and press your upper body back up to the starting position while squeezing your chest, arms, and abdominal muscles.

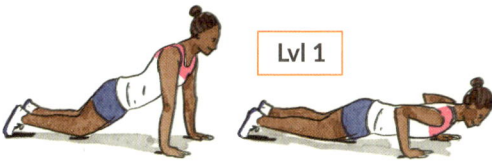

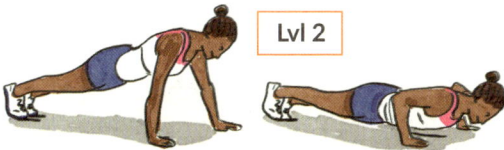

Lvl 1

Lvl 2

Rocking Feet w/ Arm Raise

1. Stand straight up, comfortably, with your arms by your side.

2. In one motion, lift your straight arms as high as you can above your head, while coming up onto the balls of your feet to your tippy toes.

3. Then, in one motion, lower your straight arms and stretch them as far back behind you as you can while rotating your feet back onto your heels. Do this VERY slowly to make sure you can actually balance on your heels!

4. Repeat the exercise in each direction 10-15 times for a total of 20-30 repetitions.

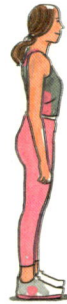

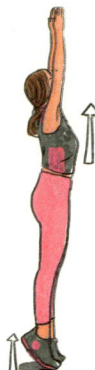

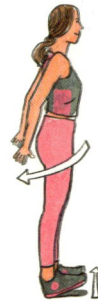

Start

Step 1

Step 2

Dynamic Warm-Ups

Roundhouse Kick to Squat

1. Get into a squat position by bending your knees, keeping your spine in a straight line, tucking your pelvis in, engaging your abdominal muscles, and pushing your glutes and hips down and out behind you as if you were trying to sit in a chair.

2. Stand up from the squat position, and as you do, shift your body to the right, raise your left foot, and kick out to the left.

3. As you're bringing your leg back to the floor, enter into the original squat position.

4. Perform 10-15 repetitions on each side for a total of 20-30 repetitions.

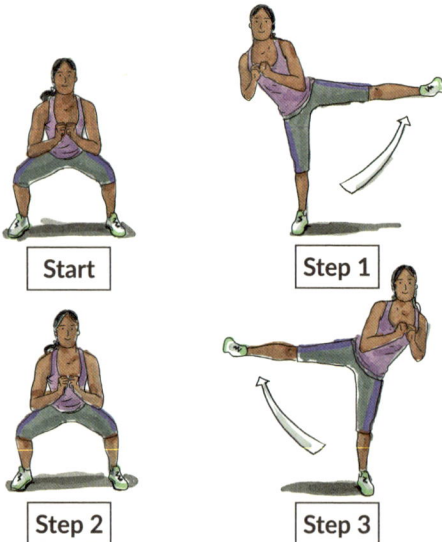

Side Plank w/ Twist

1. Position yourself in a side plank, left shoulder over left elbow and body in a strong, straight line.

2. Reach the fingertips of your right hand toward the ceiling.

3. Engage your core and turn your torso forward. Bring your right hand down and position it between your torso and the floor, as though you were trying to twist and reach the rest of the room behind you.

4. Slowly rotate back to starting position. Repeat on the other side to complete one rep.

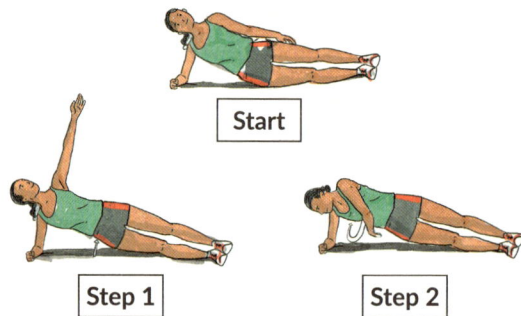

Start

Step 1

Step 2

Step 3

Start

Step 1

Step 2

Dynamic Warm-Ups

Speed Skater Arms

1. Stand with legs shoulder-width apart and your knees bent, so your legs are making about a 45-degree angle (in between straight up and a 90-degree angle squat).

2. Lift your arms and hold them straight out horizontally at shoulder level, remaining in the semi-squat position.

3. Staying in this semi-squatted position with your arms up, without moving your legs at all, slowly twist your whole upper body (including the head and neck) as if you were trying to look behind you to the right side (your arms will twist as well).

4. Immediately twist and rotate the other way as if you were trying to look behind you to the left.

5. Perform 10-15 repetitions in each direction for a total of 20-30 repetitions.

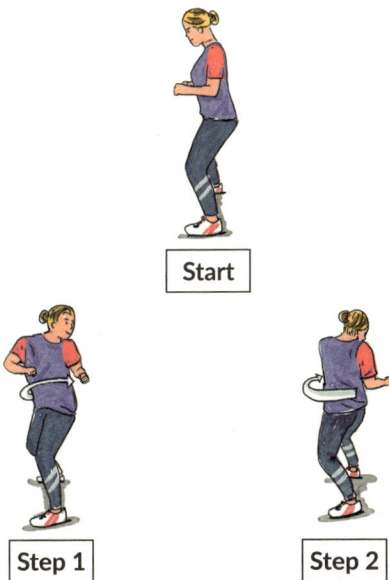

Split Squat

1. Stand with feet shoulder-width apart.

2. Step one foot forward as far as possible without losing form or balance.

3. Bend both knees and lift the heel of your back foot up off of the ground, putting weight into the heel of the front foot. Ensure that your knee in front doesn't overextend past your toes.

4. Continue lowering your weight until your back leg shin and front leg thigh are nearly parallel to the ground.

5. Pause for a count of two. Drive the heel of the front foot into the ground and stand to return to starting position.

6. Staying in the same position (without moving your feet), lift yourself up and come back down into the squat 10-15 times.

7. Switch legs and perform the same movement on the other side for another 10-15 reps.

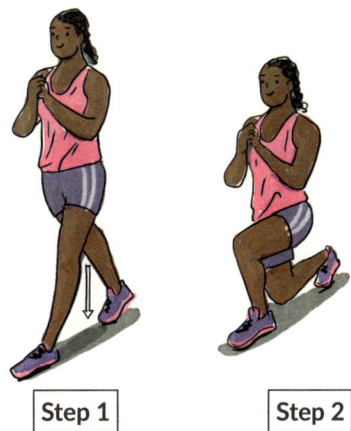

Start

Step 1

Step 2

Step 1

Step 2

Dynamic Warm-Ups

Standing Hamstring Scoop

1. Stand with your right foot forward and to the right, so that your right heel is about 6 inches in front of the toes on your left foot and 6-12 inches to the right of your left foot.

2. Lift your right foot so that it is on the heel.

3. In one motion, bend at the hip so your body folds forward towards the ground (keep the back and spine straight in one line). Keep both arms straight the whole time, stretch both arms directly down towards the ground, and make a semi-circle with your arms toward your body, as if you were scooping something off your the floor.

4. Perform the movement repeatedly 10-15 times.

5. Switch legs and perform the movement 10-15 more times, for a total of 20-30 repetitions.

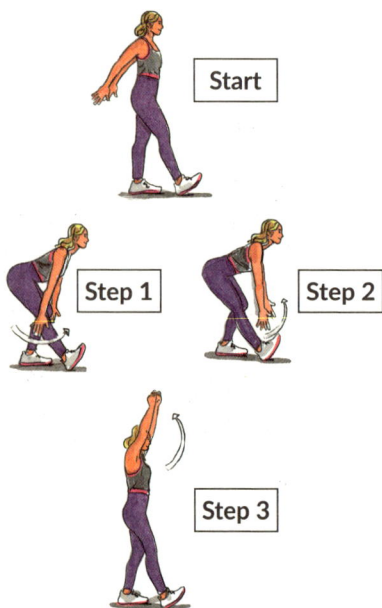

Standing Hip Circles

1. Stand straight with your feet a little wider than shoulder-width apart.

2. Slightly bend your knees and place your hands on your hips.

3. Rotating clockwise, make as big of a circle as you can with your hips, bending your torso at the waist backwards, to the side, and forwards as you rotate your hips. Perform 10-15 repetitions.

4. Then, perform 10-15 repetitions rotating your body counterclockwise.

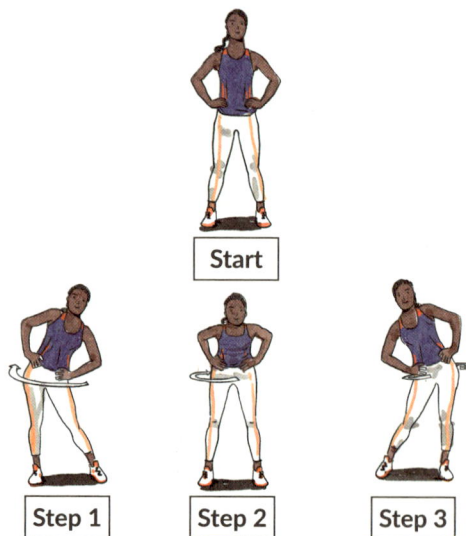

Start

Step 1

Step 2

Step 3

Start

Step 1

Step 2

Step 3

Dynamic Warm-Ups

Towel Snatch

1. Grab a towel, t-shirt, band, or any sturdy, lightly stretchable object you can pull between your hands. Hold the ends of it and let your hands naturally drop down below your waist as if you were simply holding it.

2. Bend your knees slightly to get into a high squat position.

3. Hold the object taut, as if you're attempting to rip it in half (make sure you've chosen a fabric that can withstand this).

4. As you pull it, keep your hands and arms straight and do not move your elbows. Move your hands up from your body, all the way over your head, and then bring them back towards your waist, ensuring that you are pulling the object the entire time.

5. Perform the movement 15-20 times.

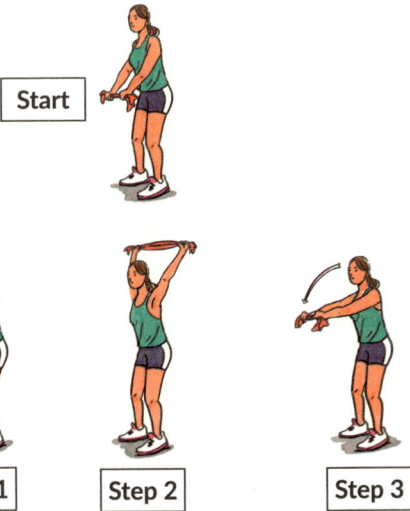

Walking Jacks (or Jumping Jacks)

1. Stand straight, with your feet shoulder-width apart.

2. As you lift both arms (arms should be straight) from your sides in a circular motion, step to the right with your right foot.

3. Bring your arms down in the same circular motion while returning the right leg to its original position.

4. Lift both arms again in a circular motion and step out to the left with your left foot.

5. Repeat 10-15 times on each side, for a total of 20-30 repetitions.

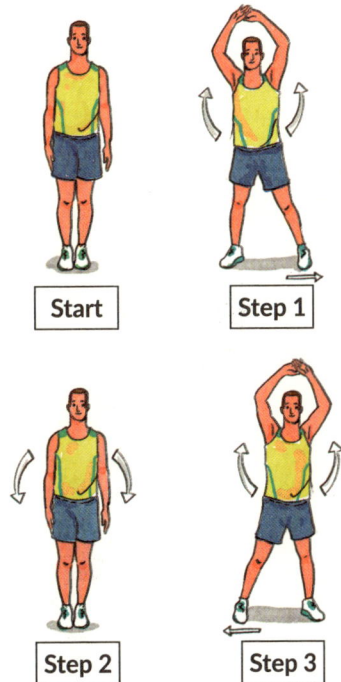

Dynamic Warm-Ups

World's Greatest Stretch

1. Start on your hands and knees in push-up position on the floor, with your wrists directly under your shoulders and your body in one straight line from the top of your head down to your heels.

2. Step your right foot forward next to your hand, and bend forward so that the right knee is over the right ankle and you feel a stretch in your left hip flexor.

3. Place your left hand on the ground inside of the right foot for stabilization, and then twist your body to the right, towards your right leg, reaching the right hand up toward the sky. Turn your neck towards your outstretched arm in the same motion and look just beyond your fingertips.

4. Return your hand to the floor, bring your right leg back so that you find yourself in the original push-up position.

5. Repeat the above on the other side.

6. Perform 5-10 repetitions on each side for a total of 10-20 repetitions.

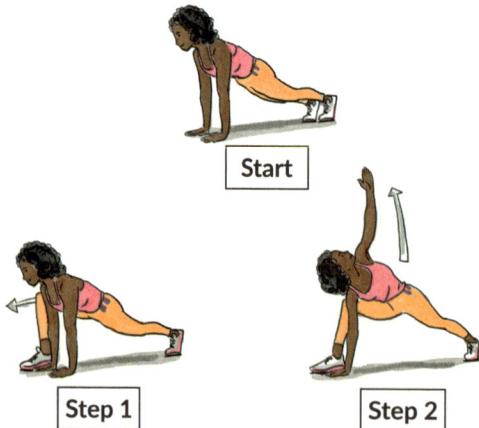

Start

Step 1

Step 2

Y Raise

1. Stand upright, feet shoulder-width apart.

2. With a slight bend in your elbows, raise your arms upward and out to the sides, making a "Y" formation until elbows are aligned with each ear. Contract shoulder muscles.

3. Slowly lower arms, maintaining control to complete one rep.

4. Remember, the point is to feel the resistance and tension. Keep your shoulder and upper back muscles flexed throughout the movement.

5. Perform 20-30 repetitions.

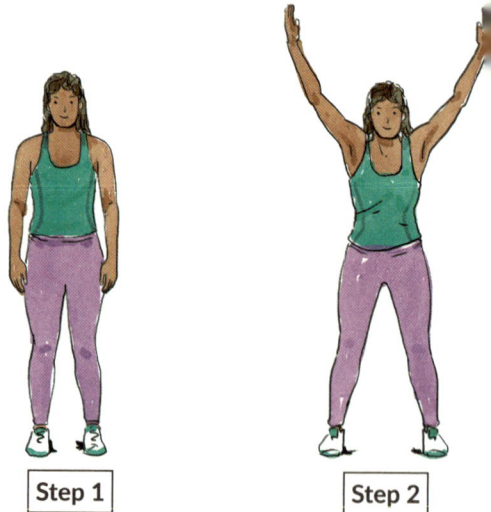

Step 1

Step 2

Upper Body Stretches

Behind the Back
Elbow to Elbow Grip

Starting position: Sitting down on the edge of a chair, or standing with your arms hanging by your sides.

1. Press your shoulders back to open up your chest by squeezing your shoulder blades together and broadening the chest.

2. Bring your arms behind your back and grab your wrists with both hands behind your back.

3. If you can, extend the stretch and grab both forearms or elbows.

4. Hold for 30 seconds.

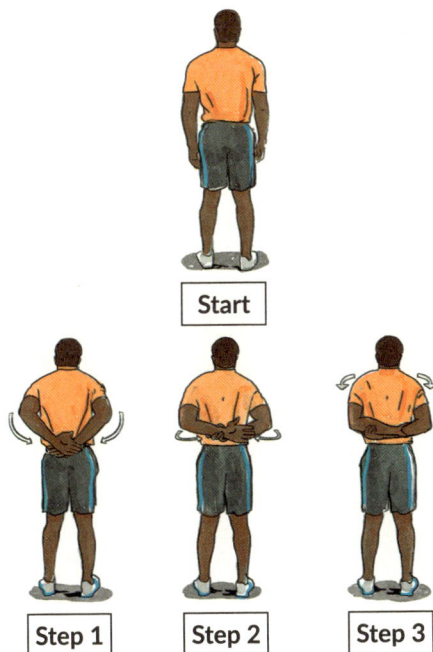

Behind the Back
Tricep Extension

Starting position: Stand comfortably, with your feet shoulder-width apart

1. Lift your right arm straight up above your body and then bend at the elbow to lower your right hand behind your back, bringing your palm down as far down your back as you can.

2. Grab your right elbow with your left hand and gently pull it to the left until you feel a comfortable stretch.

3. Hold for 15 seconds.

4. Relax, and then perform the same stretch on the left tricep.

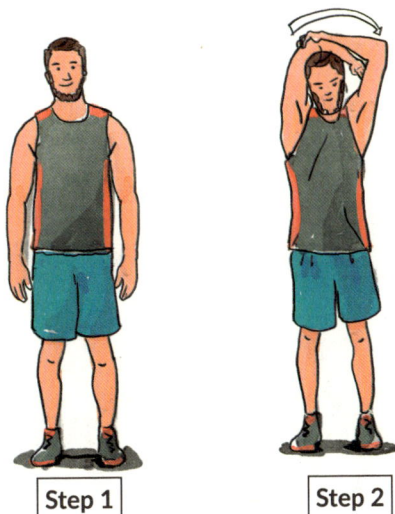

Start

Step 1   **Step 2**   **Step 3**

Step 1   **Step 2**

Upper Body Stretches

Cat-Cow

Starting position: Get into tabletop position on the floor, with your hands directly under your shoulders and your knees in line with your hips. The neck should begin neutrally, looking at the floor in front of you.

1. As you lift your head, push your chest forward towards the floor, allow your belly to sink, pull your shoulder blades back, and your butt/tailbone up towards the ceiling. (Cow)

2. Hold this pose for a few moments.

3. Then, try to do the exact opposite and round your spine while releasing your head towards the floor, pulling your tailbone/butt towards the ground, and pulling your pubic bone forward. (Cat)

4. Perform both movements in succession for 30 seconds, holding each pose for a few moments.

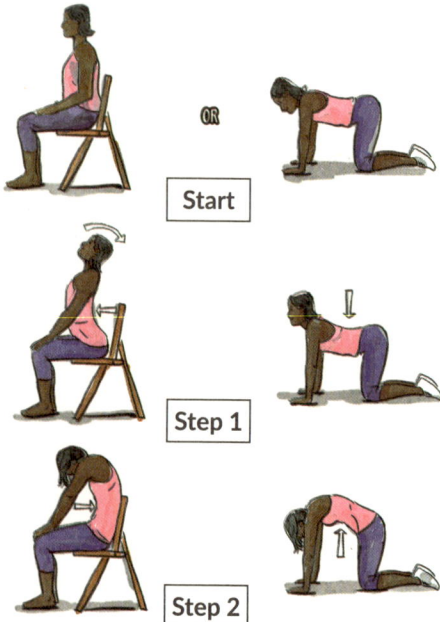

Child's Pose

Starting position: Get into a tabletop position, with your hands directly under your shoulders and your knees in line with your hips.

1. Push your butt back towards your feet as far as possible.

2. Stretch your arms out on the floor in front of you until you feel like your spine is elongating.

3. Reach forward with your fingers to further elongate the spine, to the extent that it feels good and comfortable.

4. Hold the stretch for 60 seconds and deepen the stretch when you feel it is possible by further elongating your spine.

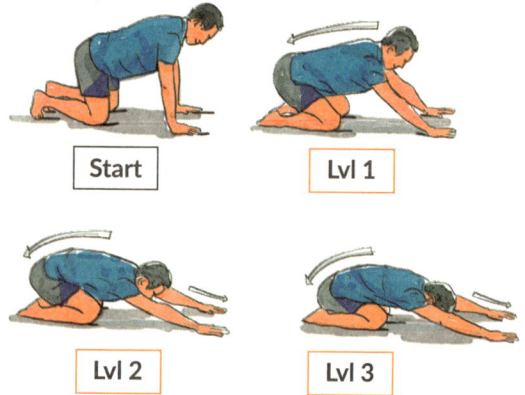

340

Upper Body Stretches

Corner Chest Stretch

Starting position: Stand at a corner between two walls, about 1 foot away from the corner of the wall.

1. Place one arm on each wall, with each forearm and palm resting comfortably on a wall.

2. Lean in towards the wall as much as possible as you feel the stretch in your chest.

3. Lean your head back as the front of your neck stretches, with your chin reaching towards the ceiling.

4. Hold for 30 seconds.

Cross Arm Shoulder Stretch

Starting position: Stand comfortably, with your feet shoulder-width apart, and hold your arms out horizontally.

1. Cross your left arm across your chest, so that your left fingers are pointing towards the right side of your body.

2. Support your left arm with the elbow crease of your right arm, or use your right hand to hold your left arm in place against your chest.

3. Use your right arm to pull your left arm in towards your body, so that you feel a stretch in your left shoulder.

4. Hold for 15 seconds.

5. Relax, and then perform the same stretch on the right shoulder.

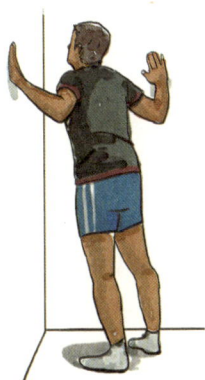

Step 1

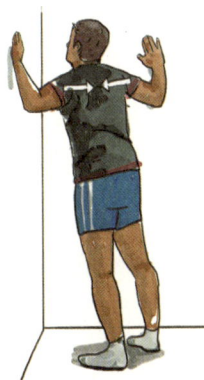

Step 2

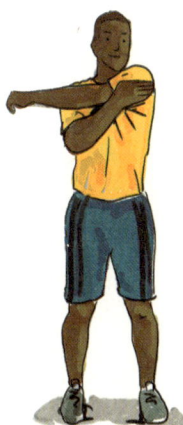

Start

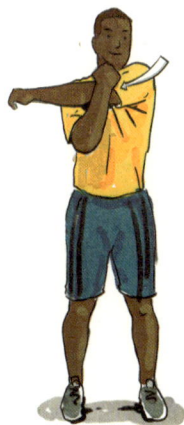

Step 1

Upper Body Stretches

Doorway Pectoral Stretch

Starting position: Stand in an open doorway.

1. Raise each arm up to the side, bent at a 90-degree angle, with palms facing forward. Rest your palms on the door frame.

2. Slowly step forward with one foot and you'll feel a stretch in your shoulders and chest.

3. Hold for 30 seconds, deepening the stretch whenever possible.

Elbow Opener

Starting position: Stand or sit comfortably with arms by your side.

1. Place your hands clasped together behind your head.

2. Pull your elbows apart as wide as comfortably possible, as if you were trying to touch your elbows together behind your back.

3. Hold for 30 seconds.

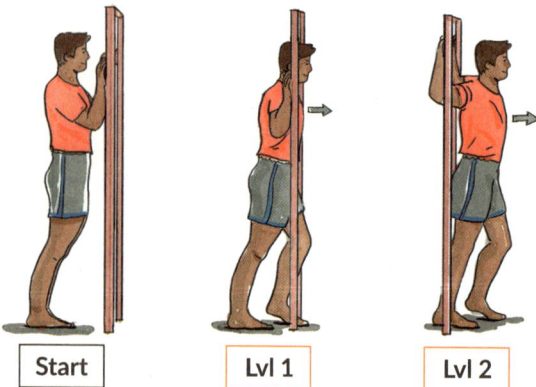

Start   **Lvl 1**   **Lvl 2**

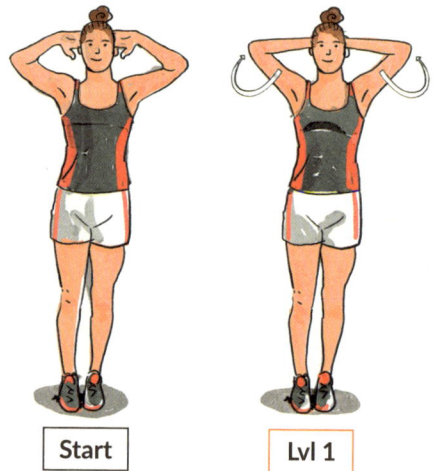

Start   **Lvl 1**

Upper Body Stretches

Floor Angel

Starting position: Lie on your back, with your knees bent and your feet flat on the ground. Legs should be comfortable, so separate them as much as feels comfortable. They're not included in the stretch!

1. Position both arms to the side of your body at a 90-degree angle, with your palms facing up towards the ceiling.

2. Try as much as feels right and comfortable to have the entirety of your arms and shoulders touching the floor behind your body.

3. Keeping your arms on the floor (or as close to it as possible for you), slowly raise your arms up over your head until they are fully extended and reach out above your head (with your arms still touching the floor) to until you feel a nice stretch for a few moments in your shoulders and chest.

4. Lower your arms back to the original position, again, while keeping them on the floor.

5. Repeat both positions sequentially for 30 seconds, switching every few moments.

Forearm Stretch w/ Hands on Surface

Starting position: Stand in front of a surface like a bench, bed, table, couch, or any surface that is about waist level or a little bit lower.

1. Place your fingers on the edge of the surface and drop your wrists down, so that your palms are facing up and your fingers are pointing towards your body.

2. Lean forward until you feel a comfortable stretch in your forearms and wrists.

3. Hold for 15 seconds.

4. Now, turn your hands over so that your palms are facing the surface and your fingers are pointing away from your body.

5. Drop your wrists down and lean forward until you feel the stretch in your forearms and wrists.

6. Hold for 15 seconds.

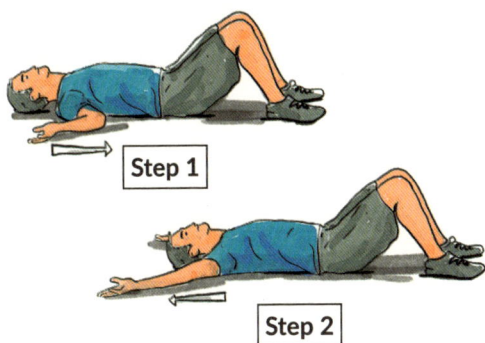

Step 1

Step 2

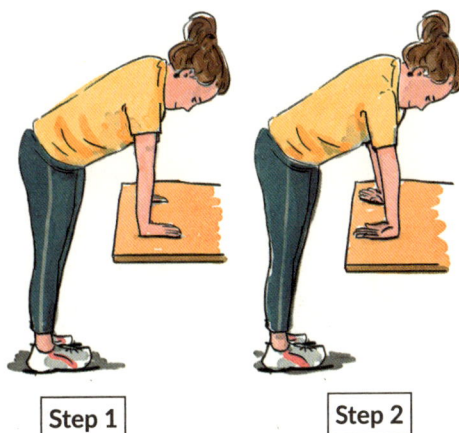

Step 1

Step 2

Upper Body Stretches

Forward & Backward Neck Tilt

Starting position: Stand, with your feet hip-width apart and arms down by your sides, or sit in a chair with your back straight up.

1. Stand straight with your feet hip-width apart and arms down by your sides.

2. Gently reach your chin directly forward in front of you as far as you can, as if you were trying to touch the wall in front of you with your chin.

3. Hold the stretch for 3-5 seconds, then return to the starting position.

4. Pull your chin inward, as if you were trying to pull it into your spine. Hold for 3-5 seconds, and return to the starting position.

5. Repeat both stretches in succession for 30 seconds.

Start

Step 1

Step 2

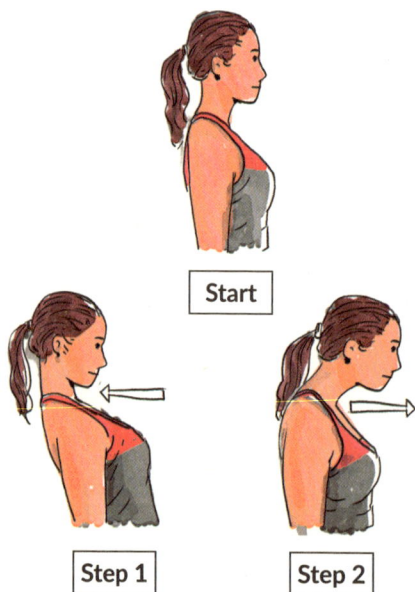

Lateral Side to Side Neck Rotation

Starting position: Stand, with your feet hip-width apart and arms down by your sides, or sit in a chair with your back straight.

1. Gently turn your head directly to the right, as if you were trying to turn around and see what was behind you. Hold the stretch for 3-5 seconds, then return to the starting position.

2. Perform the same movement on the other side, hold for 3-5 seconds, and then return to the starting position.

3. Repeat both stretches in succession for a total of 30 seconds.

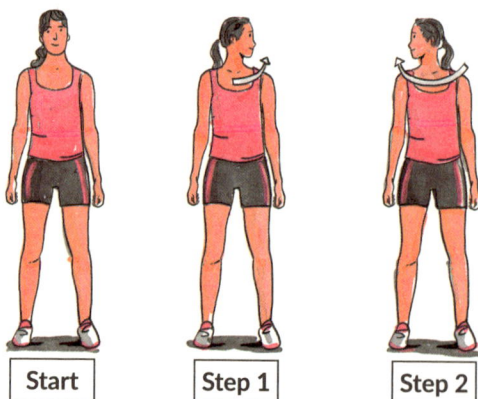

Start

Step 1

Step 2

Upper Body Stretches

Lying Full Body Extension

Starting position: Lie on your back with your arms outstretched comfortably above your head.

1. Reach your arms above your head and push through your fingertips to elongate your spine and torso.

2. At the same time, stretch the lower half of your body through your heel, also with the aim of elongating your spine and torso.

3. Hold for 30 seconds.

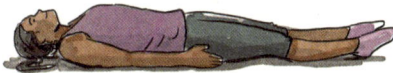

Step 1

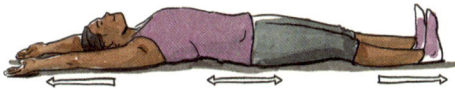

Step 2

Leaning Long Arm Shoulder Stretch

Starting position: Choose an object you can hold in front of you that is high enough for you to grab with your hands, and sturdy enough that it won't fall when you fold your body over (think: table or chair). Ideally, it should be somewhere in between belly and chest-height. Stand in front of the object and grab it with your hands.

1. Take a few steps back to give yourself space, and shift your body weight forward, bending at the waist to create a stretch in the chest and shoulder muscles.Elongate the arms and spine as much as possible while trying to open the chest and shoulder muscles by pushing your torso towards the ground.

2. Hold for 30 seconds.

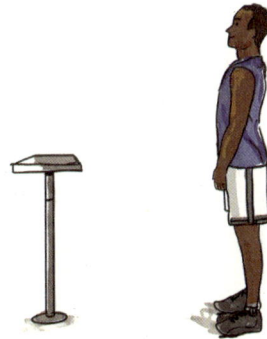

Step 1

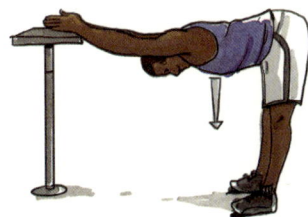

Step 2

Upper Body Stretches

Levator Scap Neck Stretch

Starting position: Stand, with your feet hip-width apart and arms down by your sides, or sit in a chair with your back straight.

1. Put your right hand on the back of your head with your fingertips reaching the base of your skull. Fingertips should be facing down your spine.

2. Bring your chin to your chest and turn the back of your head towards your right armpit.

3. Hold the stretch for 15 seconds, and then relax.

4. Repeat the same stretch on the left side for 15 seconds.

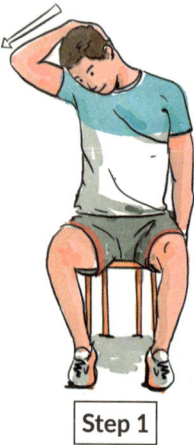

Step 1

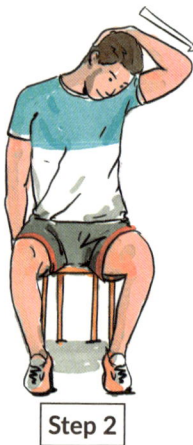

Step 2

Locust Pose

Starting position: Lie flat with your face and belly towards the ground and your arms lying comfortably beside your body.

1. Lift your chest, arms and your legs as much as possible to form a sort of boat shape, curving the inner part of your back towards the ground and the outer parts of your body and spine towards the ceiling.

2. Hold for 30 seconds.

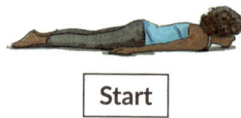

Start

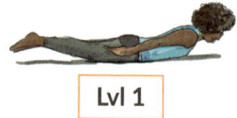

Lvl 1

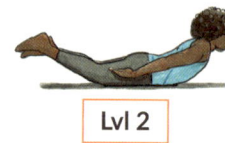

Lvl 2

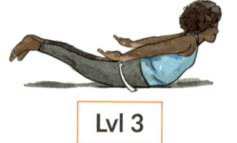

Lvl 3

Upper Body Stretches

Open Book Chest Stretch

Starting position: Lie down on your left side, with both knees bent and legs lying on top of each other on the ground.

1. Stretch your left arm out so it's extended horizontally to the side of your body, with the palm facing up.

2. Extend your right hand, and place it directly on the left hand, so now both of your arms and legs are simply lying on top of each other.

3. Without moving your legs at all, raise your right arm and, making a semi-circle, twist your head and torso to the other side as you try to place your right arm on the floor to the right side of your body, as if you were an open book.

4. Hold the stretch for 30 seconds.

5. Repeat the same stretch on the other side.

Reverse Prayer

Starting position: Stand comfortably with your arms by your side.

1. Bring your hands behind your back, with the backs of your hands facing each other and your fingers facing down.

2. From there, if possible, flip your hands in the other direction so your fingers are facing up.

3. Then, if possible, turn your palms to face each other and press them together, slightly drawing your elbows back to open your chest and shoulders.

4. Hold for 30 seconds.

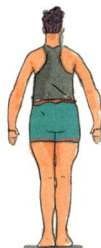
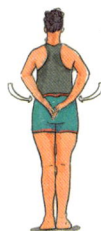
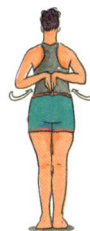
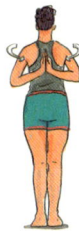

Start	Lvl 1	Lvl 2	Lvl 3

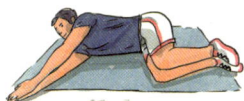

Start

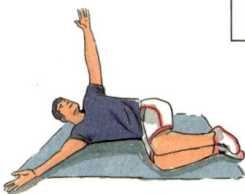

Lvl 1

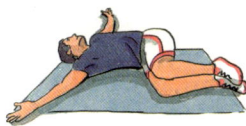

Lvl 2

Upper Body Stretches

Seated Forward Curl

Starting position: Sit in a chair with your feet flat on the ground.

1. Bending at the waist, bend your whole upper body towards the floor, as if you were trying to touch your chest to the floor.

2. Stretch and hold for 30 seconds, trying to deepen the stretch as you relax.

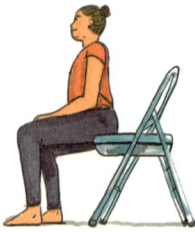

Start

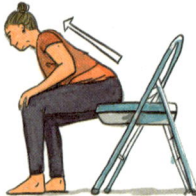

Lvl 1

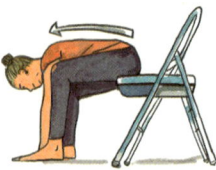

Lvl 2

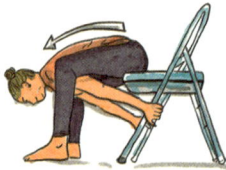

Lvl 3

Seated Spinal Twist

Starting position: Sit on the floor with one leg extended straight out in front of you, the other leg bent comfortably so that the sole of your resting foot touches the inner thigh of the straight leg, and your back straight.

1. Bend forward at the waist, making sure to keep the back straight, and reach out towards your foot with your hands as far as you can.

2. Hold for 30 seconds, deepening the stretch whenever it feels comfortable to do so.

3. Relax and perform the same stretch on the other leg.

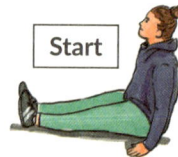

Start

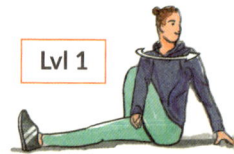

Lvl 1

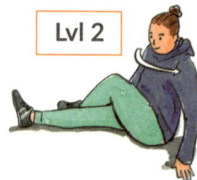

Lvl 2

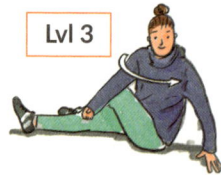

Lvl 3

Upper Body Stretches

Side Neck Stretch w/ Upside Down Palm on Wall

Starting position: Stand an arm's length away from the wall and place your right hand on the wall, arm straight with your fingertips facing towards the ground.

1. Standing straight up, bend your neck to the left, trying to touch your left shoulder with your left ear.

2. Hold for 15 seconds.

3. Repeat on the other side.

Side Neck Tilt

Starting position: Stand, with your feet hip-width apart and arms down by your sides, or sit in a chair with your back straight.

1. Gently tilt your head toward your right shoulder and try to touch it with your ear, while stretching to point the other ear to the ceiling.

2. Hold the stretch for 15 seconds, then return to the start position.

3. Perform the same stretch on your left side. Hold for 15 seconds.

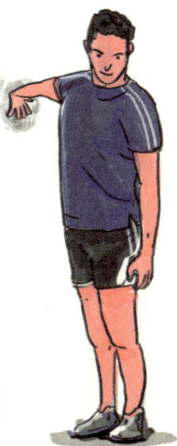

Step 1

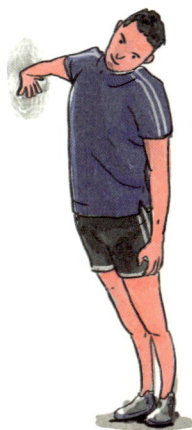

Step 2

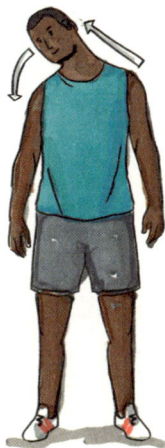

Step 1

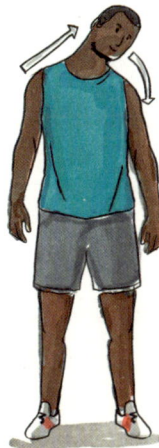

Step 2

Upper Body Stretches

Sphinx/Cobra

Starting position: Lie on your stomach on the floor, as if you were sleeping on the floor on your belly.

4. Slowly prop yourself up on your elbows, bringing the upper half of your torso up off the ground.

5. Start to straighten your elbows, further extending your back and lifting more of your torso off the ground, until you feel a gentle stretch in your spine. Only lift yourself to the extent that it feels right and comfortable.

6. Hold the stretch for 30 seconds.

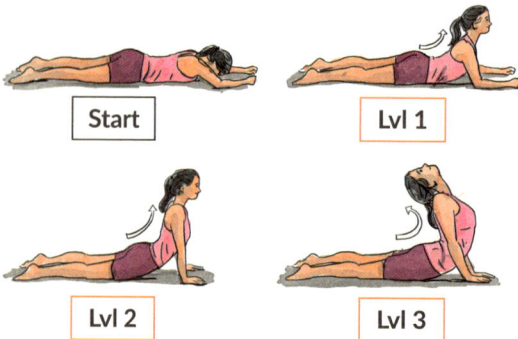

Standing Oblique Stretch

Starting position: Stand with your feet slightly wider than hip-width apart, and with a slight bend in the knees.

1. Place your right hand on your hip, and raise your left arm straight up above your body.

2. Lean your torso towards the right, bending at the right side of the waist. Keep the knee on the leg you're leaning towards slightly bent.

3. Try not to actually move your hips, but simply bend towards the right until you feel a stretch in your left obliques (the muscles on the left side of your abdomen).

4. Hold for 15 seconds.

5. Relax, and then repeat the same stretch on the other side.

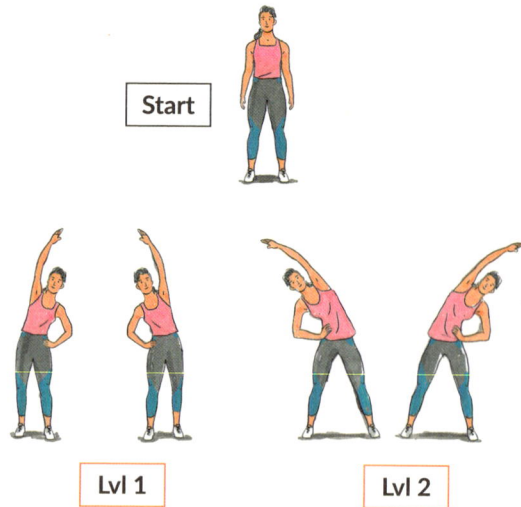

Start

Lvl 1

Lvl 2

Lvl 3

Start

Lvl 1

Lvl 2

Upper Body Stretches

Static Y Hold

Starting position: Stand straight with your arms by your side.

1. Keeping your arms completely straight, lift them above you to create a Y shape with your torso and your arms.

2. Without moving your torso, and without bending your arms at all, try to pull your arms back behind your body to open the shoulder muscles as much as feels comfortable and right.

3. Hold for 30 seconds.

Surface Tricep Stretch

Starting position: Stand with your right side next to a chest-high support structure - anything sturdy enough for you to lean a part of your weight on like a chair, or countertop. If there is no such structure available, you can also perform this stretch using a wall.

1. Place your left leg about 2 feet behind your right leg, and to the left of your right leg so that you have stable support on the ground.

2. Place your right elbow on the top of the support structure, and lower your body until you feel a stretch in your right tricep and the side of your back.

3. Hold for 15 seconds.

4. Relax, and then perform the same stretch on the left side.

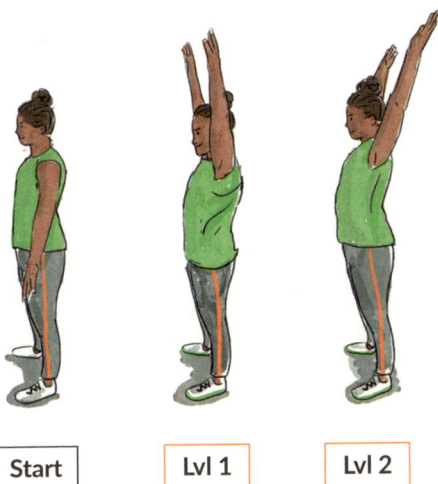

Start

Lvl 1

Lvl 2

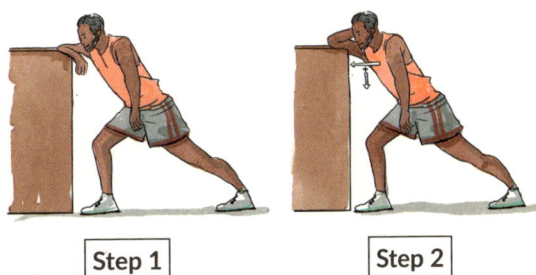

Step 1

Step 2

Upper Body Stretches

Thread the Needle Shoulder Stretch

Starting position: Start on all fours, with your hands underneath your shoulders and your knees in line with your hips.

1. Bend your legs so that your torso is supported as much as possible by your legs.

2. Hold your left arm out in front of you for stability.

3. Reach your right arm through the hole between your left arm and the floor, palm facing up.

4. Bend your left elbow as you gently lean into your right side. You should feel a stretch in the back of your right shoulder.

5. Hold for 15 seconds.

6. Perform the same stretch on the left side.

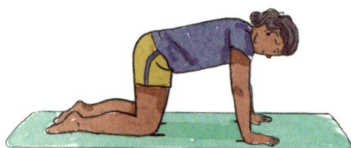

Step 1

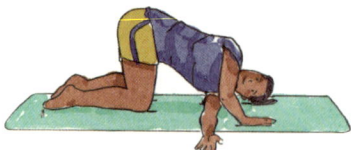

Step 2

Up & Down Neck Tilt

Starting position: This can be done while you're seated or standing.

1. Start with your head squarely over your shoulders and your back straight.

2. Lower your chin toward your chest, hold for 3-5 seconds. Relax, and slowly lift your head back up.

3. Tilt your chin up toward the ceiling and bring the base of your skull toward your back. Hold, and then alternate.

4. Repeat both motions in succession, alternating every few seconds.

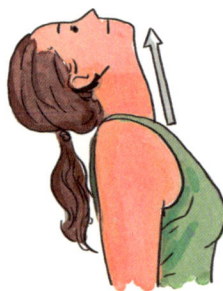

Step 1

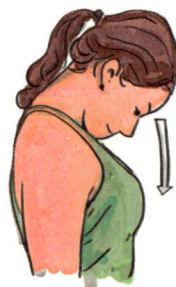

Step 2

Upper Body Stretches

Wall Lat Stretch

Starting position: Standing in front of a wall,
place your hands on the wall about shoulder level.

1. Bend at the waist and lower your torso as much
   as possible until you feel a stretch in your lats
   (the sides of your back).

2. Hold for 30 seconds, deepening the stretch
   whenever possible.

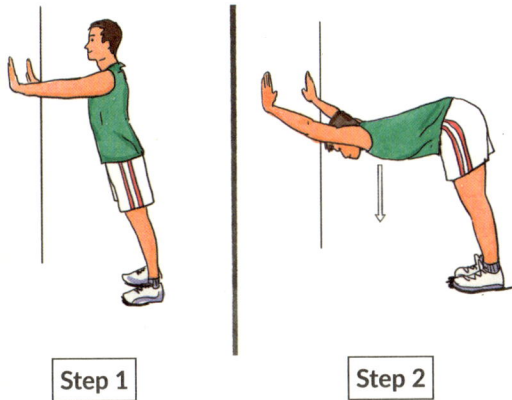

Step 1

Step 2

Lower Body Stretches

Butterfly

Starting position: Sit on the ground and place the soles of your feet together in front of you. Let your knees bend out and fall to the ground as much as gravity allows them to.

1. Place your hands on your feet and pull your heels towards you.

2. Keep your back straight and your abs engaged as you let your knees relax and inch closer to the floor. You'll feel the stretch in your groin muscles.

3. Hold for 30 seconds, deepening the stretch whenever it feels comfortable to do so.

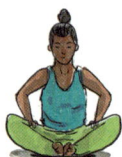

Start

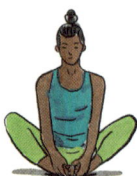

Lvl 1

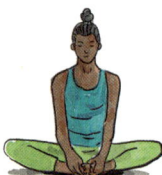

Lvl 2

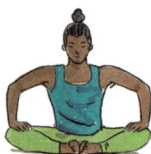

Lvl 3

Downward Dog

Starting position: Begin on all fours, with your knees hip-width apart and your hands directly below your shoulders.

1. Press back into your heels to straighten your knees and raise your butt up to the ceiling until you feel the stretch in your hamstrings. If you need to, extend your arms forward so that you can straighten your legs a bit more.

2. Keep your head, neck, and spine aligned as you press back into the feeling of the stretch in the back of your legs and calves.

3. Hold for 30 seconds, deepening the stretch whenever it feels comfortable to do so.

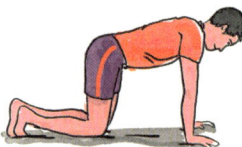

Start

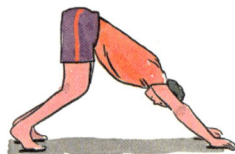

Lvl 1

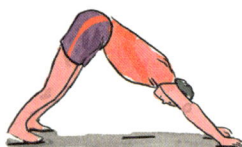

Lvl 2

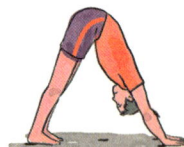

Lvl 3

Lower Body Stretches

Extended Triangle Pose

Starting position: Stand with your feet hip-width apart. Step your right leg out to the side while shifting your foot, so the toes on your right foot are facing out.

1. Stretch both arms out to your sides at shoulder height.

2. Shift your torso to the right and extend down, reaching your right arm towards your right foot as far as you can.

3. Hold for 30 seconds, deepening the stretch whenever it feels comfortable to do so.

4. Relax and perform the same stretch on the other leg.

Figure 4

Starting position: Lie down on your back, with your knees bent and feet flat on the floor in front of you.

1. Cross your left foot over your right knee.

2. Grab your right leg with both hands and pull your right knee in towards your upper body until you feel a stretch in the glute muscles on the left side of your body.

3. Hold the stretch for 30 seconds, then relax and return to the starting position.

4. Repeat the stretch on the other side. Hold for 30 seconds.

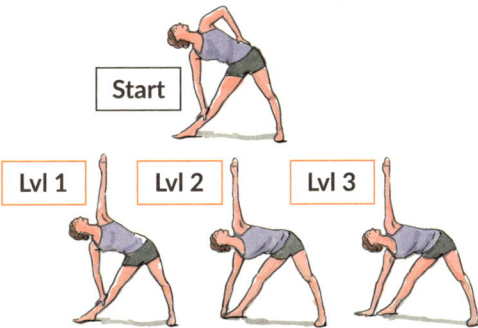

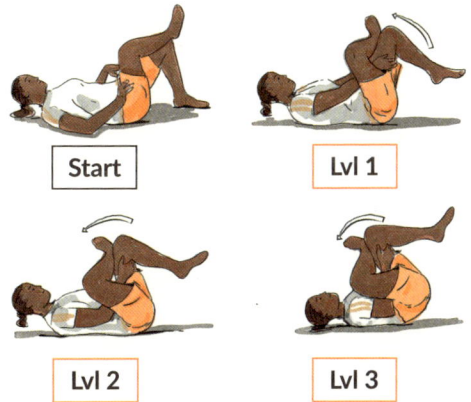

Lower Body Stretches

Frog Pose

Starting position: Lie facedown, bend your knees about 90 degrees, and spread them as wide as you can.

1. Fold your hands under your forehead to relax the upper half of the body.

2. Keeping your knees bent, sink your hips towards the floor.

3. Hold for 60 seconds, and deepen the stretch by sinking your hips more towards the floor whenever possible.

Halfway Center Split

Starting position: Stand straight up and widen your feet two shoulder-widths apart (as wide as possible).

1. Bend forward at the hips while keeping your legs as straight as possible.

2. Let your body hang down and try to place your palms on the ground. You'll feel the stretch in your inner thighs on both legs.

3. Hold for 30 seconds.

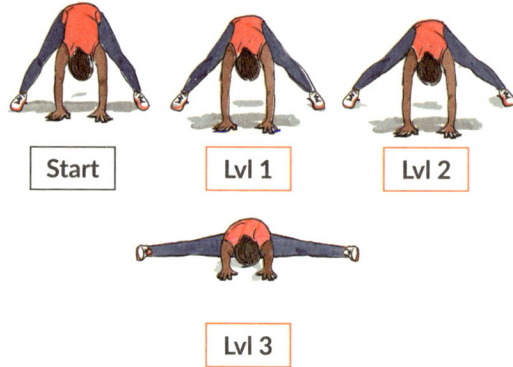

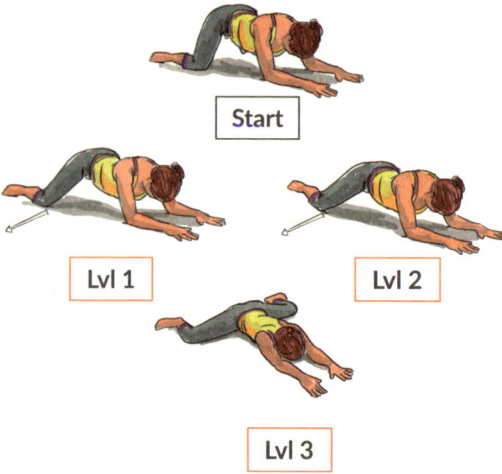

Lower Body Stretches

Hanging Calf Stretch

Starting position: Stand on the ball of your feet at the edge of a stair or step. If you don't have a stair or step, you can place a few towels on top of each other to simulate one.

1. While keeping your legs straight, allow gravity to pull your heels down towards the floor.

2. Hold the stretch for 30 seconds.

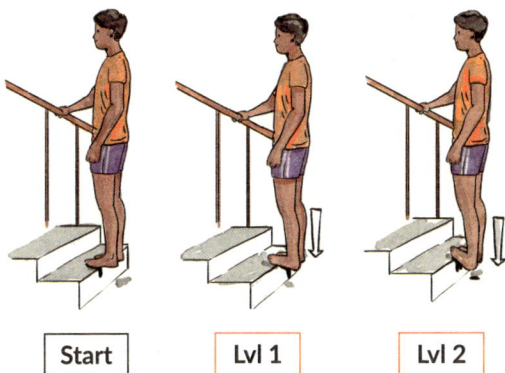

Start   Lvl 1   Lvl 2

Happy Baby Pose

Starting position: Lie on your back on the floor, with both knees bent and feet flat on the floor.

1. Lift your feet off the floor and grab the outside edges of your feet with your hands. If you can't grab your feet while keeping your whole back and head on the floor, grab the area around your knees, shins, or ankles.

2. Gently pull your feet towards your chest and let your knees lower toward the floor on both sides of your body.

3. Hold for 30 seconds.

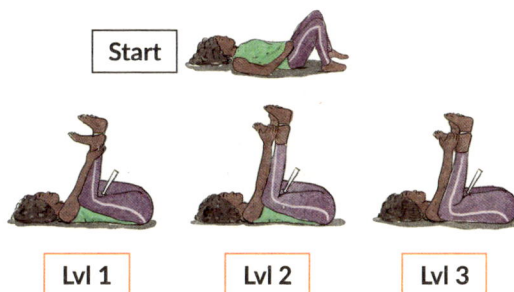

Start

Lvl 1   Lvl 2   Lvl 3

Lower Body Stretches

Knee to Chest Stretch

Starting position: Lie on your back with your whole body relaxed on the floor and your legs outstretched. Make sure your whole back is touching the floor.

1. Bring one knee towards your chest and grab your knee with both hands to pull.

2. Pull until you feel the stretch in the top of your butt and lower back.

3. Hold for 15 seconds, gently let go and relax.

4. Hold for 30 seconds, deepening the stretch whenever it feels comfortable to do so.

5. Relax and perform the same stretch on the other leg.

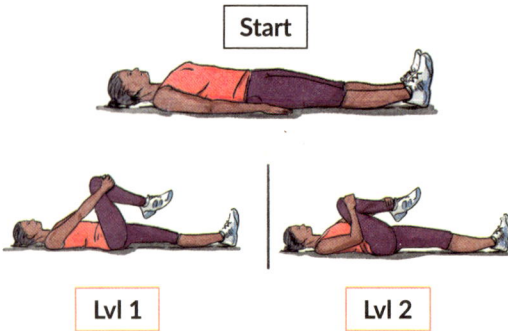

Kneeling Quad Stretch

Starting position: Place your right knee on the ground and your left in a kneeling position, at a 90 angle.

1. Take a moment to find your balance, and once you're ready, reach back with your right arm, and grab your ankle, or middle of your shin, depending on what's easiest.

2. Pull the right leg towards your butt.

3. Hold for 30 seconds, deepening the stretch whenever it feels comfortable to do so.

4. Relax and perform the same stretch on the other leg.

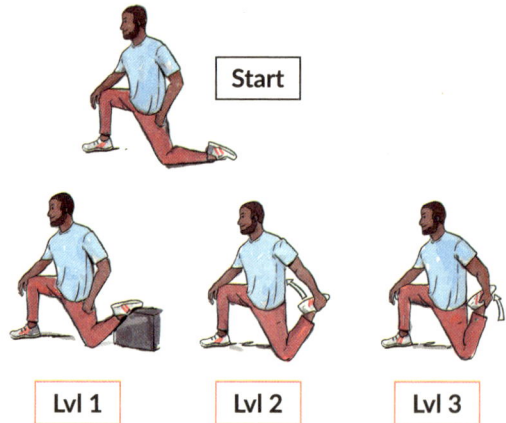

Lower Body Stretches

Lateral Squat

Starting position: Stand straight up with your feet very widely apart (double shoulder-width).

1. Shift your weight to your right leg, bend your right knee, and push your hips back as if you're going to sit down. This results in a slight squat towards your right leg. Keep your chest, back, and spine straight without curling or bending forward.

2. Drop as low as possible towards your right foot while keeping your left leg straight and your left foot flat on the ground, with your toes on your left leg pointing directly in front of you.

3. Hold for 30 seconds, deepening the stretch whenever it feels comfortable to do so.

4. Relax, and repeat the same stretch on the other leg.

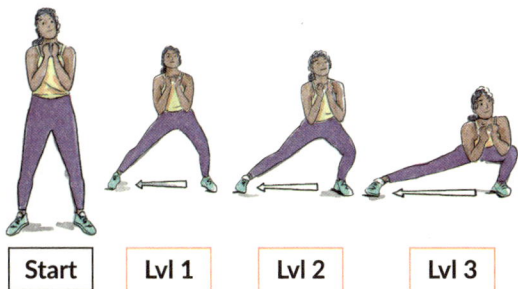

| Start | Lvl 1 | Lvl 2 | Lvl 3 |

Lateral Squat w/ Toe Raise

Starting position: Stand straight up with your feet very widely apart (double shoulder-width).

1. Shift your weight to your right leg, bend your right knee, and push your hips back as if you're going to sit down. This results in a slight squat towards your right leg.

2. Twist your left foot so that only your heel is on the ground and your toes are pointing straight up towards the ceiling.

3. Turn your body so that you're facing your left leg.

4. Drop as low as possible towards your right foot while keeping your left leg straight with toes pointed to the ceiling. Find your balance in this position and place your hands on the floor as needed to stabilize.

5. If possible, reach towards your left foot while bending only at the hip/waist, curling your back as little as necessary.

6. Hold for 30 seconds, deepening the stretch whenever it feels comfortable to do so.

7. Relax and perform the same stretch on the other leg.

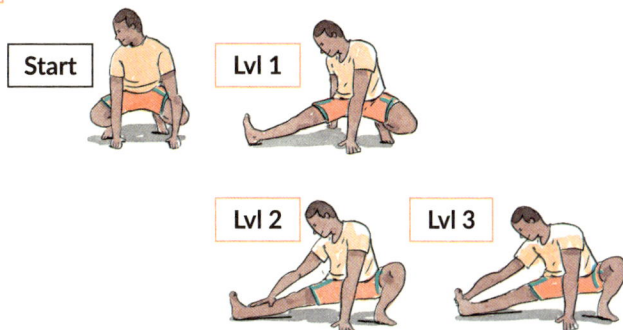

| Start | Lvl 1 |
| Lvl 2 | Lvl 3 |

Lower Body Stretches

Lying Hamstring Extension

Starting position: Lie flat on the ground with both your legs fully stretched out.

8. Hold the back of the knee with both hands and pull the leg up towards your chest while the knee is bent.

9. Slowly straighten the knee until you feel a stretch as you continue to hold the leg for stabilization.

10. Lift your straight leg towards your chest as much as possible.

11. Hold for 30 seconds, deepening the stretch whenever it feels comfortable to do so.

12. Relax and perform the same stretch on the other leg.

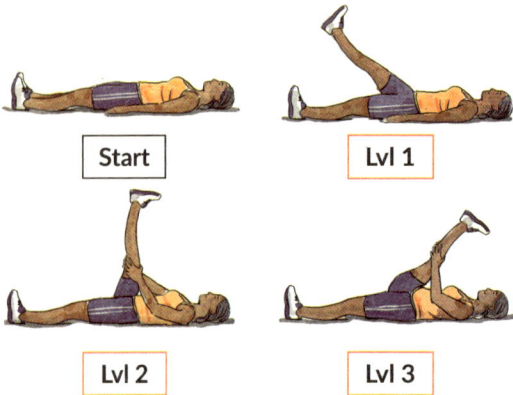

Lying Hip Extension

Starting position: Lay on the floor on your back with your arms outstretched into a 'Y' shape above your head. Arms should be resting comfortably on the floor. Feet flat on the floor with legs shoulder-width apart.

13. Lift your right leg and cross it over your left knee so that your right leg is resting, open, on your left leg.

14. Without moving your torso, bend your left leg down towards the ground until the whole left side of your left leg is resting on the ground.

15. Open your right hip by pulling your right leg towards the ground.

16. Hold for 30 seconds, and then perform the same stretch on the other side.

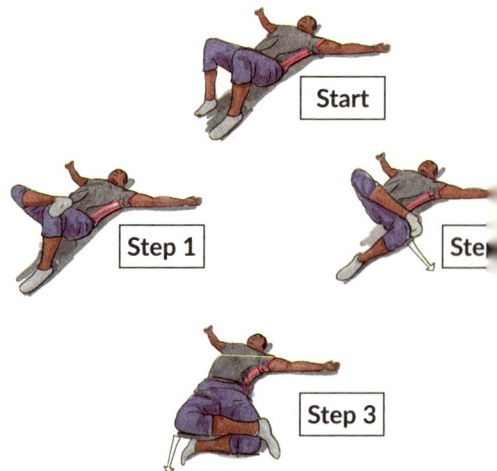

Start

Lvl 1

Lvl 2

Lvl 3

Start

Step 1

Ste

Step 3

Lower Body Stretches

Lying Quad Stretch

Starting position: Lie on the left side of your body and hold your head up with your hand so that you're laying on your left side with your head propped up and supported by your left hand. Your right knee can be slightly bent for stability and comfort (whatever feels right).

1. With your free, right hand, grab your right foot while bending the leg behind you so that your right knee is in a straight line with the rest of your body as you stretch and pull your right foot towards your butt.

2. Hold for 30 seconds, deepening the stretch whenever it feels comfortable to do so.

3. Relax and perform the same stretch on the other leg.

Pigeon Stretch

Starting position: Start by getting into a tabletop position on your hands and knees.

1. Bring your right knee forward and place it behind your wrist while shifting the leg so that your right ankle is in front of your left hip or left elbow.

2. Straighten your left leg behind you, making sure your left knee is straight and your toes are pointed out behind you.

3. Keeping your hips square, lower your torso towards the ground until you feel the maximum possible stretch that feels comfortable for you.

4. Hold the position for 30 seconds.

5. Repeat the same stretch on the left leg.

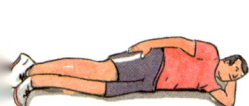
Start

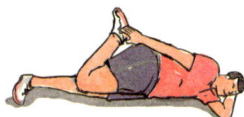
Lvl 1

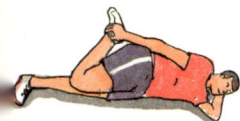
Lvl 2

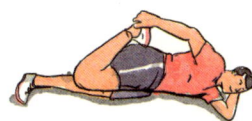
Lvl 3

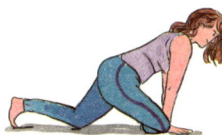
Start

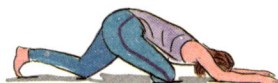
Lvl 1

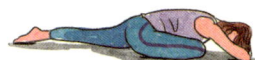
Lvl 2

Lower Body Stretches

Prone Quad Stretch

Starting position: Begin by lying on your stomach with your arms laying in front of you. All limbs should be relaxed, with your head facing directly in front of you.

1. Lift your right leg towards your glutes while reaching behind with your right arm to grab your foot.

2. Gently turn back to face the wall as you hold your ankle and stretch your right quadriceps.

3. Hold for 30 seconds, deepening the stretch whenever it feels comfortable to do so.

4. Relax and perform the same stretch on the other leg.

Pry Squat

Starting position: Stand with feet about 1.5 shoulder-distance apart with your feet comfortably pointed outwards away from your body

1. Sit into a squat and place your elbows on the inside of your knees. Feet should be pointed outwards away from your body. If you can't do this, get into a comfortable squat, and lean your hands on your elbows for support.

2. While trying to make sure both feet are completely flat on the ground, deepen the squat as much as you can by lowering closer to the floor.

3. Use your arms to press your knees as far out as is comfortable while still maintaining a tight core and proper squat form with your spine as straight as possible, without arching your spine.

4. Hold for 30 seconds and deepen the stretch whenever possible.

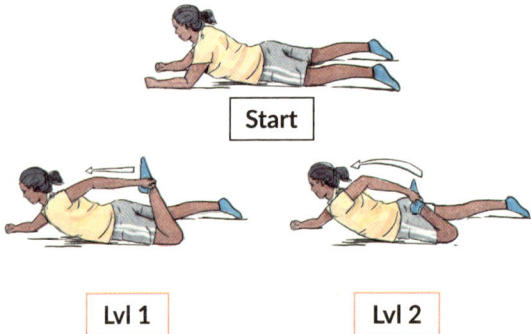

Start

Lvl 1   Lvl 2

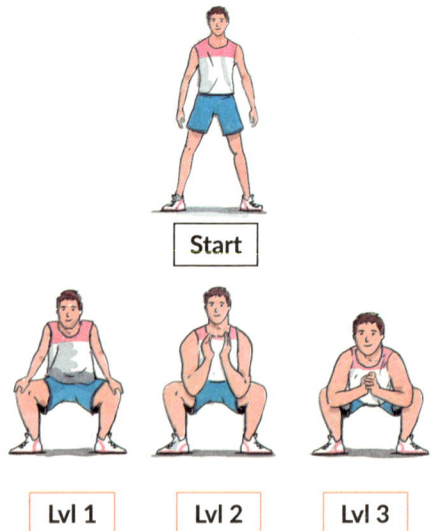

Start

Lvl 1   Lvl 2   Lvl 3

Lower Body Stretches

Reclining Angle Bound Pose

Starting position: Lie flat on your back with your knees bent and your feet flat on the ground.

1. Turn your feet so now the sides of your feet are on the ground and there is an open space between your knees.

2. Bring the soles of your feet together, pull them up towards your butt as much as you can.

3. Allow your knees to open up and drop closer to the floor.

4. Hold for 30 seconds.

Reverse Tabletop

Starting position: Sit on the floor with your feet shoulder-width apart and place your hands about shoulder-width apart as close to your shoulders as possible, with fingers facing away from your face.

1. Flatten your fleet on the ground, and lift your whole body off the ground using your palms and feet glutes, and back muscles.

2. Try to reach your hips towards the ceiling as high as you can, as you relax your head and neck and look up towards the ceiling.

3. Hold for 30 seconds.

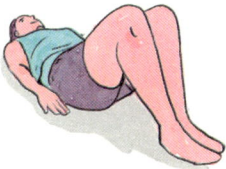

Start

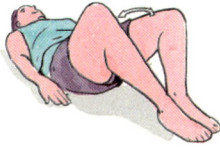

Lvl 1

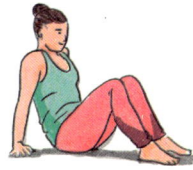

Start

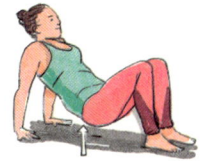

Lvl 1

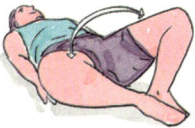

Lvl 2

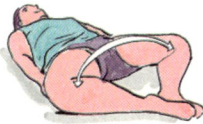

Lvl 3

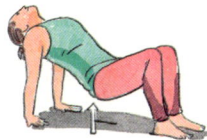

Lvl 2

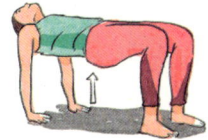

Lvl 3

Lower Body Stretches

Runner's Lunge

Starting position: Get into a push-up position with your hands and the balls of your feet on the floor, both shoulder-width apart, and a straight line running through your head down to your feet.

1. Step your right foot to a point just outside your right hand. You should feel a stretch in your hip and groin area on the left side.

2. If you feel comfortable and want a deeper stretch you can stretch more, lower your elbows closer to the floor instead of using your hands for stability.

3. Hold for 30 seconds.

4. Return to the starting position, and repeat with the left leg forward.

Scorpion Pose

Starting position: Sit on the floor with one leg extended straight out in front of you, the other leg bent comfortably so that the sole of your resting foot touches the inner thigh of the straight leg, and your back straight.

1. Bend forward at the waist, making sure to keep the back straight and reach out towards your foot with your hands as far as you can.

2. Hold for 30 seconds, deepening the stretch whenever it feels comfortable to do so.

3. Relax and perform the same stretch on the other leg.

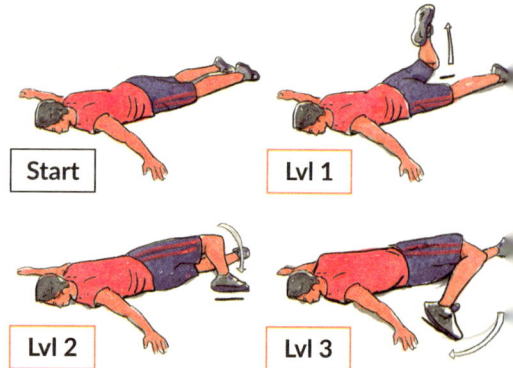

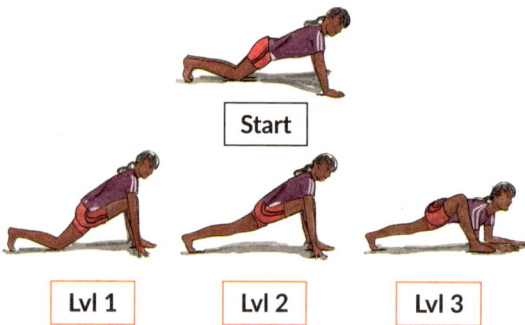

Lower Body Stretches

Seated Forward Fold Hamstring Stretch

Starting position: Sit down on the floor and straighten both legs in front of you while sitting upright.

1. With both arms, reach towards your feet as far as you can while only bending the upper body at the waist and keeping your spine straight.

2. Hold for 30 seconds, deepening the stretch whenever it feels comfortable to do so.

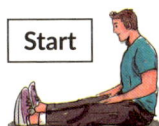

Start

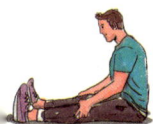 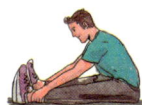 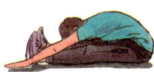

Lvl 1   **Lvl 2**   **Lvl 3**

Seated Single Leg Hamstring Stretch

Starting position: Sit on the floor with one leg extended straight out in front of you, the other leg bent comfortably so that the sole of your resting foot touches the inner thigh of the straight leg, and your back straight.

1. Bend forward at the waist, making sure to keep the back straight and reach out towards your foot with your hands as far as you can.

2. Hold for 30 seconds, deepening the stretch whenever it feels comfortable to do so.

3. Relax and perform the same stretch on the other leg.

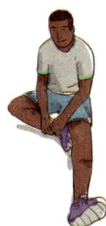 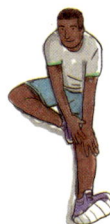 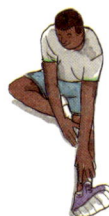 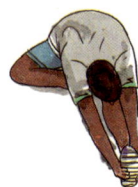

Start   **Lvl 1**   **Lvl 2**   **Lvl 3**

Lower Body Stretches

Standing Quad Stretch

Starting position: Stand with your whole body relaxed.

1. While balancing on your left foot, grab the bottom of your right shin, where it meets your foot, by bending your leg behind you.

2. Tuck your pelvis in, and pull your shin toward your butt (glutes), making sure your knee is pointing to the ground, or as close to the ground as possible.

3. Hold for 30 seconds, deepening the stretch whenever it feels comfortable to do so.

4. Relax and perform the same stretch on the other leg.

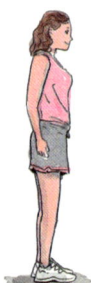

Start

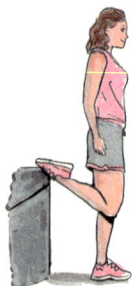

Lvl 1

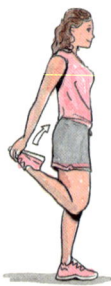

Lvl 2

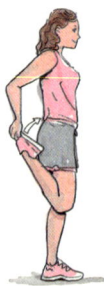

Lvl 3

Standing Wall Calf Stretch

Starting position: Stand directly in front of a wall, about 1–2 feet away from it depending on how long your arms are.

1. Put your hands on the wall and slightly bend your knees.

2. Lift your left foot, and place it behind your body so that your right foot is in front of your left foot with reasonable distance between them.

3. Straighten your left leg completely, and keep the whole foot on the ground until you feel a comfortable stretch in your left calf.

4. Hold for 15 seconds, deepening the stretch whenever it feels comfortable to do so.

5. Relax and perform the same stretch on the other leg.

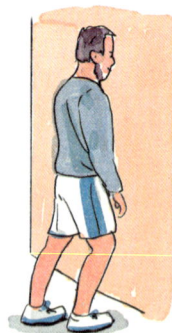

Start

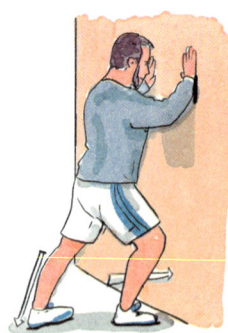

Lvl 1

Lower Body Stretches

Standing Wall Calf Stretch w/ Achilles Focus

Starting position: Stand directly in front of a wall, about 6 inches to 1 foot away from it.

1. Put your hands on the wall and slightly bend your knees.

2. Place the left foot a tiny bit back from your right foot, and flex your left foot so that it's on the left toes.

3. Bend your right knee so that it inches closer to the wall so you feel a stretch in the bottom of your right calf, where the Achilles tendon is. Bend as far forward as possible while keeping the right heel on the ground.

4. Hold for 15 seconds, deepening the stretch whenever it feels comfortable to do so.

5. Relax and perform the same stretch on the other leg.

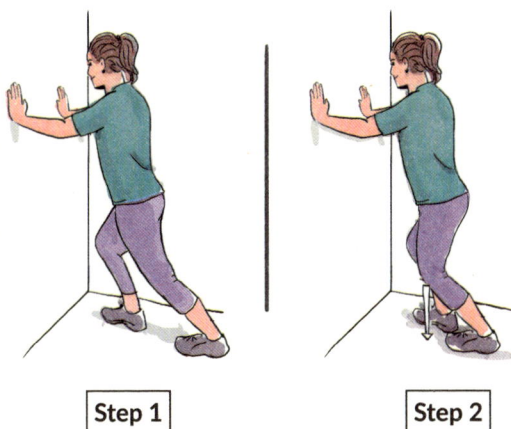

Warrior II Pose

Starting position: Stand with your feet double shoulder length apart and your arms extended horizontally with your palms facing down.

1. Turn your left foot our about 90 degrees, and then bend your left knee into a lunge. Your right foot should still be pointing forwards. If this feels too comfortable, try to widen the distance between your legs by swiveling your left leg further away from the right foot.

2. Turn your head to the left and look over your fingers.

3. Hold for 30 seconds, and then return to the starting position.

4. Perform the same sequence with your right side and hold for 30 seconds.

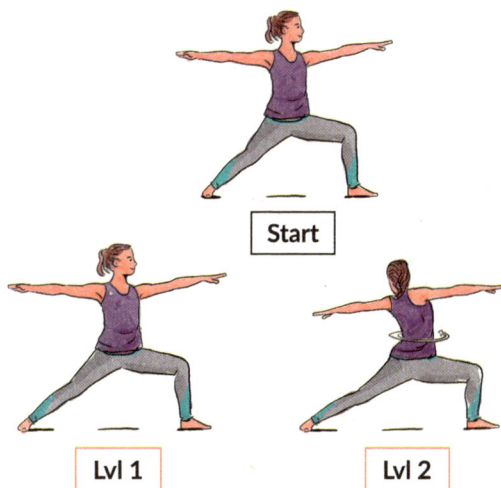

Step 1

Step 2

Start

Lvl 1

Lvl 2

Lower Body Stretches

Wig Wag

Starting position: Lie on your back, with your knees bent on the floor and your arms to the side.

1. Pull your right leg towards your chest and twist your body to the left, trying to touch your right knee to the floor on the left side of your body.

2. Use your left arm to pull your leg and deepen the stretch to the extent it feels good and comfortable.

3. Hold for 30 seconds, deepening the stretch whenever possible.

4. Return to the starting position, and then perform the same stretch on the other side.

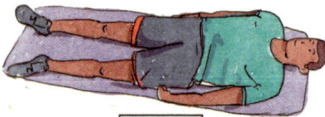
Step 1

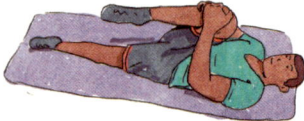
Step 2

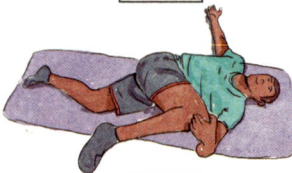
Step 3